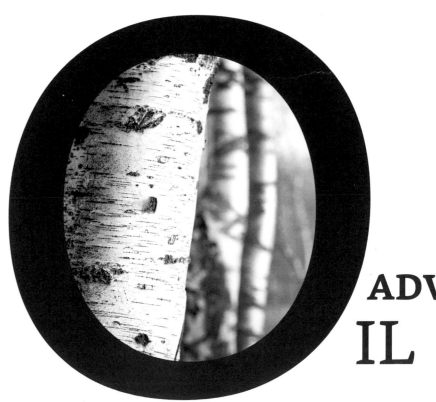

ADVANCED
OIL MAGIC

Advanced Oil Magic
Advanced Oil Guidebook, Lifestyle Protocols, & QR Video Blips

April 2019
(first printing updated)

©2018 Oil Magic Publishing, LLC
All rights reserved.

ISBN: 978-0-9993689-2-3

Published by:

Oil Magic Publishing
Cheyenne, WY
contact@oilmagicbook.com

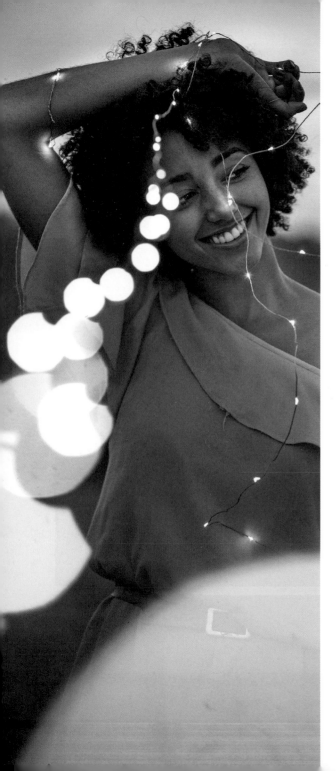

About this book

Advanced Oil Magic brings the balance of essential magic and science. The magic is in the protocols. The science backs it up.

The contents of this book have been compiled with influence from the best resources, researchers, doctors, naturopaths, and holistic specialists. While a true relationship with essential oils and natural remedies comes from discovering what works best for your body, following the recommendations in this book will get you off to a perfect start.

Advanced Oil Magic features gorgeous artwork from up-and-coming photographers featured on Unsplash. Visit www.oilmagicbook.com to learn more and find your favorite featured artists.

A most common complaint among essential oil users is that they want more specific instruction. Many people are used to explicit usage instructions from traditional healthcare providers. Advanced Oil Magic provides similar guidance for the natural world.

Use this guide as your first go-to. Turn to nature as your first resort, and remember that you also have the power of western medicine when needed.

Enjoy all the things your oils can do for you. Enjoy the aromas, and have fun blending oils to make your own experiences. Try creative DIY projects found on the individual oil pages. Discover how unlimited the possibilities are.

Most importantly, see what happens to your confidence as you learn to trust nature and yourself with your family's wellness.

Use the Ailments section as a quick reference guide for your health concerns. Discover the top uses of popular essential oils in the Single Oils and Oil Blends sections. Use the Protocols section to get serious results. Once you've become accustomed to solving health challenges with natural solutions first, uplevel your experience with Emotions & Energy and Lifestyle Protocols!

Here's to all the magic you'll create.

Table of *Contents*

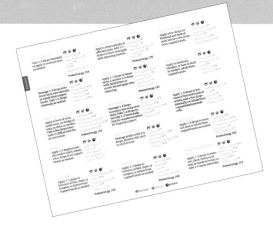

Start by looking up quick suggestions for your health challenges & needs.

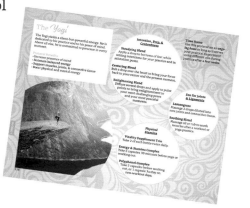

Then get to know your essential oils a bit more.

Commit to a Protocol or a Lifestyle Protocol to get big, long-term results.

QR Video Blips!
Simply flash your smart phone's camera at the QR code on a single oil page to pull up a cool video on that essential oil.

Oil Magic does not provide technical support for QR codes. Please refer to your smart phone manufacturer for help scanning codes.

"We do not need magic to transform our world. We carry all of the power we need inside ourselves already."

-J.K. Rowling

Section 1

Advanced
Usage Guide

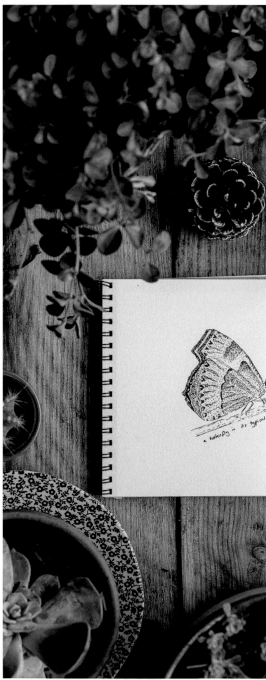

a butterfly in its typical

What is an Essential Oil?

Volatile Aromatic Compounds
Essential oils are volatile compounds naturally occurring in certain plants. They are extracted from seeds, flowers, bark, resins, leaves, rinds, and roots. The word "volatile" means they easily evaporate at normal temperatures.

Distillation
While many essential oils on the market are extracted using practices that render the oil impure and non-therapeutic, a true essential oil is carefully distilled using either steam distillation or cold pressing (citrus oils).

Benefits
Essential oils provide a number of benefits to plants, and many of those benefits are passed onto the human body with appropriate application:

• Anti-bacterial, anti-fungal, anti-viral, and anti-parasitic protection
• Restoration and regeneration from physical damage
• Communication via chemical signals

Misconceptions
Contrary to occasional misconception, essential oils do not contain vitamins or minerals. The health benefits they provide occur from the interactions of their naturally occurring chemical constituents with the human body in various ways.

Another misconception is that essential oils are the "lifeblood of the plant." Oils contribute significantly to a plant's well-being, but they do not keep the plant alive.

Original Medicine
While the term "alternative medicine" is a buzz word frequently used to describe remedies like herbs and essential oils, plant medicine is indeed *original* medicine.

Plants have been used for medicinal purposes for thousands of years in every culture. Modern science is quickly recognizing and validating the usefulness of plants as medicine (see the Science and Research section).

The Power of Aroma
Essential oils affect the body quickly and powerfully. When used aromatically, aromatic compounds interact with the olfactory system and limbic system to effectively instigate therapeutic chemical changes in the body. When used internally or topically, they interact directly with cells, organs, and entire body systems for health benefits.

Uses

It's hard to go wrong when using essential oils. This book suggests ways to use your oils for specific conditions, but you can try what feels best for your body.

Over time you'll discover your favorite ways to use your oils.

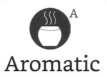

Aromatic

Diffuse

Put 4-8 drops in a diffuser to spread the oil throughout the room.

From Hands

Inhale a couple drops from cupped hands.

From Bottle

Enjoy the aroma directly from the bottle.

Not sure *what to do?*

Apply oils in ways that make sense for your needs. For example, use oils topically on location for a rash. If it's digestive upset, use them internally (though some people rub oils outside their tummy area!)

Again, you won't do it wrong. Discover and enjoy.

Topical

Neat

Apply certain oils directly to skin without dilution.

Dilute

Dilute with Fractionated Coconut Oil or other carrier oil/lotion as needed.

Roller Bottle

Put 10-20 drops in a roller bottle. Fill the rest with Fractionated Coconut Oil.

Internal

Veggie Capsule

Put oils in an empty veggie cap, and take with water.

Drink with Water

Drink 1-2 drops with water (for oils with a friendly taste).

Sublingually

Place a drop under the tongue for rapid absorption.

Most brands of oils are not safe for internal use. Be sure yours has undergone strict gas chromatography and mass spectrometry to ensure purity and chemical soundness.

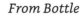

9

Safety

Children

Essential oils are safe to use with children in smaller amounts. The smaller the child, the less essential oil needed. Use this chart as a general guideline for use with children.

Age	Topical Dilution Ratio*	Internal Use
Birth - 12 months	1:30	1 drop (3-12 drops in 12 hours)
1-5 years	1:20	1 drop (3-12 drops in 12 hours)
6-11 years	1:15	1-2 drops (3-12 drops in 12 hours)

*essential oil : carrier oil

Medication

Always consult with a physician if you have questions about using an essential oil with a medication. While certain foods may interact with medications, essential oils frequently require less restraint because of the chemical makeup of the oil vs. the food.

Pregnancy

Essential oils are wonderful for pregnancy support. Some women wish to use oils only aromatically during their first trimester.

Oils can be used in smaller doses, and certain oils should be avoided: Birch[ATI], Cassia[TI], Cinnamon[TI], Cypress[I], Eucalyptus[I], Rosemary[ATI], Thyme[ATI], Wintergreen[TI].

Sensitive Skin

Dilute as needed for sensitive skin. Apply to the bottoms of feet to avoid sensitivity.

What to Keep in Mind

If it Burns
If an oil causes burning or irritation to the skin, immediately dilute it with a carrier oil. You can also use soap to wash the oil off.

Mixing with Water
Oil and water don't mix, and water will usually make discomfort from an essential oil worse.

Avoid Sensitive Areas
Do not put essential oils in your eyes, nose, ears, or other sensitive areas.

If You Use Too Much
If too much oil comes out of the bottle, simply wipe up the excess with a napkin (or give it to someone near you!)

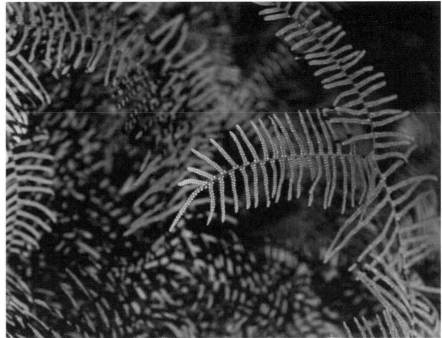

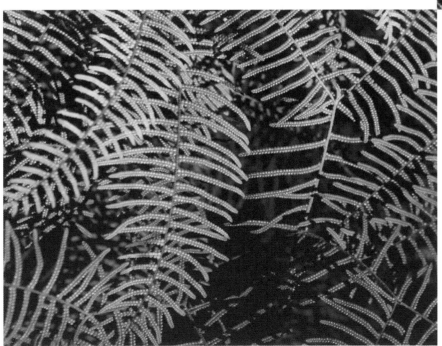

Photosensitivity
Certain oils, like citrus oils, can cause photosensitivity. This means that the skin can be more sensitive in sunlight, and that sunlight can even cause unsightly temporary hyper-pigmentation. Heed photosensitivity warnings in this book.

Lifestyle Habits
Keep your oils accessible. Have favorite ones in your bag, in high-traffic areas of the home, in the car, and at work. The easier they are to find, the more benefit you'll get from them.

How Much Should You Use?
Discover what works best for your body. Take heed of the safety warnings for each oil in this book.

Remember - small amounts more frequently tend to produce the best results.

Reflexology

Reflexology refers to contact points on the feet where nerve endings connect to other parts of the body. This is an ideal way to apply essential oils when the area of concern isn't accessible or when sensitivities limit application methods. It is also an ideal way to expose energy pathways such as those studied in Chinese medicine to the effects of essential oils.

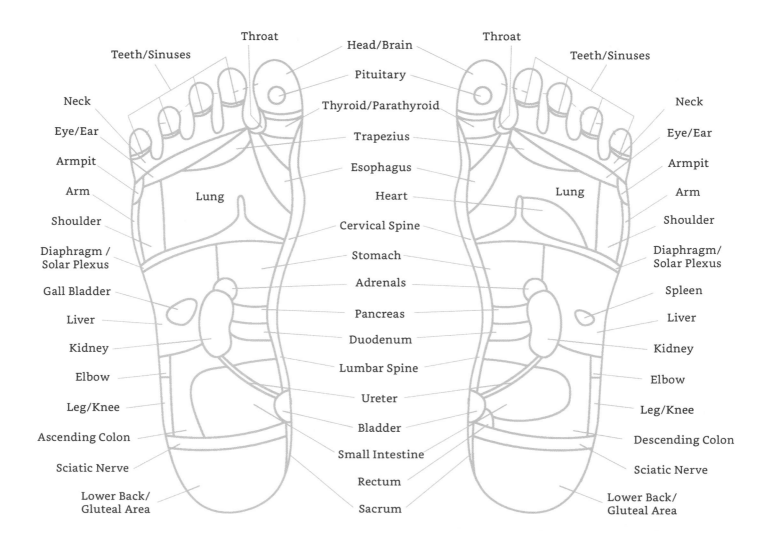

Preferences & Blending

Find the Right Solution for You

Remember that while essential oils have a most useful purpose, you should also enjoy what you use! Enjoying the use of oils makes it easier to create lifestyle habits with them.

If you love the smell of an essential oil, use away! If you don't love the smell, try an application method that limits exposure to the fragrance (like in a veggie cap or on the bottoms of feet), or look for a different oil that has similar properties.

Use oils you have on hand. Sometimes you'll find an oil in this book that you don't have, but that you do have in a blend. Sometimes you'll need to use an oil that has similar chemical properties to another oil you're missing. That's fine!

Blending

You can't break your oils. If you experiment with blending, but don't succeed, try again. You'll learn the smells that resonate best with you.

If you find yourself in need of an oil you may not love, try combining it with another oil to create a new fragrance.

Here are some blending tips:

• Pay attention to low, mid, and high notes in your oils for a well-rounded fragrance. (e.g. Vetiver is a low note, Lavender is a mid note, and Lemon is a high note.)

• Add FCO to your blends to help the fragrance last longer.

• When layering oils topically (using multiple oils one on top of the other), the oils on top will generally smell the strongest.

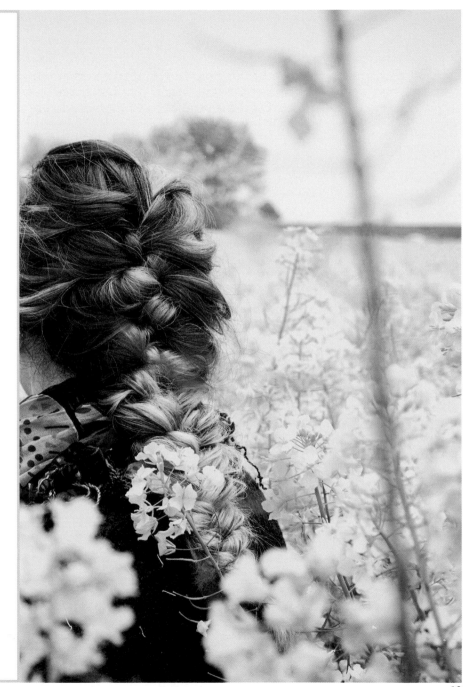

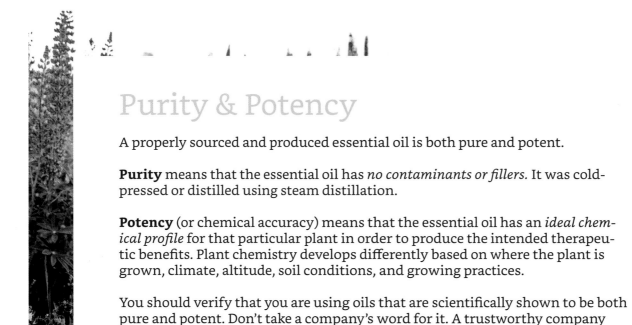

Purity & Potency

A properly sourced and produced essential oil is both pure and potent.

Purity means that the essential oil has *no contaminants or fillers.* It was cold-pressed or distilled using steam distillation.

Potency (or chemical accuracy) means that the essential oil has an *ideal chemical profile* for that particular plant in order to produce the intended therapeutic benefits. Plant chemistry develops differently based on where the plant is grown, climate, altitude, soil conditions, and growing practices.

You should verify that you are using oils that are scientifically shown to be both pure and potent. Don't take a company's word for it. A trustworthy company will make available the tests performed on every essential oil.

Know what you are putting in, on, and around your body.

Adulteration & Testing

The complexity of essential oils makes adulterating them too easy sometimes. Because some constituents appear in such small amounts, only sophisticated lab equipment with sufficiently comprehensive databases are able to detect skillful adulteration.

Unethical essential oil manufacturers use synthetic agents, fillers, and look-alike oils to produce inferior oils at cheaper costs.

Examples of Adulteration
(Tisserand, 2014)

Grapefruit Orange terpenes, purified limonene

Jasmine Absolute Indole, α-amyl cinnamic aldehyde, Ylang Ylang fractions

Lavender Lavandin, Spike Lavender, Spanish Sage, White Camphor fractions, rectified Ho, acetylated Lavandin

Lemon Synthetic citral or limonene

Peppermint Cornmint

Rose Ethanol, 2-phenylethanol, Geranium fractions, Rhodinol

Sandalwood Australian Sandalwood, Sandalwood terpenes and fragrance chemicals

Ylang Ylang Gurjun Balsam, Cananga oil, Benzyl Acetate, ρ-cresyl methyl ether

Standard Tests to Verify Purity & Potency

- Gas Chromatography
- Mass Spectrometry
- High Performance Liquid Chromatography
- Nuclear Magnetic Resonance Spectroscopy
- Fourier Transform Infrared Spectroscopy
- Chiral GC Testing
- Isotope Carbon 14
- Total Plate or Bacterial Count (TPC)/Microbial

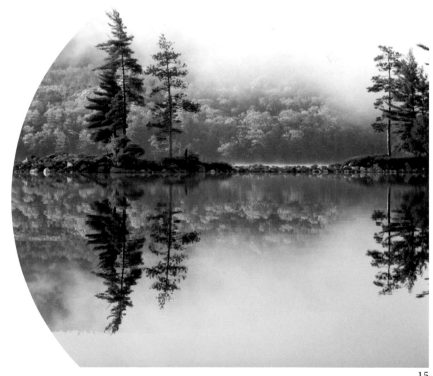

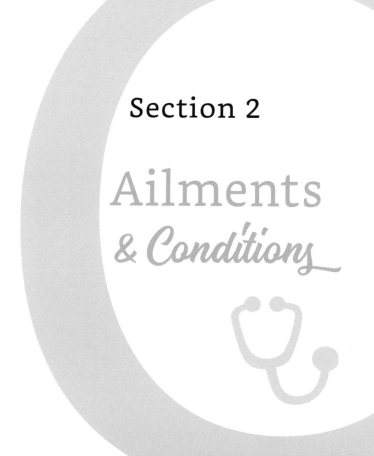

Section 2

Ailments
& Conditions

How to Use *Ailments & Conditions*

Using plant-based medicine is simple:

1. Look up your ailment.
2. Try one or a few oils from the suggested list.
3. Decide what works best for your body.

Each ailment includes the primary oils and supplements that are beneficial for that ailment. You don't need to use all five products listed. Try the ones you have on hand, and consider trying some new ones in the near future.

Every solution listed here is only a recommendation. You may learn of other oils that help with your ailment as well!

Remember that trying essential oils is the same process as trying any remedy; you may go through a few oils, or combinations of oils, before you find what your body responds best to.

Many of the ailments listed reference a protocol found later in the book. While this section is intended to provide quick answers, the protocols give detailed instructions for serious results.

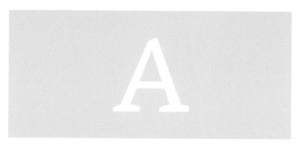

A

Abscess

Apply 2-4 drops 3x daily over affected area.

Lavender ᵀ
Melaleuca ᵀ
Roman Chamomile ᵀ
Arborvitae ᵀ
Neroli ᵀ

Absentmindedness

Massage 1-3 drops into forehead, temples, back of neck, and chest as needed; inhale from cupped hands.

Rosemary ᴬᵀ
Peppermint ᴬᵀ
Bergamot ᴬᵀ
Lavender ᴬᵀ
Frankincense ᴬᵀ

Protocol on pg. 218

Abuse Recovery

Apply 1-3 drops to top of head, forehead, and back of neck 3x daily.

Hopeful Blend ᴬᵀ
Women's Monthly Blend ᴬᵀ
Rose ᴬᵀ
Bergamot ᴬᵀ
Lavender ᴬᵀ

Protocol on pg. 233

Aches

Massage 2-4 drops into affected muscles and joints as needed.

Marjoram ᴬᵀᴵ
Lemongrass ᴬᵀᴵ
Soothing Blend ᴬᵀ
Massage Blend ᴬᵀ
Helichrysum ᴬᵀᴵ

Protocol on pg. 197

Acid Reflux

Take 2-4 drops internally or rub over stomach as needed.

Peppermint ᵀᴵ
Digestive Blend ᵀᴵ
Ginger ᵀᴵ
Cardamom ᵀᴵ
Digestion Tablets ᴵ

Protocol on pg. 180

Acne/Blemishes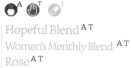

Apply a drop topically to affected areas 1-2x daily. Add 2-3 drops to facial lotion and apply after cleansing routine.

Melaleuca ᵀ
Skin Clearing Blend ᵀ
Juniper Berry ᵀ
Neroli ᵀ
Lavender ᵀ

Protocol on pg. 180

Actinic Keratosis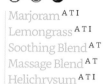

Apply 3-5 drops to affected area 4x daily.

Frankincense ᵀ
Lavender ᵀ
Melaleuca ᵀ
Neroli ᵀ
Myrrh ᵀ

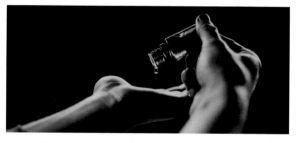

ADD/ADHD

Apply a few drops on forehead and back of neck; inhale a few drops from cupped hands.

Focus Blend ᴬᵀ
Vetiver ᴬᵀᴵ
Reassuring Blend ᴬᵀ
Frankincense ᴬᵀᴵ
Grounding Blend ᴬᵀ

Protocol on pg. 181

Addiction: Alcohol

Apply a couple drops to back of neck, temples, ears, and below chest as often as needed.

Bergamot ᴬᵀᴵ
Hopeful Blend ᴬᵀ
Encouraging Blend ᴬᵀ
Black Pepper ᴬᵀᴵ
Lemon ᴬᵀᴵ

Protocol on pg. 210

Addiction: Caffeine

Apply a couple drops to back of neck, temples, ears, and below chest as often as needed.

Peppermint ᴬᵀᴵ
Wild Orange ᴬᵀᴵ
Jasmine ᴬᵀ
Encouraging Blend ᴬᵀ
Lavender ᴬᵀᴵ

Protocol on pg. 210

Addiction: Drugs

Apply a couple drops to chest, temples, and bottoms of feet daily; inhale from cupped hands as needed.

Copaiba ᴬᵀᴵ
Detoxification Blend ᴬᵀᴵ
Cleansing Blend ᴬᵀ
Black Pepper ᴬᵀᴵ
Frankincense ᴬᵀᴵ

Protocol on pg. 210

Addiction: Food

Apply 3-5 drops as needed to abdomen and inside of legs from knees to ankles.

Bergamot ᴬᵀᴵ
Lemon ᴬᵀᴵ
Cinnamon ᴬᵀᴵ
Ginger ᴬᵀᴵ
Coriander ᴬᵀᴵ

Protocol on pg. 210

Addiction: Internet/Video Games

Apply 3-5 drops to bottom of feet and outside of legs from knees to ankles.

Lavender ᴬᵀ
Wild Orange ᴬᵀ
Bergamot ᴬᵀ
Cedarwood ᴬᵀ
Vetiver ᴬᵀ

Protocol on pg. 210

Addiction: Pain Medication

Apply a couple drops to back of neck, temples, and outside of ears as often as needed.

Lavender ᴬᵀᴵ
Ylang Ylang ᴬᵀᴵ
Cinnamon ᴬᵀᴵ
Hopeful Blend ᴬᵀ
Eucalyptus ᴬᵀ

Protocol on pg. 210

Addiction: Sugar

Apply 3-5 drops as needed to abdomen and inside of legs from knees to ankles. Also add a few drops to water throughout the day.

Metabolic Blend ᴬᵀᴵ
Ginger ᴬᵀᴵ
Coriander ᴬᵀᴵ
Encouraging Blend ᴬᵀᴵ
Joyful Blend ᴬᵀᴵ

Protocol on pg. 210

Addison's Disease

Apply 3-5 drops 3x daily to lower back and front of legs near the shins and knees.

Women's Perfume Blend ᴬᵀ
Ylang Ylang ᴬᵀ
Lavender ᴬᵀ
Cinnamon ᴬᵀ
Bergamot ᴬᵀ

Age Spots

Apply 3-5 drops diluted to face at bed time.

Frankincense ᵀ
Sandalwood ᵀ
Helichrysum ᵀ
Anti-Aging Blend ᵀ
Neroli ᵀ

Protocol on pg. 211

AIDS

Apply 3-5 drops to lower back, back of neck, and bottoms of feet. Also combine a few drops in a veggie cap 2-3x daily.

Oregano ᴬᵀᴵ
Sandalwood ᴬᵀᴵ
Myrrh ᴬᵀᴵ
Frankincense ᴬᵀᴵ
Melaleuca ᴬᵀᴵ

Protocol on pg. 181

Addiction: Sex/ Pornography

Apply 3-5 drops to back of neck, forehead, and crown of head as often as needed.

Bergamot ᴬᵀ
Lavender ᴬᵀ
Cedarwood ᴬᵀ
Vetiver ᴬᵀ
Siberian Fir ᴬᵀ

Protocol on pg. 210

Adenitis

Apply 3-5 drops to the lower right quadrant of the abdomen and take internally.

Protective Blend ᴬᵀᴵ
Oregano ᴬᵀᴵ
Melaleuca ᴬᵀᴵ
Frankincense ᴬᵀᴵ
Lavender ᴬᵀᴵ

Aging

Apply 1-3 drops to target areas. Combine 2-8 drops with facial lotion or carrier oil and apply after cleansing.

Anti-Aging Blend ᵀ
Frankincense ᵀ
Cedarwood ᵀ
Sandalwood ᵀ
Vitality Trio ᴵ

Protocol on pg. 211

Air Pollution

Diffuse several drops or apply 3-5 drops over the lungs and nose as often as needed.

Neroli ᴬᵀ
Litsea ᴬᵀ
Patchouli ᴬᵀ
Basil ᴬᵀ
Lavender ᴬᵀ

Addiction: Smoking

Ingest 2-4 drops daily; inhale from cupped hands as needed when experiencing cravings.

Black Pepper ᴬᵀᴵ
Grapefruit ᴬᵀᴵ
Basil ᴬᵀᴵ
Bergamot ᴬᵀᴵ
Detoxification Blend ᴬᵀᴵ

Protocol on pg. 202

Addiction: Work

Apply 3-5 drops to bottoms of feet and outside of legs from knees to ankles.

Lavender ᴬᵀ
Wild Orange ᴬᵀ
Bergamot ᴬᵀ
Cedarwood ᴬᵀ
Vetiver ᴬᵀ

Protocol on pg. 237

Adrenal Fatigue

Massage 1-3 drops onto lower back over adrenals, or inhale from cupped hands. Ingest 1-3 drops as needed.

Basil ᴬᵀᴵ
Juniper Berry ᴬᵀᴵ
Rosemary ᴬᵀᴵ
Geranium ᴬᵀᴵ
Peppermint ᴬᵀᴵ

Protocol on pg. 181

Agitation

Apply 3-5 drops 3x daily over forehead, back of neck, and top of the head. Also use a drop under the tongue.

Bergamot ᴬᵀᴵ
Lavender ᴬᵀᴵ
Restful Blend ᴬᵀ
Roman Chamomile ᴬᵀᴵ
Reassuring Blend ᴬᵀ

Protocol on pg. 202

Airborne Bacteria

Apply 3-5 drops 3x daily over chest and around the nose. Also diffuse several drops throughout the day.

Protective Blend ᴬᵀ
Respiratory Blend ᴬᵀ
Pink Pepper ᴬᵀ
Eucalyptus ᴬᵀ
Melaleuca ᴬᵀ

Alertness

Apply 1-2 drops to forehead, temples, or base of skull as needed; inhale a few drops from cupped hands.

Peppermint ᴬᵀᴵ
Frankincense ᴬᵀᴵ
Basil ᴬᵀᴵ
Rosemary ᴬᵀᴵ
Focus Blend ᴬᵀ

Alkalosis

Apply 3 drops of the oils on hand (preferably all 5 listed) over the chest and ribs.

Lavender ᵀ
Vetiver ᵀ
Roman Chamomile ᵀ
Rose ᵀ
Rosemary ᵀ

Allergies (Seasonal, Pet Dander)

Apply to back of neck, on bridge of nose, or chest as needed; use a drop under the tongue; diffuse several drops.

Lavender ᴬᵀᴵ
Respiratory Blend ᴬᵀ
Cleansing Blend ᴬᵀ
Peppermint ᴬᵀᴵ
Detoxification Blend ᴬᵀᴵ

Protocol on pg. 182

Alzheimer's/ Dementia

Massage 1-2 drops into scalp daily; ingest 2-4 drops 1-2x daily; supplement daily.

Frankincense ᴬᵀᴵ
Rosemary ᴬᵀᴵ
Cellular Complex ᴬᵀᴵ
Rose ᴬᵀ
Vitality Trio ᵀ

Protocol on pg. 182

Amnesia

Diffuse several drops daily and apply 3 -5 drops 3x daily to forehead and top of head.

Rosemary ᴬᵀ
Peppermint ᴬᵀ
Bergamot ᴬᵀ
Wild Orange ᴬᵀ
Frankincense ᴬᵀ

Analgesic

Apply 3-5 drops as needed over the affected area. Also use a drop under the tongue.

Frankincense ᴬᵀᴵ
Lavender ᴬᵀᴵ
Marjoram ᴬᵀᴵ
Peppermint ᴬᵀᴵ
Rosemary ᴬᵀᴵ

Anemia

Apply 1-3 drops to bottoms of feet and inside of wrists; take a few drops internally; inhale from cupped hands periodically.

Protective Blend ᴬᵀᴵ
Basil ᴬᵀᴵ
Lemon ᴬᵀᴵ
Lavender ᴬᵀᴵ
Vitality Trio ᵀ

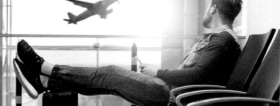

Aneurysm

Diffuse several drops and apply 3-5 drops 3x daily to forehead and top of head.

Frankincense ᴬᵀ
Rosemary ᴬᵀ
Helichrysum ᴬᵀ
Vetiver ᴬᵀ
Myrrh ᴬᵀ

Anger

Apply 1-3 drops to temples and chest; inhale a few drops from cupped hands as needed.

Grounding Blend ᴬᵀ
Renewing Blend ᴬᵀ
Reassuring Blend ᴬᵀ
Melissa ᴬᵀ
Magnolia ᴬᵀ

Protocol on pg. 221

Angina

Apply 3-5 drops over the chest as needed.

Rose ᵀ
Lavender ᵀ
Bergamot ᵀ
Vetiver ᵀ
Siberian Fir ᵀ

Anguish

Apply 3-5 drops 3x daily over forehead, back of neck, and top of the head.

Hopeful Blend ᴬᵀ
Reassuring Blend ᴬᵀ
Comforting Blend ᴬᵀ
Vetiver ᴬᵀ
Siberian Fir ᴬᵀ

Protocol on pg. 235

Animals: Bleeding

Apply 1-2 drops to affected area every 15-30 minutes until bleeding stops. Dilute for sensitive/small animals.

Helichrysum ᵀ
Geranium ᵀ
Rose ᵀ
Lavender ᵀ
Melaleuca ᵀ

Animals: Bone Pain
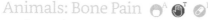

Apply 2-5 drops over the affected area. Dilute for sensitive/small animals.

Wintergreen ᵀ
Eucalyptus ᵀ
Peppermint ᵀ
Rosemary ᵀ
Sandalwood ᵀ

Animals: Cancer (skin)

Apply 2-5 drops to affected area 4-5x daily. Dilute for sensitive/small animals.

Frankincense ᵀ
Lavender ᵀ
Sandalwood ᵀ
Hopeful Blend ᵀ
Geranium ᵀ

Animals: Colds & Cough
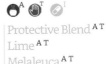

Apply 2-5 drops over chest, and around ears and throat 3x daily. Dilute for sensitive/small animals.

Protective Blend ᴬᵀ
Lime ᴬᵀ
Melaleuca ᴬᵀ
Rosemary ᴬᵀ
Oregano ᴬᵀ

Animals: Stress & Anxiety

Apply 2-5 drops over the forehead, back of neck, and top of head as needed. Dilute for sensitive/small animals.

Reassuring Blend ᴬᵀ
Rose ᴬᵀ
Lavender ᴬᵀ
Restful Blend ᴬᵀ
Neroli ᴬᵀ

Ankle Swelling

Massage ankles with 2-4 drops diluted with carrier oil if desired.

Juniper Berry ᵀ
Grapefruit ᵀ
Lemongrass ᵀ
Soothing Blend ᵀ
Tension Blend ᵀ

Ankylosing Spondylitis

Apply 2 drops of each to spine, back of the neck, and other affected areas.

Ginger ᵀ
Frankincense ᵀ
Myrrh ᵀ
Wintergreen ᵀ
Bergamot ᵀ

Anorexia

Apply 1-3 drops to stomach area or inhale from cupped hands as needed.

Grapefruit ᴬᵀ
Ginger ᴬᵀ
Invigorating Blend ᴬᵀ
Joyful Blend ᴬᵀ
Uplifting Blend ᴬᵀ

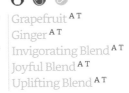
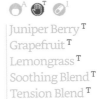
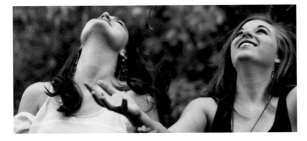

Antibacterial

Combine 3 drops of oils on hand into a capsule and take internally 4x daily; apply topically or diffuse as needed.

Protective Blend ᴬᵀᴵ
Oregano ᴬᵀᴵ
Cinnamon ᴬᵀᴵ
Melaleuca ᴬᵀᴵ
Melissa ᴬᵀᴵ

Anticoagulant

Add 2 drops of each to a capsule and take internally 2x daily.

Basil ᵀᴵ
Oregano ᵀᴵ
Wintergreen ᵀᴵ
Birch ᵀᴵ
Cassia ᵀᴵ

Antidepressant

Apply 3-5 drops over the forehead, back of neck, and top of head 3x daily. Also diffuse several drops.

Joyful Blend ᴬᵀᴵ
Magnolia ᴬᵀᴵ
Rose ᴬᵀᴵ
Frankincense ᴬᵀᴵ
Melaleuca ᴬᵀᴵ

Protocol on pg. 189

Antifungal

Combine 3-5 drops of oils on hand with carrier oil and rub into affected area.

Melaleuca ᵀ
Oregano ᵀ
Thyme ᵀ
Clove ᵀ
Geranium ᵀ

Antioxidant

Apply 3-5 drops to outside of legs and feet. Use a few drops in a capsule.

Clove ᵀᴵ
Blue Tansy ᵀ
Yarrow ᵀᴵ
Rosemary ᵀᴵ
Oregano ᵀᴵ

Antisocial

Apply 3-5 drops over the forehead and back of neck. Also diffuse several drops.

Encouraging Blend ᴬᵀ
Siberian Fir ᴬᵀ
Spearmint ᴬᵀ
Lime ᴬᵀ
Ginger ᴬᵀ

Antiviral

Combine 3 drops of oils on hand into a capsule and take internally 4x daily. Rub 2-3 drops on bottoms of feet. Also diffuse several drops.

Melissa ᴬᵀᴵ
Oregano ᴬᵀᴵ
Protective Blend ᴬᵀᴵ
Melaleuca ᴬᵀᴵ
Green Mandarin ᴬᵀᴵ

Anxiety

Apply 1-3 drops to bottoms of feet, chest, or temples, or inhale from cupped hands as needed; use a drop under the tongue.

Grounding Blend ᴬᵀ
Vetiver ᴬᵀᴵ
Reassuring Blend ᴬᵀ
Bergamot ᴬᵀᴵ
Frankincense ᴬᵀᴵ

Protocol on pg. 182

Apathy

Apply 1-3 drops to bottoms of feet, chest, or temples, or inhale from cupped hands as needed. Also diffuse several drops.

Patchouli ᴬᵀ
Neroli ᴬᵀ
Peppermint ᴬᵀ
Ylang Ylang ᴬᵀ
Renewing Blend ᴬᵀ

Aphrodisiac

Apply 2-4 drops to wrists and neck. Also diffuse several drops.

Inspiring Blend [AT]
Jasmine [AT]
Cinnamon [AT]
Sandalwood [AT]
Rose [AT]

Protocol on pg. 227

Appetite Stimulant

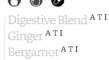

Apply 3-5 drops over the abdomen or drink a couple drops in water. Also diffuse several drops.

Digestive Blend [ATI]
Ginger [ATI]
Bergamot [ATI]
Coriander [ATI]
Fennel [ATI]

Appetite Suppressant

Apply 1-3 drops to stomach, chest, bottoms of feet, or inside of wrists or take 2-4 drops internally.

Metabolic blend [ATI]
Peppermint [ATI]
Grapefruit [ATI]
Ginger [ATI]
Wild Orange [ATI]

Arrhythmia

Apply 3-5 drops to inside of arms and chest 3x daily.

Lemon [T]
Lavender [T]
Ylang Ylang [T]
Marjoram [T]
Cypress [T]

Artery Issues

Apply 3-5 drops to inside of arms and chest 2x daily.

Basil [T]
Clary Sage [T]
Cypress [T]
Cassia [T]
Eucalyptus [T]

Arteriosclerosis

Place 2 drops of oils on hand in a capsule and take internally 3x daily.

Frankincense [I]
Ginger [I]
Clary Sage [I]
Cinnamon [I]
Melaleuca [I]

Arthritic Pain

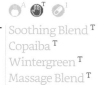

Apply 1-3 drops and massage into affected areas with lotion or carrier oil as needed.

Soothing Blend [T]
Copaiba [T]
Wintergreen [T]
Massage Blend [T]
Cellular Complex [T]

Protocol on pg. 183

Asthma

Apply 1-3 drops topically to chest, neck, under nose, and on bridge of nose, or inhale from cupped hands as needed.

Respiratory Blend [AT]
Eucalyptus [AT]
Peppermint [AT]
Roman Chamomile [AT]
Lavender [AT]

Protocol on pg. 183

Atherosclerosis

Place 2 drops of oils on hand in a capsule and take internally 3x daily.

Lemon [I]
Ginger [I]
Clary Sage [I]
Cinnamon [I]
Grapefruit [I]

Athlete's Foot

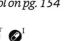

Apply 1-3 drops to area between toes and around toenails 2-3x daily. Ingest 1-3 drops of melaleuca or oregano once a day (no more than 10 days).

Melaleuca [TI]
Oregano [TI]
Skin Clearing Blend [T]
Geranium [TI]
Lemon [TI]

Protocol on pg. 154

Autism/Asperger's

Apply 1-3 drops to bottoms of feet and back of neck. Ingest 1-3 drops of Cilantro or Cellular Complex 1-2x daily.

Frankincense [ATI]
Focus Blend [AT]
Cilantro [ATI]
Rose [AT]
Cellular Complex [ATI]

Protocol on pg. 183

Autoimmune Disorders

Apply 1-3 drops to stomach, chest, bottoms of feet, or inside of wrists. Ingest 2-4 drops 3x daily.

Cellular Complex [TI]
Detoxification Blend [TI]
Frankincense [TI]
Anti-Aging Blend [T]
Vitality Trio [I]

Protocol on pg. 184

Autointoxication

Apply 1-3 drops to stomach, chest, bottoms of feet, or inside of wrists. Ingest 1-3 drops 2-3x daily for additional support.

Detoxification Blend [ATI]
Cilantro [ATI]
Thyme [ATI]
Grapefruit [ATI]
Geranium [ATI]

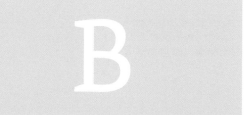

Back Pain

Apply 1-3 drops and massage into affected areas as needed. Use a carrier oil or lotion for increased efficacy. Take 2 capsules of Cellular Complex 2-3x daily.

Soothing Blend [AT]
Massage Blend [AT]
Turmeric [ATI]
Copaiba [ATI]
Polyphenol Complex [I]

Protocol on pg. 184

Back Stiffness

Combine 3-5 drops of oils on hand and massage into affected area as often as needed.

Soothing Blend ^T — Soothing Blend ᵀ
Wintergreen ᵀ
Ylang Ylang ᵀ
Peppermint ᵀ
Cypress ᵀ

Protocol on pg. 184

Bacterial Infection

Apply 1-3 drops with a carrier oil to affected areas as needed. Ingest 1-3 drops every 2-3 hours for systemic/internal infections.

Oregano ᴬᵀᴵ
Thyme ᴬᵀᴵ
Protective Blend ᴬᵀᴵ
Melaleuca ᴬᵀᴵ
Pink Pepper ᴬᵀᴵ

Bags Under Eyes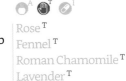

Combine 2 drops with carrier oil and gently rub under eyes at bedtime.

Rose ᵀ
Fennel ᵀ
Roman Chamomile ᵀ
Lavender ᵀ
Cypress ᵀ

Balance Problems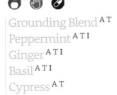

Apply 1-3 drops topically to forehead, temples, back of neck, and behind the ears or inhale from cupped hands. Ingest 1-3 drops of Ginger as needed.

Grounding Blend ᴬᵀ
Peppermint ᴬᵀᴵ
Ginger ᴬᵀᴵ
Basil ᴬᵀᴵ
Cypress ᴬᵀ

Balding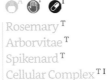

Dilute 5 drops in 20 drops of carrier oil. Massage into scalp every night. Supplement with Cellular Complex and Vitality Trio daily.

Rosemary ᵀ
Arborvitae ᵀ
Spikenard ᵀ
Cellular Complex ᵀᴵ
Vitality Trio ᵀᴵ

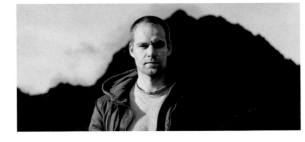

Basal Cell Carcinoma

Combine 3-5 drops of oils on hand and apply directly to affected area.

Frankincense ᵀ
Cellular Complex ᵀ
Sandalwood ᵀ
Myrrh ᵀ
Vetiver ᵀ

Protocol on pg. 186

Bed Bugs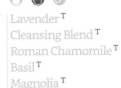

Combine 10 drops of oils on hand (preferably all 5 listed oils) into 20 oz glass spray bottle of water and spray on bed or upholstery.

Melaleuca ᵀ
Lemon ᵀ
Lavender ᵀ
Sandalwood ᵀ
Cinnamon ᵀ

Bed Sores

Apply 3-6 drops with carrier oil to affected area 3x daily.

Frankincense ᵀ
Melaleuca ᵀ
Lavender ᵀ
Neroli ᵀ
Helichrysum ᵀ

Bed-wetting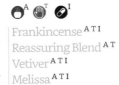

Massage 2-4 drops over bladder and kidneys before bedtime.

Cypress ᵀ
Black Pepper ᵀ
Ylang Ylang ᵀ
Lemongrass ᵀ
Roman Chamomile ᵀ

Bee Sting

Apply 1-2 drops topically to sting or bite several times daily until symptoms cease.

Lavender ᵀ
Cleansing Blend ᵀ
Roman Chamomile ᵀ
Basil ᵀ
Magnolia ᵀ

Bell's Palsy

Ingest 2-4 drops every 2-3 hours as needed.

Clove ᴵ
Melissa ᴵ
Frankincense ᴵ
Thyme ᴵ
Vitality Trio ᴵ

Bipolar Disorder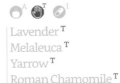

Apply 1-3 drops to bottoms of feet, chest, or temples, or inhale from cupped hands as needed.

Frankincense ᴬᵀᴵ
Reassuring Blend ᴬᵀ
Vetiver ᴬᵀᴵ
Melissa ᴬᵀᴵ
Vitality Trio ᴵ

Protocol on pg. 184

Bites

Apply 2-4 drops to affected area as often as needed.

Lavender ᵀ
Melaleuca ᵀ
Yarrow ᵀ
Roman Chamomile ᵀ
Petitgrain ᵀ

Bladder Control

Apply 1-3 drops topically over bladder and kidneys as needed. Add 1-2 drops to drinking water and sip throughout the day.

Rosemary ᵀᴵ
Juniper Berry ᵀᴵ
Cypress ᵀᴵ
Marjoram ᵀᴵ
Sandalwood ᵀᴵ

Bladder Infection

Rub 3-4 drops over bladder. Take 3-5 drops in a capsule after food 3x daily.

Cypress ᵀ
Oregano ᵀ ᴵ
Clove ᵀ ᴵ
Eucalyptus ᵀ
Melaleuca ᵀ ᴵ

Protocol on pg. 204

Bleeding

Apply a drop topically to affected area as needed.

Helichrysum ᵀ
Geranium ᵀ
Myrrh ᵀ
Lemon ᵀ
Melaleuca ᵀ

Blisters from Sun

Apply a few drops liberally to affected area.

Frankincense ᵀ
Lavender ᵀ
Patchouli ᵀ
Melaleuca ᵀ
Myrrh ᵀ

Protocol on pg. 203

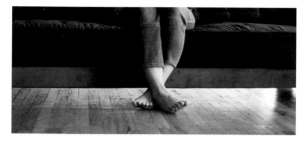

Blisters on Feet

Apply a few drops topically to affected area.

Lavender ᵀ
Frankincense ᵀ
Patchouli ᵀ
Melaleuca ᵀ
Myrrh ᵀ

Bloating
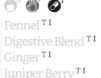

Apply 1-3 drops to stomach, rubbing in a clockwise direction. Use 1-3 drops internally as needed.

Fennel ᵀ ᴵ
Digestive Blend ᵀ ᴵ
Ginger ᵀ ᴵ
Juniper Berry ᵀ ᴵ
Peppermint ᵀ ᴵ

Protocol on pg. 190

Blocked Tear Ducts

Apply 1-2 drops to bridge of nose; avoid getting in the eyes; dilute if using on an infant.

Lavender ᵀ
Clary Sage ᵀ
Melaleuca ᵀ

Blood Clotting

Apply 1-3 drops to affected area or ingest a few drops internally as needed.

Wintergreen ᵀ
Helichrysum ᵀ ᴵ
Birch ᵀ
Peppermint ᵀ ᴵ
Ginger ᵀ ᴵ

Blood Pressure (High)

Apply 2-4 drops to stomach, chest, bottoms of feet, or inside of wrists; ingest 2-4 drops 2x daily.

Cypress ᴬ ᵀ
Marjoram ᴬ ᵀ ᴵ
Lemon ᴬ ᵀ ᴵ
Ylang Ylang ᴬ ᵀ ᴵ
Jasmine ᴬ ᵀ

Protocol on pg. 184

Blood Pressure (Low)

Apply 1-3 drops to stomach, chest, bottoms of feet, or inside of wrists, or ingest a few drops as needed.

Helichrysum ᴬ ᵀ ᴵ
Frankincense ᴬ ᵀ ᴵ
Jasmine ᴬ ᵀ
Cedarwood ᴬ ᵀ
Vitality Trio ᴵ

Blood Sugar (High)

Apply 2-4 drops over pancreas and bottoms of feet daily; take a few drops internally.

Protective Blend ᵀ ᴵ
Metabolic Blend ᵀ ᴵ
Cinnamon ᵀ ᴵ
Coriander ᵀ ᴵ
Ginger ᵀ ᴵ

Blood Sugar (Low)

Apply 1-3 drops to stomach, chest, bottoms of feet, or inside of wrists, or ingest 1-3 drops as needed.

Cinnamon ᵀ ᴵ
Melissa ᵀ ᴵ
Cassia ᵀ ᴵ
Wild Orange ᵀ ᴵ
Vitality Trio ᴵ

Blurred Vision

Mix oils in a roller bottle with carrier oil and carefully apply around eyes 2-4x daily.

Clary Sage ᵀ
Helichrysum ᵀ
Anti-Aging Blend ᵀ
Cellular Complex ᵀ
Lavender ᵀ

Body Odor

Take 3-5 drops of Cilantro, Detoxification Blend, or Dill at least once daily. Apply 1-3 drops on bottoms of feet.

Cilantro ᵀ ᴵ
Detoxification Blend ᵀ ᴵ
Dill ᵀ ᴵ
Melaleuca ᵀ ᴵ
Petitgrain ᵀ ᴵ

Protocol on pg. 188

Boils

Apply 1-3 drops topically to affected areas several times daily.

Melaleuca ᵀ
Skin Clearing Blend ᵀ
Lavender ᵀ
Myrrh ᵀ
Bergamot ᵀ

Bone Pain/Break

Apply 3-5 drops topically to affected areas as needed. Massage with lotion or carrier oil to improve efficacy.

Soothing Blend [T]
Wintergreen [T]
Birch [T]
Helichrysum [T]
Bone Nutrient Complex [I]

Bone Spurs

Add 10 drops of oils on hand to a roller bottle and apply to affected area as often as needed.

Eucalyptus [T]
Myrrh [T]
Frankincense [T]
Wintergreen [T]
Peppermint [T]

Protocol on pg. 185

Brain Fog
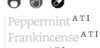

Apply 1-3 drops to forehead, temples, back of neck, and behind ears or inhale from cupped hands as needed.

Peppermint [ATI]
Frankincense [ATI]
Lemon [ATI]
Rosemary [ATI]
Vitality Trio [I]

Protocol on pg. 191

Brain Injury

Apply a few drops to forehead, temples, base of skull, and behind the ears. Diffuse several drops. Take 3-5 drops in a capsule 3x daily.

Frankincense [ATI]
Cellular Complex [ATI]
Cedarwood [AT]
Sandalwood [ATI]
Vitality Trio [I]

Brain Support

Apply 3-5 drops to the back of neck and backside of legs. Diffuse Several Drops. Take 3-5 drops in a capsule 3x daily.

Rosemary [ATI]
Frankincense [ATI]
Basil [ATI]
Grapefruit [ATI]
Lemon [ATI]

Breastfeeding (Increase Milk)

Massage 1-3 drops with carrier oil over breasts and apply to bottoms of feet or take internally when needed.

Fennel [TI]
Clary Sage [TI]
Basil [TI]
Vitality Trio [I]
Bone Nutrient Complex [I]

Brittle Nails

Apply 1-2 drops to nail bed once daily. Use supplements consistently for long-term benefits.

Lemon [T]
Helichrysum [T]
Frankincense [T]
Bone Nutrient Complex [I]
Vitality Trio [I]

Broken Bones

Apply 3-5 drops to the affected area 5x daily.

Cypress [T]
Wintergreen [T]
Helichrysum [T]
Frankincense [T]
Vetiver [T]

Bronchitis

Apply 2-4 drops to chest and neck area, gargle hourly, or inhale from cupped hands as needed.

Respiratory Blend [AT]
Cardamom [ATI]
Lime [ATI]
Roman Chamomile [ATI]
Eucalyptus [AT]

Protocol on pg. 185

Bruising

Apply 2-4 drops to bruise area. Use carrier oil if desired. Reapply 2-4x daily.

Tension Blend [T]
Soothing Blend [T]
Helichrysum [T]
Cypress [T]
Anti-Aging Blend [T]

Bulimia

Apply 3-5 drops to back of neck and back 2x daily.

Basil [T]
Bergamot [T]
Melaleuca [T]
Eucalyptus [T]
Lavender [T]

Bunions

Apply 2-4 drops with carrier oil to affected area or joint as needed.

Lemon [T]
Soothing Blend [T]
Copaiba [T]
Peppermint [T]
Cypress [T]

Burns

Apply 2-4 drops to affected area hourly or as needed. For more severe, mix 2-8 drops with 4 oz witch hazel and apply as needed.

Lavender [T]
Frankincense [T]
Helichrysum [T]
Anti-Aging Blend [T]
Cedarwood [T]

Burping
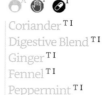

Apply 3-5 drops to upper abdomen as often as needed. Drink a couple drops in water if desired.

Coriander ᵀ ᴵ
Digestive Blend ᵀ ᴵ
Ginger ᵀ ᴵ
Fennel ᵀ ᴵ
Peppermint ᵀ ᴵ

Bursitis

Combine 5 drops of oils on hand to carrier oil and apply liberally to affected area as often as desired.

Wintergreen ᵀ
Soothing Blend ᵀ
Ylang Ylang ᵀ
Helichrysum ᵀ
Blue Tansy ᵀ

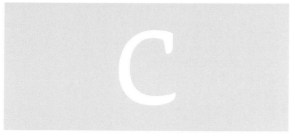

C

Calluses
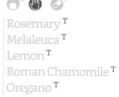

Rub 3-5 drops onto affected area, followed by a pumice stone to remove.

Rosemary ᵀ
Melaleuca ᵀ
Lemon ᵀ
Roman Chamomile ᵀ
Oregano ᵀ

Cancer
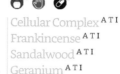

Ingest 3-5 drops 3-5x daily. Apply topically if appropriate. Diffuse several drops. Supplement for added support.

Cellular Complex ᴬ ᵀ ᴵ
Frankincense ᴬ ᵀ ᴵ
Sandalwood ᴬ ᵀ ᴵ
Geranium ᴬ ᵀ ᴵ
Vitality Trio ᴵ

Protocol on pg. 186

Candida
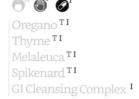

Apply 2-4 drops over abdomen and bottoms of feet. Take 3-5 drops in a capsule at least twice daily until symptoms subside.

Oregano ᵀ ᴵ
Thyme ᵀ ᴵ
Melaleuca ᵀ ᴵ
Spikenard ᵀ ᴵ
GI Cleansing Complex ᴵ

Protocol on pg. 186

Canker Sores
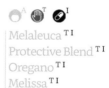

Apply a drop diluted with carrier oil directly to canker sore or gargle several times daily until sore is gone.

Melaleuca ᵀ ᴵ
Protective Blend ᵀ ᴵ
Oregano ᵀ ᴵ
Melissa ᵀ ᴵ
Frankincense ᵀ ᴵ

Protocol on pg. 186

Cardiovascular Disease

Apply 2-4 drops over chest 3x daily. Ingest 3-5 drops as needed.

Cellular Complex ᵀ ᴵ
Geranium ᵀ ᴵ
Black Pepper ᵀ ᴵ
Coriander ᵀ ᴵ
Cypress ᵀ

Carpal Tunnel

Apply 2-4 drops to affected area several times daily. Massage with carrier oil or lotion for improved efficacy.

Soothing Blend ᵀ
Wintergreen ᵀ
Lemongrass ᵀ
Marjoram ᵀ
Oregano ᵀ

Cartilage Injury

Apply 1-3 drops to affected area several times daily. Massage with carrier oil or lotion for improved efficacy.

Soothing Blend ᵀ
Lemongrass ᵀ
Frankincense ᵀ
Helichrysum ᵀ
Copaiba ᵀ

Cataracts

Apply 1-3 drops under eyes, lower back and temples 3x daily.

Frankincense ᵀ
Rosemary ᵀ
Cypress ᵀ
Vitality Trio ᴵ

Cats (General Health)

Heavily dilute 1-2 drops and apply topically to paws daily.

Jasmine ᵀ
Basil ᵀ
Rose ᵀ
Clary Sage ᵀ
Thyme ᵀ

Cavities

Apply 1-2 drops directly on tooth 2x daily. Dilute with carrier oil if necessary.

Clove ᵀ ᴵ
Protective Blend ᵀ ᴵ
Melaleuca ᵀ ᴵ
Bone Nutrient Complex ᴵ
Vitality Trio ᴵ

Celiac Disease

Apply 2-4 drops to abdomen as often as needed. Also take 2-5 drops in a capsule.

Ginger ᵀ ᴵ
Peppermint ᵀ ᴵ
Fennel ᵀ ᴵ
Coriander ᵀ ᴵ
Digestive Blend ᵀ ᴵ

Protocol on pg. 187

Cellulite

Massage 4-8 drops onto target areas daily, especially before exercising. Add to drinking water and consume throughout the day.

Metabolic Blend ᵀ ᴵ
Grapefruit ᵀ ᴵ
Lemon ᵀ ᴵ
Juniper Berry ᵀ ᴵ
Cinnamon ᵀ ᴵ

Protocol on pg. 205

Cellulitis

Apply 3-5 drops liberally to affected areas 3x daily. Dilute with carrier oil if needed.

Lavender ᵀ
Melaleuca ᵀ
Helichrysum ᵀ
Roman Chamomile ᵀ
Lemon ᵀ

Chapped Skin

Apply a drop or two to affected area as often as needed. Use a carrier oil to increase efficacy.

Myrrh ᵀ
Roman Chamomile ᵀ
Anti-Aging Blend ᵀ
Cedarwood ᵀ
Magnolia ᵀ

Charley Horse

Massage 1-3 drops onto area of concern. Use a carrier oil or lotion for improved efficacy.

Massage Blend ᵀ
Soothing Blend ᵀ
Marjoram ᵀ
Black Pepper ᵀ
Bergamot ᵀ

Chest Pain

Apply 1-3 drops topically to chest or ingest at least twice daily.

Cellular Complex ᵀ ᴵ
Protective Blend ᵀ ᴵ
Lemon ᵀ ᴵ
Wild Orange ᵀ ᴵ
Marjoram ᵀ ᴵ

Chicken Pox

Dilute 2-4 drops with a carrier oil and dab lightly on spots a couple times a day or ingest for immune support.

Lavender ᵀ ᴵ
Thyme ᵀ ᴵ
Melaleuca ᵀ ᴵ
Cellular Complex ᵀ ᴵ
Melissa ᵀ ᴵ

Chiggers

Dilute 2-4 drops with a carrier oil and dab lightly on bites a couple times a day.

Outdoor Blend ᵀ
Lemongrass ᵀ
Melaleuca ᵀ
Detoxification Blend ᵀ
Arborvitae ᵀ

Cholera

Apply 1-3 drops with a carrier oil to the affected areas as needed. Ingest 1-3 drops every 2-3 hours for systemic/internal infections.

Thyme ᵀ ᴵ
Oregano ᵀ ᴵ
Protective Blend ᵀ ᴵ
Melaleuca ᵀ ᴵ
Arborvitae ᵀ ᴵ

Cholesterol (High)

Apply 2-4 drops to chest area, bottoms of feet, or inside of wrists; ingest 2-4 drops once daily.

Cellular Complex ᵀ ᴵ
Lemon ᵀ ᴵ
Rosemary ᵀ ᴵ
Detoxification Blend ᵀ ᴵ
Vitality Trio ᴵ

Protocol on pg. 187

Chronic Fatigue

Apply 2-4 drops to chest area, bottoms of feet, or inside of wrists; inhale 1-3 drops from cupped hands; supplement regularly for long-term benefits.

Lemon ᴬ ᵀ ᴵ
Melissa ᴬ ᵀ ᴵ
Basil ᴬ ᵀ ᴵ
Energy & Stamina Complex ᴵ
Vitality Trio ᴵ

Protocol on pg. 191

Chronic Pain

Apply 1-3 drops to affected areas as needed, using carrier oil for improved efficacy; supplement regularly for long-term care.

Soothing Blend ᴬ ᵀ
Copaiba ᴬ ᵀ ᴵ
Cellular Complex ᴬ ᵀ ᴵ
Turmeric ᴬ ᵀ ᴵ
Vitality Trio ᴵ

Circulation (Poor)

Apply 1-3 drops to bottoms of feet; ingest 1-3 drops twice daily or as needed.

Cypress ᵀ ᴵ
Ginger ᵀ ᴵ
Black Pepper ᵀ ᴵ
Cellular Complex ᵀ ᴵ
Energy & Stamina Complex ᴵ

Cirrhosis of the Liver

Apply 3 drops of oils on hand (preferably all 5 listed) with carrier oil over the liver 3x daily.

Clove ᵀ
Grapefruit ᵀ
Geranium ᵀ
Rosemary ᵀ
Frankincense ᵀ

Cold (Common)

Ingest 3-5 drops 3-4x daily until symptoms subside. Diffuse several drops. Supplement regularly for long-term benefits.

Protective Blend ᴬ ᵀ ᴵ
Respiratory Blend ᴬ ᵀ
Oregano ᴬ ᵀ ᴵ
Melissa ᴬ ᵀ ᴵ
Thyme ᴬ ᵀ ᴵ

Protocol on pg. 187

Cold Extremities

Apply 2-4 drops to bottoms of feet, chest area, and inside of wrists; ingest 2-4 drops daily as needed.

Cypress ^{ATI}
Black Pepper ^{ATI}
Cinnamon ^{ATI}
Protective Blend ^{ATI}
Energy & Stamina Complex ^I

Cold Sores

Dilute with carrier oil and apply a drop to affected area as needed.

Melissa ^T
Protective Blend ^T
Melaleuca ^T
Clove ^T
Frankincense ^T

Protocol on pg. 193

Colic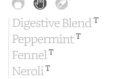

Dilute 1-2 drops with a carrier oil and apply topically to stomach and back before baby goes to sleep.

Digestive Blend ^T
Peppermint ^T
Fennel ^T
Neroli ^T
Roman Chamomile ^T

Colitis

Add 2 drops of oils on hand to capsule and take after eating 3x daily.

Lemon ^I
Clove ^I
Fennel ^I
Ginger ^I
Frankincense ^I

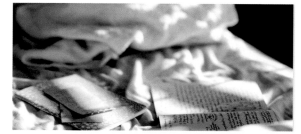

Coma

Massage 3-5 drops onto temples and base of skull 3x daily. Also diffuse several drops.

Bergamot ^{AT}
Lavender ^{AT}
Wintergreen ^{AT}
Wild Orange ^{AT}
Siberian Fir ^{AT}

Concentration

Apply 3 drops to back of neck and temples. Also diffuse several drops.

Frankincense ^{AT}
Peppermint ^{AT}
Focus Blend ^{AT}
Vetiver ^{AT}
Rosemary ^{AT}

Protocol on pg. 191

Concussion

Apply 2-4 drops to forehead, temples, base of skull, and behind the ears; inhale 1-3 drops from cupped hands; take 2-5 drops internally for a few days.

Frankincense ^{ATI}
Bergamot ^{ATI}
Cypress ^{AT}
Copaiba ^{ATI}
Rosemary ^{ATI}

Confusion

Apply 3 drops to back of neck and temples. Also diffuse several drops.

Lavender ^{AT}
Peppermint ^{AT}
Rosemary ^{AT}
Bergamot ^{AT}
Lemon ^{AT}

Congenital Heart Disease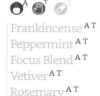

Place 2 drops of oils on hand (preferably all 5 listed) in a capsule and take internally 3x daily. Rub 2-4 drops over chest.

Frankincense ^{TI}
Ginger ^{TI}
Clary Sage ^{TI}
Cinnamon ^{TI}
Melaleuca ^{TI}

Congestion

Apply 1-3 drops to back of neck, under nose, on bridge of nose, or chest; inhale 1-3 drops from cupped hands as needed. Also gargle a drop.

Respiratory Blend ^{AT}
Lemon ^{ATI}
Rosemary ^{ATI}
Cardamom ^{ATI}
Lime ^{ATI}

Conjunctivitis (Pink Eye)

Apply 1-3 drops around the eye 4x daily. Do not get directly in eye.

Melaleuca ^T
Myrrh ^T
Eucalyptus ^T
Litsea ^T
Lavender ^T

Connective Tissue Injury

Combine 5 drops to carrier oil and apply liberally to affected area as often as desired.

Wintergreen ^T
Ylang Ylang ^T
Soothing Blend ^T
Helichrysum ^T
Blue Tansy ^T

Constipation

Massage 2-4 drops over abdomen, moving in a clockwise fashion. Repeat as desired every 5-10 minutes as needed. Ingest 2-4 drops for additional support.

Digestive Blend ^{TI}
Ginger ^{TI}
Marjoram ^{TI}
Cilantro ^{TI}
Fennel ^{TI}

Protocol on pg. 190

Control Issues

Apply a few drops as often as needed to back of the neck, temples and ears (not inside ears).

Vetiver ^{AT}
Siberian Fir ^{AT}
Lavender ^{AT}
Cedarwood ^{AT}
Oregano ^{AT}

Protocol on pg. 221

Convulsions

Apply 2-4 drops to bottoms of feet, spine, and back of neck as needed. Also diffuse several drops.

Frankincense ^{AT}
Wintergreen ^{AT}
Vetiver ^{AT}
Sandalwood ^{AT}
Rosemary ^{AT}

Corns

Apply 3-5 drops to affected area 3x daily for a few days, then use pumice stone to remove.

Rosemary ^T
Melaleuca ^T
Peppermint ^T
Roman Chamomile ^T
Oregano ^T

Cortisol (Heightened)

Apply 1-3 drops to back of neck, under nose, on bridge of nose, or chest as needed; ingest 2-4 drops; inhale from cupped hands.

Lavender ^{ATI}
Basil ^{ATI}
Bergamot ^{ATI}
Marjoram ^{ATI}
Neroli ^{AT}

Protocol on pg. 202

Cough

Apply 1-3 drops to chest, back of neck, under nose, or on bridge of nose, as needed; inhale from cupped hands; gargle a drop.

Respiratory Blend ^{AT}
Rosemary ^{ATI}
Peppermint ^{ATI}
Lemon ^{ATI}
Cardamom ^{ATI}

Protocol on pg. 188

Cows (insect repellent)

Apply or spray 10 drops 3x daily as needed for insect repellent.

Outdoor Blend ^T
Rosemary ^T
Siberian Fir ^T
Eucalyptus ^T
Cedarwood ^T

Cradle Cap

Add 3-5 drops to 30 drops of carrier oil and apply 2x daily.

Melaleuca ^T
Lavender ^T
Frankincense ^T
Lemongrass ^T
Helichrysum ^T

Cramps

Massage 2-4 drops into affected areas as needed. Use with carrier oil to improve efficacy.

Soothing Blend ^T
Massage Blend ^T
Arborvitae ^T
Women's Monthly Blend ^T
Peppermint ^T

Cramps (Menstrual)

Massage 2-4 drops into abdomen, lower back, and shoulders; apply to a warm compress over uterus area; ingest 2-4 drops as needed.

Women's Monthly Blend ^T
Clary Sage ^T
Frankincense ^T
Peppermint ^T
Massage Blend ^T

Protocol on pg. 195

Crohn's Disease

Apply 2-5 drops with carrier oil over abdomen as often as needed.

Peppermint ^T
Basil ^T
Ginger ^T
Fennel ^T
Cardamom ^T

Protocol on pg. 188

Croup

Dilute with carrier oil and apply 1-3 drops to baby's chest and back as needed. Diffuse several drops.

Respiratory Blend ^{AT}
Roman Chamomile ^{AT}
Lemon ^{AT}
Sandalwood ^{AT}
Wild Orange ^{AT}

Crying

Apply 1-2 drops to front of shirt or sleeve, or diffuse several drops.

Lavender ^{AT}
Wild Orange ^{AT}
Reassuring Blend ^{AT}
Roman Chamomile ^{AT}
Restful Blend ^{AT}

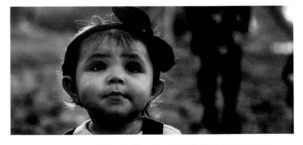

Cushing's Syndrome

Apply 3-5 drops 3x daily over the lower back and back of neck.

Clary Sage ^T
Fennel ^T
Frankincense ^T
Juniper Berry ^T
Helichrysum ^T

Cuts

Dilute 1-2 drops with a carrier oil and apply to affected area a couple times daily.

Melaleuca ^T
Lavender ^T
Helichrysum ^T
Myrrh ^T
Cedarwood ^T

Cutting/Self-Harm

Gargle a few drops. Apply 2-4 drops as often as needed to back of the neck, temples and ears (not inside ears).

Lavender ^{AT}
Vetiver ^{AT}
Ylang Ylang ^{AT}
Bergamot ^{AT}
Comforting Blend ^{AT}

Protocol on pg. 235

Cyst (Ganglion)

Massage 3-5 drops into affected area 3x daily.

Frankincense[T]
Oregano[T]
Thyme[T]
Lemongrass[T]
Cypress[T]

Protocol on pg. 188

Cystic Fibrosis

Apply 1-3 drops to chest and under nose; inhale from cupped hands as needed.

Frankincense[AT]
Respiratory Blend[AT]
Arborvitae[AT]
Eucalyptus[AT]
Melaleuca[AT]

Cystitis/Infection

Add 3-5 drops of each to an empty capsule and take after food 3x daily.

Clove[TI]
Melaleuca[TI]
Oregano[TI]
Eucalyptus[TI]
Cinnamon[TI]

Cysts

Apply 2-4 drops to affected area 3x daily or as needed.

Oregano[T]
Frankincense[T]
Thyme[T]
Tangerine[T]
Cellular Complex[T]

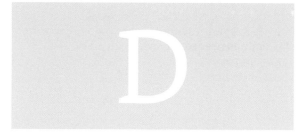

Dandruff

Dilute 2-6 drops in carrier oil and massage into scalp. Rinse after 60 minutes.

Melaleuca[T]
Cedarwood[T]
Rosemary[T]
Myrrh[T]
Petitgrain[T]

Dehydrated Skin

Apply 2-4 drops with carrier oil to affected area as needed. Use with lotion for improved efficacy.

Cedarwood[T]
Captivating Blend[T]
Myrrh[T]
Sandalwood[T]
Anti-Aging Blend[T]

Dehydration

Apply 2-4 drops to bottom of feet, spine and back of neck.

Ylang Ylang[T]
Neroli[T]
Roman Chamomile[T]
Sandalwood[T]
Lavender[T]

Dementia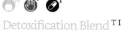

Apply 2-4 drops to forehead, temples, base of skull, and behind the ears; take internally as needed; inhale from cupped hands as needed.

Frankincense[ATI]
Cellular Complex[ATI]
Rose[ATI]
Rosemary[ATI]
Peppermint[ATI]

Protocol on pg. 182

Deodorant

Add 10 drops with carrier oil to roller bottle or apply a dab with carrier oil to underarms.

Melaleuca[T]
Arborvitae[T]
Lavender[T]
Lemongrass[T]
Rosemary[T]

Protocol on pg. 188

Depression

Apply 2-4 drops to forehead and temples; place a drop of Frankincense on thumb and press to roof of mouth; inhale from cupped hands as needed.

Joyful Blend[AT]
Frankincense[ATI]
Uplifting Blend[AT]
Melissa[ATI]
Vitality Trio[I]

Protocol on pg. 189

Detoxification

Apply 3-5 drops to bottoms of feet and inside of wrists; ingest 2-4 drops a few times daily; supplement regularly for improved cleansing.

Detoxification Blend[TI]
Cilantro[TI]
Lemon[TI]
Grapefruit[TI]
Detox Herbal Complex[I]

Protocol on pg. 189

Diabetes

Apply a couple drops over pancreas and bottoms of feet daily; take a few drops internally.

Protective Blend[TI]
Metabolic Blend[TI]
Cinnamon[TI]
Coriander[TI]
Ginger[TI]

Protocol on pg. 189

Diabetes (Gestational)

Apply a couple drops over pancreas and bottoms of feet daily; take a few drops internally.

Protective Blend[TI]
Metabolic Blend[TI]
Cinnamon[TI]
Coriander[TI]
Ginger[TI]

Diaper Rash

Dilute 1-3 drops with carrier oil and apply to affected area several times daily until rash disappears.

Lavender[T]
Roman Chamomile[T]
Ylang Ylang[T]
Coriander[T]
Cedarwood[T]

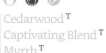

Diarrhea

Ingest 2-4 drops; massage 1-3 drops into abdomen clockwise hourly as needed.

Digestive Blend ᵀ ᴵ
Lemon ᵀ ᴵ
Ginger ᵀ ᴵ
Lavender ᵀ ᴵ
Spearmint ᵀ ᴵ

Digestion Issues

Ingest 2-4 drops; massage 1-3 drops into abdomen clockwise hourly as needed.

Coriander ᵀ ᴵ
Fennel ᵀ ᴵ
Ginger ᵀ ᴵ
Lavender ᵀ ᴵ
Cinnamon ᵀ ᴵ

Protocol on pg. 190

Disinfectant

Add 20 drops to glass spray bottle.

Melaleuca ᵀ
Protective Blend ᵀ
Cleansing Blend ᵀ
Lime ᵀ
Cilantro ᵀ

Diuretic

Add 3-5 drops with carrier oil and apply over the lower back.

Juniper Berry ᵀ
Cypress ᵀ
Rosemary ᵀ
Cedarwood ᵀ
Arborvitae ᵀ

Diverticulitis

Ingest 2-4 drops twice daily for ongoing support; massage 1-3 drops into abdomen clockwise as needed.

Digestive Blend ᵀ ᴵ
Cypress ᵀ ᴵ
Lemon ᵀ ᴵ
Cellular Complex ᵀ ᴵ
Digestive Enzymes ᴵ

Dizziness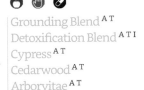

Apply 1-3 drops to back of neck, under nose, or on temples; inhale from cupped hands; ingest 2-4 drops of Detoxification Blend as needed.

Grounding Blend ᴬ ᵀ
Detoxification Blend ᴬ ᵀ ᴵ
Cypress ᴬ ᵀ
Cedarwood ᴬ ᵀ
Arborvitae ᴬ ᵀ

Dogs: Anxiety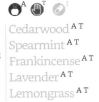

Apply 1-2 drops diluted to pads of paws or outside of ears 2x daily as needed.

Cedarwood ᴬ ᵀ
Spearmint ᴬ ᵀ
Frankincense ᴬ ᵀ
Lavender ᴬ ᵀ
Lemongrass ᴬ ᵀ

Dogs: Arthritis

Apply 1-2 drops diluted to affected areas 2x daily as needed.

Copaiba ᵀ
Clove ᵀ
Lemongrass ᵀ
Wintergreen ᵀ
Rosemary ᵀ

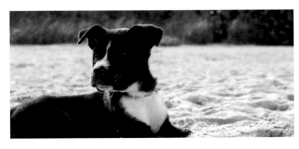

Dogs: Bone Injury

Apply 1-2 drops diluted to affected areas 2x daily as needed.

Copaiba ᵀ
Clove ᵀ
Lemongrass ᵀ
Wintergreen ᵀ
Rosemary ᵀ

Dogs: Dermatitis

Apply 1-2 drops diluted to affected areas 2x daily as needed.

Peppermint ᵀ
Cedarwood ᵀ
Roman Chamomile ᵀ
Lavender ᵀ
Neroli ᵀ

Dogs: Ear Infection

Apply 1-2 drops diluted to outside of ears 2x daily as needed.

Copaiba ᵀ
Lavender ᵀ
Spearmint ᵀ
Rosemary ᵀ
Wintergreen ᵀ

Dogs: Earache

Apply 1-2 drops diluted to outside of ears 2x daily as needed.

Copaiba ᵀ
Lavender ᵀ
Spearmint ᵀ
Rosemary ᵀ
Wintergreen ᵀ

Dogs: Fleas

Add 2-4 drops to dog shampoo and wash 2x daily as needed.

Outdoor Blend ᵀ
Melaleuca ᵀ
Lavender ᵀ
Neroli ᵀ
Rosemary ᵀ

Dogs: Heart Issues

Apply 1-2 drops diluted over chest 2x daily as needed.

Cedarwood ᵀ
Lavender ᵀ
Frankincense ᵀ
Rosemary ᵀ
Roman Chamomile ᵀ

Dogs: Sleep

Apply 1-2 drops diluted to pads of paws or outside of ears 2x daily as needed.

- Lavender A T
- Lemongrass A T
- Roman Chamomile A T
- Cedarwood A T
- Rosemary A T

Dogs: Stroke

Apply 1-2 drops diluted to pads of paws and back of neck 2x daily as needed.

- Cedarwood A T
- Lavender A T
- Frankincense A T
- Rosemary A T
- Roman Chamomile A T

Dry Eyes

Dab a drop diluted with a carrier oil around eyes (do not put directly in eyes). Also apply 2 drops to eye reflex points on bottoms of feet.

- Lavender T
- Lemon T
- Rose T
- Rosemary T
- Marjoram T

Dry Mouth

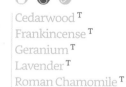

Place 1-2 drops on tongue 2x daily.

- Peppermint I
- Lime I
- Siberian Fir I
- Lemon I
- Ginger I

Dry Skin

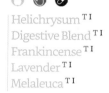

Add 3-5 drops to carrier oil and apply to affected area 2-4x daily.

- Cedarwood T
- Frankincense T
- Geranium T
- Lavender T
- Roman Chamomile T

Dysentery

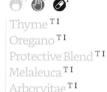

Massage 1-3 drops into abdomen; ingest 2-4 drops as needed.

- Helichrysum T I
- Digestive Blend T I
- Frankincense T I
- Lavender T I
- Melaleuca T I

Dysphagia

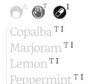

Apply 1-3 drops to neck or ingest a few drops as needed.

- Copaiba T I
- Marjoram T I
- Lemon T I
- Peppermint T I
- Frankincense T I

E

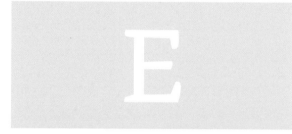

E. Coli

Ingest 1-3 drops every 2-3 hours for systemic and/or internal infections.

- Thyme T I
- Oregano T I
- Protective Blend T I
- Melaleuca T I
- Arborvitae T I

Ear Infection

Apply 1-3 drops around the opening of the ear or apply to a cotton ball and place over ear opening overnight. Do NOT use essential oils in ear. Ingest 2-4 drops as needed.

- Melaleuca T I
- Lavender T I
- Basil T I
- Helichrysum T I
- Melaleuca T I

Protocol on pg. 192

Ear Mites

Apply 2 drops with carrier oil around ear.

- Lemon T
- Lavender T
- Melaleuca T
- Sandalwood T
- Cinnamon T

Earache

Apply 1-3 drops around the opening of the ear or apply to a cotton ball and place over ear opening overnight. Do NOT use essential oils in ear.

- Helichrysum T
- Basil T
- Lavender T
- Melaleuca T
- Frankincense T

Protocol on pg. 192

Eating Disorder

Apply 3-5 drops as needed to abdomen and inside of legs from knees to ankles.

- Bergamot A T
- Lemon A T
- Cinnamon A T
- Ginger A T
- Coriander A T

Ebola Virus

Apply 3-5 drops to back of neck and spine 3x daily; take 3-5 drops in a capsule 2-3x daily as needed.

- Oregano T I
- Clove T I
- Frankincense T I
- Melaleuca T I
- Arborvitae T I

Eczema

Apply 2-4 drops to affected area as needed. For improved efficacy, dilute with carrier oil.

- Skin Clearing Blend T
- Helichrysum T
- Cedarwood T
- Anti-Aging Blend T
- Magnolia T

Protocol on pg. 190

Edema

Massage 2-4 drops into affected area and on bottoms of feet; ingest a couple times daily or as needed.

Lemon ᵀ ᴵ
Eucalyptus ᵀ ᴵ
Peppermint ᵀ ᴵ
Metabolic Blend ᵀ ᴵ
Grapefruit ᵀ ᴵ

Emphysema

Apply 1-3 drops to back of neck, under nose, chest, or on bridge of nose as needed; ingest 3-5 drops; inhale from cupped hands.

Respiratory Blend ᴬ ᵀ
Frankincense ᴬ ᵀ ᴵ
Rose ᴬ ᵀ
Eucalyptus ᴬ ᵀ
Lavender ᴬ ᵀ ᴵ

Endometriosis

Apply 3-5 drops to lower abdomen 3x daily.

Clary Sage ᵀ
Eucalyptus ᵀ
Frankincense ᵀ
Ylang Ylang ᵀ
Patchouli ᵀ

Protocol on pg. 190

Endurance

Massage 2-4 drops on lower back over adrenals, or inhale from cupped hands. Ingest 2-4 drops as needed.

Basil ᴬ ᵀ ᴵ
Juniper Berry ᴬ ᵀ ᴵ
Rosemary ᴬ ᵀ ᴵ
Geranium ᴬ ᵀ ᴵ
Ylang Ylang ᴬ ᵀ ᴵ

Protocol on pg. 212

Energy (low)

Apply 2-4 drops to bottoms of feet, under nose, on bridge of nose, or chest as needed; inhale from cupped hands as needed.

Wild Orange ᴬ ᵀ ᴵ
Peppermint ᴬ ᵀ ᴵ
Spearmint ᴬ ᵀ ᴵ
Energy & Stamina Complex ᴵ
Vitality Trio ᴵ

Protocol on pg. 191

Epilepsy

Apply 1-3 drops to back of neck, under nose, or on temples; inhale from cupped hands; ingest 2-4 drops of Frankincense or Cellular Complex blend 3-5x daily.

Frankincense ᴬ ᵀ ᴵ
Spikenard ᴬ ᵀ ᴵ
Copaiba ᴬ ᵀ ᴵ
Cellular Complex ᴬ ᵀ ᴵ
Vitality Trio ᴵ

Epstein-Barr Virus

Apply 3-5 drops 3x daily to outside of legs, spine and back of neck. Also take in a capsule 2x daily.

Bergamot ᵀ ᴵ
Ylang Ylang ᵀ ᴵ
Lavender ᵀ ᴵ
Marjoram ᵀ ᴵ
Rosemary ᵀ ᴵ

Erectile Dysfunction

Apply 2-4 drops to temples, wrists, and back of neck as needed; inhale from cupped hands; add a drop to personal lubricant.

Rose ᴬ ᵀ
Ylang Ylang ᴬ ᵀ
Inspiring Blend ᴬ ᵀ
Ginger ᴬ ᵀ
Cellular Complex ᴬ ᵀ

Estrogen Imbalance

Apply 2-4 drops to feet, abdomen, and lower back; inhale from cupped hands; take 2-4 drops of Clary Sage in a capsule 2x daily.

Clary Sage ᴬ ᵀ ᴵ
Lavender ᴬ ᵀ ᴵ
Basil ᴬ ᵀ ᴵ
Women's Perfume Blend ᴬ ᵀ
Phytoestrogen Complex ᴵ

Exhaustion

Inhale 1-3 drops from cupped hands; apply a couple drops to feet and back; ingest 2-4 drops Ylang Ylang or Tangerine as needed.

Ylang Ylang ᴬ ᵀ ᴵ
Tangerine ᴬ ᵀ ᴵ
Uplifting Blend ᴬ ᵀ
Encouraging Blend ᴬ ᵀ
Peppermint ᴬ ᵀ ᴵ

Protocol on pg. 191

Eye Support

Apply 2-4 drops diluted around eyes (do not get directly in eyes), lower back, and eye reflex points.

Clary Sage ᵀ
Frankincense ᵀ
Helichrysum ᵀ
Cypress ᵀ
Vetiver ᵀ

Eyes (swollen)

Apply 1-3 drops around eyes (do not get directly in eyes).

Geranium ᵀ
Frankincense ᵀ
Rose ᵀ
Eucalyptus ᵀ
Juniper Berry ᵀ

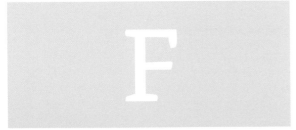

Fainting

Inhale 1-3 drops from cupped hands as needed; apply a drop onto ears and under nose; diffuse several drops.

Peppermint ᴬ ᵀ
Frankincense ᴬ ᵀ
Wild Orange ᴬ ᵀ
Neroli ᴬ ᵀ
Respiratory Blend ᴬ ᵀ

Fear

Inhale from cupped hands; apply a couple drops to feet and back.

Black Pepper ᴬ ᵀ
Juniper Berry ᴬ ᵀ
Grounding Blend ᴬ ᵀ
Frankincense ᴬ ᵀ
Encouraging Blend ᴬ ᵀ

Fever

Apply 2-4 drops to back of neck, under nose, on bridge of nose, or chest; ingest 2-4 drops Oregano every 2-4 hours until symptoms subside.

Peppermint ^{A T I}
Oregano ^{A T I}
Roman Chamomile ^{A T I}
Lavender ^{A T I}
Frankincense ^{A T I}

Fibrocystic Breasts

Massage 1-3 drops into breasts as needed; ingest 3-5 drops 3x daily.

Frankincense ^{T I}
Clary Sage ^{T I}
Sandalwood ^{T I}
Rose ^T
Cellular Complex ^{T I}

Fibroids (Uterine)
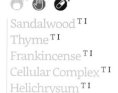

Apply 2-4 drops to abdomen 3x daily; ingest 3-5 drops.

Sandalwood ^{T I}
Thyme ^{T I}
Frankincense ^{T I}
Cellular Complex ^{T I}
Helichrysum ^{T I}

Fibromyalgia

Apply 2-4 drops to affected area; ingest 2-4 drops 3x daily; use full protocol for most profound results.

Cellular Complex ^{A T I}
Soothing Blend ^{A T}
Copaiba ^{A T I}
Frankincense ^{A T I}
Turmeric ^{A T I}

Protocol on pg. 191

Flu (Influenza)

Apply 2-4 drops to chest, bottoms of feet, and back over lungs; ingest 2-4 drops every 2-3 hours as desired for antiviral and immune-boosting support.

Respiratory Blend ^{A T}
Protective Blend ^{A T I}
Oregano ^{A T I}
Thyme ^{A T I}
Black Pepper ^{A T I}

Protocol on pg. 191

Focus

Apply 1-3 drops to forehead, temples, back of neck, and behind the ears; inhale from cupped hands; diffuse several drops.

Peppermint ^{A T}
Focus Blend ^{A T}
Rosemary ^{A T}
Frankincense ^{A T}
Green Mandarin ^{A T}

Protocol on pg. 191

Food Poisoning

Apply 1-3 drops to stomach and rub clockwise; ingest 2-4 drops every 2-4 hours as needed.

Oregano ^{T I}
Digestive Blend ^{T I}
Pink Pepper ^{T I}
Protective Blend ^{T I}
GI Cleansing Complex ^I

Fragile Hair

Apply 3-5 drops to a carrier oil and apply to hair at bedtime or 30 minutes before showering.

Lavender ^T
Peppermint ^T
Rosemary ^T
Cedarwood ^T
Lemongrass ^T

Frozen Shoulder

Apply 2-4 drops to affected area. Massage with carrier oil for improved efficacy.

Soothing Blend ^T
Massage Blend ^T
Cypress ^T
Siberian Fir ^T
Lemongrass ^T

Fungal Skin

Apply 1-3 drops to affected area several times daily.

Melaleuca ^T
Skin Clearing Blend ^T
Oregano ^T
Arborvitae ^T
Cedarwood ^T

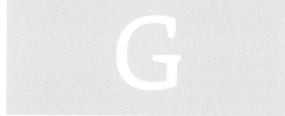

Gallbladder Issues

Massage 2-4 drops over gallbladder several times daily; ingest 2-4 drops as needed.

Juniper Berry ^{T I}
Detoxification Blend ^{T I}
Melaleuca ^{T I}
Helichrysum ^{T I}
Tangerine ^{T I}

Gallbladder Stones

Apply 2-4 drops over gallbladder several times daily; ingest 2-4 drops as needed.

Lemon ^{T I}
Cilantro ^{T I}
Rosemary ^{T I}
Bergamot ^{T I}
Detoxification Blend ^{T I}

Gangrene

Combine 3-5 drops with a carrier oil and apply to affected area hourly.

Lavender ^T
Melaleuca ^T
Frankincense ^T
Copaiba ^T
Arborvitae ^T

Gas (Flatulence)

Massage 1-3 drops into stomach area; ingest 1-3 drops as needed.

Digestive Blend ^{T I}
Fennel ^{T I}
Peppermint ^{T I}
Ginger ^{T I}
Tangerine ^{T I}

Protocol on pg. 190

Gastritis

Massage 1-3 drops into stomach area; ingest 2-4 drops diluted in carrier oil inside a veggie cap as needed.

Lavender^{T I}
Peppermint^{T I}
Roman Chamomile^{T I}
Lemon^{T I}
Coriander^{T I}

Protocol on pg. 190

Gastroesophageal Reflux Disease

Apply 3 -5 drops to upper chest and back before meals.

Lavender^T
Lemon^T
Peppermint^T
Ginger^T
Fennel^T

Genital Warts

Dilute heavily with a carrier oil and apply 1-3 drops to affected area 3x daily.

Oregano^T
Frankincense^T
Melissa^T
Melaleuca^T
Lemon^T

Giardia

Massage 1-3 drops clockwise onto stomach and chest area; ingest 1-3 drops as needed.

Digestive Blend^{T I}
Oregano^{T I}
Rosemary^{T I}
Spearmint^{T I}
Melaleuca^{T I}

Gingivitis

Gargle 1-3 drops mixed with water several times daily; ingest 1-3 drops as needed.

Protective Blend^I
Myrrh^I
Clove^I
Melaleuca^I
Arborvitae^T

Glaucoma

Dab a drop diluted around eye (do not get directly in eyes); combine 2-5 drops into a capsule and take 3x daily.

Rosemary^{T I}
Clary Sage^{T I}
Cypress^T
Lemon^{T I}
Eucalyptus^T

Gluten Sensitivity

Ingest 1-3 drops as needed. Ingest digestive enzymes 20-30 minutes before eating, or immediately after or during consumption. Rub 2-4 drops over stomach.

Digestive Enzymes^I
Digestive Blend^{T I}
Lemon^{T I}
Detoxification Blend^{T I}
Seasonal Blend^{T I}

Gout

Ingest 2-4 drops twice a day; massage 1-3 drops gently into affected joints as needed.

Lemongrass^{T I}
Birch^T
Soothing Blend^T
Peppermint^{T I}
Lavender^{T I}

Protocol on pg. 183

Grave's Disease

Apply 1-3 drops to front of neck. Dilute with carrier oil for easier application. Ingest 1-3 drops a few times daily or as needed.

Frankincense^{T I}
Myrrh^{T I}
Cellular Complex^{T I}
Detoxification Blend^{T I}
Vitality Trio^I

Protocol on pg. 203

Greasy/Oily Hair

Apply 3-5 drops to a carrier oil and apply to hair at bedtime or 30 minutes before showering.

Basil^T
Roman Chamomile^T
Cedarwood^T
Eucalyptus^T
Lemongrass^T

Growing Pains

Massage 2-4 drops into affected areas as needed.

Soothing Blend^T
Marjoram^T
Lemongrass^T
Wintergreen^T
Spikenard^T

Gum Disease

Apply 1-3 drops to gums; gargle a few drops in water as needed.

Protective blend^I
Myrrh^I
Clove^I
Melaleuca^I
Lavender^I

Gums (Bleeding)
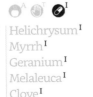

Apply 1-3 drops to gums; gargle a few drops in water as needed.

Helichrysum^I
Myrrh^I
Geranium^I
Melaleuca^I
Clove^I

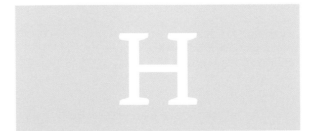

H. Pylori
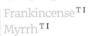

Massage 2-4 drops into stomach area; ingest 1-3 drops as needed.

Fennel^{T I}
Peppermint^{T I}
Digestive Blend^{T I}
Ginger^{T I}
Tangerine^{T I}

Hair Loss

Dilute 5 drops in 20 drops of carrier oil. Massage into scalp every night or 30 minutes before showering.

Rosemary ^T
Peppermint ^T
Geranium ^T
Spikenard ^T
Vitality Trio ^I

Halitosis

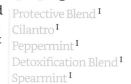

Gargle a few drops mixed with water several times daily or as needed; ingest 1-3 drops Cilantro twice daily.

Protective Blend ^I
Cilantro ^I
Peppermint ^I
Detoxification Blend ^I
Spearmint ^I

Hand, Foot, & Mouth

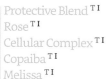

Apply 1-3 drops to affected areas (dilute for increased effectiveness); ingest as needed.

Protective Blend ^{T I}
Rose ^{T I}
Cellular Complex ^{T I}
Copaiba ^{T I}
Melissa ^{T I}

Hands Tingling

Apply 3-5 drops to the affected area, lower back, and spine.

Peppermint ^T
Eucalyptus ^T
Rosemary ^T
Frankincense ^T
Lavender ^T

Hangover

Add 4-6 drops to warm bath; massage into back of neck and over liver; ingest 2-4 drops as needed.

Digestive Blend ^{A T I}
Tension Blend ^{A T}
Grapefruit ^{A T I}
Detoxification Blend ^{A T I}
Lemon ^{A T I}

Hashimoto's

Apply 1-3 drops to front of neck. Dilute with carrier oil for easier application. Ingest 1-3 drops a few times daily or as needed.

Clove ^{T I}
Lemongrass ^{T I}
Myrrh ^{T I}
Peppermint ^{T I}
Rosemary ^{T I}

Protocol on pg. 203

Hay Fever

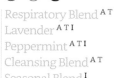

Apply 1-3 drops to bridge of nose and over sinuses or chest as needed; use a drop of Lavender under the tongue; inhale from cupped hands; diffuse several drops.

Respiratory Blend ^{A T}
Lavender ^{A T I}
Peppermint ^{A T I}
Cleansing Blend ^{A T}
Seasonal Blend ^I

Protocol on pg. 182

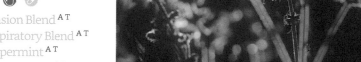

Head Lice

Dilute 1-3 drops and apply to entire scalp, shampoo, and rinse 30 minutes later. Repeat daily for several days.

Melaleuca ^T
Arborvitae ^T
Outdoor Blend ^T
Rosemary ^T
Eucalyptus ^T

Headache (Sinus)

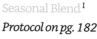

Massage 2-4 drops into forehead, temples, and back of neck; inhale from cupped hands.

Tension Blend ^{A T}
Respiratory Blend ^{A T}
Peppermint ^{A T}
Frankincense ^{A T}
Rosemary ^{A T}

Protocol on pg. 201

Headache (Tension)

Massage 1-3 drops into forehead, temples, and back of neck; inhale from cupped hands.

Tension Blend ^{A T}
Peppermint ^{A T}
Frankincense ^{A T}
Lavender ^{A T}
Massage Blend ^{A T}

Protocol on pg. 192

Hearing Issues

Apply 1-3 drops to temples and around the opening of the ear; apply to a cotton ball and place over ear opening overnight. Do not apply into ear.

Helichrysum ^T
Basil ^T
Frankincense ^T
Rose ^T
Melaleuca ^T

Heart Disease

Apply 2-4 drops over chest; ingest 3-5 drops as a daily supplement.

Geranium ^{T I}
Helichrysum ^{T I}
Marjoram ^{T I}
Cellular Complex ^{T I}
Vitality Trio ^I

Heartburn

Massage 1-3 drops into abdomen; ingest 1-3 drops as needed.

Digestive Blend ^{T I}
Peppermint ^{T I}
Metabolic Blend ^{T I}
Ginger ^{T I}
Fennel ^{T I}

Protocol on pg. 192

Heat Exhaustion

Apply 1-3 drops to forehead, back of neck, inside of wrists, and bottom of feet; add Lemon or Peppermint to mineral water and sip slowly.

Peppermint^{ATI}
Lemon^{ATI}
Tension Blend^{AT}
Siberian Fir^{ATI}
Lavender^{ATI}

Heatstroke

Apply 1-3 drops to forehead, temples, back of neck, and chest; ingest 1-3 drops as needed.

Peppermint^{ATI}
Frankincense^{ATI}
Tension Blend^{AT}
Spearmint^{ATI}
Copaiba^{ATI}

Heavy Metal Detox

Ingest 2-4 drops 2x daily; massage 2-4 drops into bottoms of feet.

Cilantro^{TI}
Frankincense^{TI}
Cellular Complex^{TI}
Detox Herbal Complex^I
Lemon^{TI}

Hematoma

Apply 1-3 drops to affected areas 2-3x daily or as needed; take 3-5 drops in a capsule 2x daily.

Cypress^T
Massage Blend^T
Geranium^T
Marjoram^{TI}
Lemon^{TI}

Hemorrhoids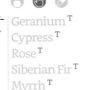

Dilute 2-4 drops with carrier oil and apply directly to affected areas daily or as needed.

Geranium^T
Cypress^T
Rose^T
Siberian Fir^T
Myrrh^T

Protocol on pg. 192

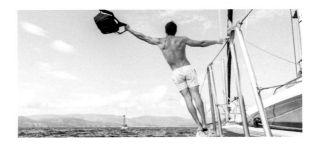

Hepatitis

Ingest 1-3 drops; use several drops topically with a warm compress over the liver area.

Copaiba^{TI}
Myrrh^{TI}
Detoxification Blend^{TI}
Helichrysum^{TI}
Lavender^{TI}

Protocol on pg. 193

Hernia (Hiatal)

Massage 1-3 drops into affected area as needed.

Helichrysum^T
Frankincense^T
Arborvitae^T
Digestive Blend^T
Digestive Enzymes^I

Herniated Disc

Massage 2-4 drops into affected area as often as needed (at least 3x daily).

Soothing Blend^T
Massage Blend^T
Lemongrass^T
Copaiba^T
Wintergreen^T

Protocol on pg. 193

Herpes Simplex

Ingest 1-3 drops; use topically with a warm compress over the kidney area; apply on the right and left side of throat daily.

Melaleuca^{TI}
Melissa^{TI}
Protective Blend^{TI}
Oregano^{TI}
Rose^T

Protocol on pg. 193

Hiccups

Inhale 1-3 drops from cupped hands; massage into chest and stomach area as needed.

Arborvitae^{AT}
Lemon^{AT}
Copaiba^{AT}
Digestive Blend^{AT}
Neroli^{AT}

HIV

Apply 1-3 drops to bottoms of feet; ingest 3-5 drops 3x daily; inhale from cupped hands for emotional support.

Melissa^{ATI}
Oregano^{ATI}
Helichrysum^{ATI}
Cellular Complex^{ATI}
Thyme^{ATI}

Protocol on pg. 181

Hives

Apply 1-3 drops diluted to affected area; ingest 2-4 drops twice daily as needed.

Melaleuca^{TI}
Frankincense^{TI}
Lavender^{TI}
Men's Blend^T
Magnolia^T

Hoarse Voice

Gargle 1-3 drops in water as needed; apply diluted to outside of throat.

Lemon^{TI}
Myrrh^{TI}
Lavender^{TI}
Protective Blend^{TI}
Arborvitae^T

Hormone Balance (Female)

Massage 2-4 drops into abdomen, temples, and bottoms of feet; ingest as needed; inhale from cupped hands.

Women's Monthly Blend^{AT}
Clary Sage^{ATI}
Ylang Ylang^{ATI}
Frankincense^{ATI}
Sandalwood^{ATI}

Hormone Balance (Male)
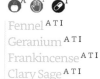

Combine 2-5 drops and apply to bottom of feet and inside of legs; take a few drops in a capsule daily.

Fennel ᴬ ᵀ ᴵ
Geranium ᴬ ᵀ ᴵ
Frankincense ᴬ ᵀ ᴵ
Clary Sage ᴬ ᵀ ᴵ
Sandalwood ᴬ ᵀ ᴵ

Horse: Anxiety/Nervousness

Allow horse to smell the oil. Massage 3-5 drops into coat.

Lavender ᴬ ᵀ
Bergamot ᴬ ᵀ
Basil ᴬ ᵀ
Roman Chamomile ᴬ ᵀ
Vetiver ᴬ ᵀ

Horse: Hoof Rot

Mix 3-5 drops in a spray bottle with 16 oz of water. Shake well and spray on hoof 5x daily.

Patchouli ᵀ
Melaleuca ᵀ
Helichrysum ᵀ
Thyme ᵀ
Vetiver ᵀ

Horse: Infection

Apply 3-5 drops to the affected area 5x daily. Dilute for sensitive skin.

Protective Blend ᵀ
Melaleuca ᵀ
Lavender ᵀ
Rosemary ᵀ
Thyme ᵀ

Horse: Leg Fracture

Apply 3-5 drops to the affected area 5x daily. Dilute for sensitive skin.

Cypress ᵀ
Soothing Blend ᵀ
Siberian Fir ᵀ
Helichrysum ᵀ
Frankincense ᵀ

Horse: Muscle Tissue

Massage 3-5 drops to the affected area 3x daily. Dilute for sensitive skin.

Lavender ᵀ
Roman Chamomile ᵀ
Eucalyptus ᵀ
Rosemary ᵀ
Soothing Blend ᵀ

Horse: Wounds

Allow horse to smell the oil. Apply 3-5 drops to the affected area 2-3x daily. Dilute for sensitive skin.

Melaleuca ᴬ ᵀ
Lavender ᴬ ᵀ
Helichrysum ᴬ ᵀ
Roman Chamomile ᴬ ᵀ
Myrrh ᴬ ᵀ

Hot Flashes

Massage 2-4 drops into chest, neck, and face as needed; ingest 2-5 drops Clary Sage and Ylang Ylang 2x daily.

Women's Monthly Blend ᴬ ᵀ
Peppermint ᴬ ᵀ ᴵ
Clary Sage ᴬ ᵀ ᴵ
Ylang Ylang ᴬ ᵀ ᴵ
Women's Perfume Blend ᴬ ᵀ

Protocol on pg. 195

Hyperactivity

Apply 1-3 drops on back of neck and bottoms of feet; inhale from cupped hands; diffuse several drops.

Focus Blend ᴬ ᵀ
Grounding Blend ᴬ ᵀ
Vetiver ᴬ ᵀ
Frankincense ᴬ ᵀ
Lavender ᴬ ᵀ

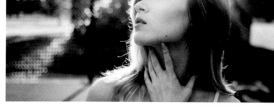

Hypersomnia

Apply 2-4 drops to chest area, bottoms of feet, or inside of wrists; inhale 1-3 drops from cupped hands; supplement regularly for long-term benefits.

Melissa ᴬ ᵀ ᴵ
Lemon ᴬ ᵀ ᴵ
Basil ᴬ ᵀ ᴵ
Energy & Stamina Complex ᴵ
Vitality Trio ᴵ

Hypertension

Apply 1-2 drops behind ears; inhale from cupped hands; use a drop under the tongue; diffuse several drops.

Grounding Blend ᴬ ᵀ
Lemon ᴬ ᵀ ᴵ
Yarrow ᴬ ᵀ ᴵ
Rose ᴬ ᵀ
Manuka ᴬ ᵀ

Hyperthyroid

Apply 1-3 drops to front of neck. Dilute with carrier oil for easier application. Ingest 3-5 drops a few times daily or as needed.

Myrrh ᵀ ᴵ
Frankincense ᵀ ᴵ
Cellular Complex ᵀ ᴵ
Detoxification Blend ᵀ ᴵ
Vitality Trio ᴵ

Protocol on pg. 203

Hypoglycemia

Apply 1-3 drops to chest, bottoms of feet, and inside of wrists; ingest 2-4 drops a few times daily or as needed.

Metabolic Blend ᵀ ᴵ
Cinnamon ᵀ ᴵ
Coriander ᵀ ᴵ
Detoxification Blend ᵀ ᴵ
Cellular Complex ᵀ ᴵ

Hypothyroid

Apply 1-3 drops to front of neck. Dilute with carrier oil for easier application. Ingest 3-5 drops a few times daily or as needed.

Peppermint ᵀ ᴵ
Lemongrass ᵀ ᴵ
Clove ᵀ ᴵ
Myrrh ᵀ ᴵ
Vitality Trio ᴵ

Protocol on pg. 203

Hysteria

Apply 3-5 drops of each with carrier oil to back of neck, temples and spine; inhale a few drops from cupped hands; diffuse several drops.

Vetiver ᴬ ᵀ
Lavender ᴬ ᵀ
Comforting Blend ᴬ ᵀ
Sandalwood ᴬ ᵀ
Cypress ᴬ ᵀ

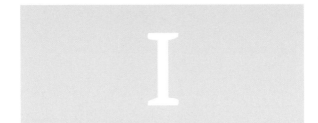

Immune Boost
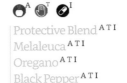

Apply 2-4 drops to bottoms of feet; ingest 3-5 drops 2x daily; inhale from cupped hands as needed.

Protective Blend ᴬ ᵀ ᴵ
Melaleuca ᴬ ᵀ ᴵ
Oregano ᴬ ᵀ ᴵ
Black Pepper ᴬ ᵀ ᴵ
Clove ᴬ ᵀ ᴵ

Impetigo

Combine 2 drops of each with carrier oil and apply to affected area 5x daily.

Lavender ᵀ
Melaleuca ᵀ
Myrrh ᵀ
Helichrysum ᵀ
Sandalwood ᵀ

Impotence

Rub 3-5 drops on lower back and outside of legs; add 1-2 drops to personal lubricant; diffuse several drops.

Ylang Ylang ᴬ ᵀ
Inspiring Blend ᴬ ᵀ
Rosemary ᴬ ᵀ
Lavender ᴬ ᵀ
Cinnamon ᴬ ᵀ

Protocol on pg. 194

Incontinence

Massage 2-4 drops over bladder and kidneys before bedtime as needed.

Cypress ᵀ
Black Pepper ᵀ
Ylang Ylang ᵀ
Lemongrass ᵀ
Roman Chamomile ᵀ

Indigestion
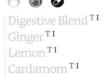

Massage 1-3 drops into stomach area clockwise as needed; drink 1-3 drops with water or in a capsule.

Digestive Blend ᵀ ᴵ
Ginger ᵀ ᴵ
Lemon ᵀ ᴵ
Cardamom ᵀ ᴵ
Digestive Tablets ᴵ

Protocol on pg. 154

Infant Reflux

Apply 1-2 drops diluted to stomach area and chest as needed.

Digestive Blend ᵀ
Lavender ᵀ
Fennel ᵀ
Frankincense ᵀ
Ginger ᵀ

Protocol on pg. 154

Infected Wounds

Apply 1-3 drops to affected areas 2-3x daily as needed; dilute for sensitive skin.

Melaleuca ᵀ
Helichrysum ᵀ
Frankincense ᵀ
Lavender ᵀ
Protective Blend ᵀ

Protocol on pg. 154

Infertility

Apply 2-4 drops to abdomen, wrists, and lower back daily; ingest 2-4 drops 2x daily.

Clary Sage ᴬ ᵀ ᴵ
Cellular Complex ᴬ ᵀ ᴵ
Ylang Ylang ᴬ ᵀ ᴵ
Fennel ᴬ ᵀ ᴵ
Vitality Trio ᴵ

Protocol on pg. 192

Inflammation

Apply 2-4 drops to affected areas as needed. For systemic inflammation, ingest 2-4 drops 2x daily.

Soothing Blend ᴬ ᵀ
Frankincense ᴬ ᵀ ᴵ
Copaiba ᴬ ᵀ ᴵ
Turmeric ᴬ ᵀ ᴵ
Wintergreen ᴬ ᵀ

Inflammatory Bowel Disease

Massage 1-3 drops onto stomach; ingest 2-4 drops 2-3x daily.

Digestive Blend ᵀ ᴵ
Frankincense ᵀ ᴵ
Lavender ᵀ ᴵ
Digestive Enzymes ᴵ
Probiotic Complex ᴵ

Protocol on pg. 194

Ingrown Toenail

Apply 1-3 drops to affected toenail 3x daily.

Melaleuca ᵀ
Protective Blend ᵀ
Detoxification Blend ᵀ
Lavender ᵀ
Oregano ᵀ

Injury (Muscle, Bone)

Apply 3-5 drops liberally to affected area as often as desired. Dilute for sensitive tissues.

Wintergreen ᵀ
Ylang Ylang ᵀ
Soothing Blend ᵀ
Helichrysum ᵀ
Blue Tansy ᵀ

Insect Bites

Apply 1-2 drops to insect bite hourly or as needed.

Lavender ᵀ
Melaleuca ᵀ
Cleansing Blend ᵀ
Roman Chamomile ᵀ
Frankincense ᵀ

Insect Repellent

Apply liberally over exposed skin areas; combine with carrier oil to spread easily.

Outdoor Blend [T]
Arborvitae [T]
Peppermint [T]
Renewing Blend [T]
Cedarwood [T]

Insomnia

Apply 1-3 drops to forehead, temples, base of skull, and behind the ear; diffuse several drops.

Restful Blend [A T]
Vetiver [A T]
Lavender [A T]
Cedarwood [A T]
Petitgrain [A T]

Protocol on pg. 201

Insulin Imbalance

Apply 2-4 drops to bottoms of feet; take 3-5 drops internally 2x daily.

Cinnamon [T I]
Protective Blend [T I]
Lavender [T I]
Clove [T I]
Metabolic Blend [T I]

Protocol on pg. 189

Irritable Bowel Syndrome

Apply 1-3 drops to bottoms of feet or over stomach; take 2-4 drops internally as needed.

Digestive Blend [T I]
Ginger [T I]
Turmeric [T I]
Frankincense [T I]
Peppermint [T I]

Protocol on pg. 194

Itchy Skin

Apply 1-3 drops to affected areas as needed. Use with carrier oil or lotion for improved efficacy.

Melaleuca [T]
Lavender [T]
Skin Clearing Blend [T]
Cedarwood [T]
Frankincense [T]

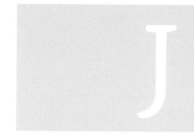

Jaundice

Massage 1-3 drops diluted over the liver; diffuse several drops nearby.

Lavender [A T]
Myrrh [A T]
Neroli [A T]
Rose [A T]
Grapefruit [A T]

Jet Lag

Apply 1-3 drops to forehead, temples, back of neck, and chest; inhale from cupped hands as needed.

Peppermint [A T]
Tangerine [A T]
Lemon [A T]
Protective Blend [A T]
Cellular Complex [A T]

Jock Itch

Apply 1-3 drops to affected areas as needed with carrier oil; ingest 3-4 drops 3x daily.

Melaleuca [T I]
Skin Clearing Blend [T]
Lavender [T I]
Cleansing Blend [T]
Thyme [T I]

Joint Pain

Massage 1-3 drops into affected areas as needed; use carrier oil for improved efficacy.

Soothing Blend [T]
Lemongrass [T]
Wintergreen [T]
Copaiba [T]
Frankincense [T]

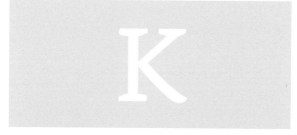

Kidney Infection

Apply 2-4 drops over kidneys 3-5x daily; ingest 1-3 drops 3-5x daily.

Juniper Berry [T I]
Lemongrass [T I]
Oregano [T I]
Protective Blend [T I]
Clove [T I]

Kidney Stones

Massage 2-4 drops over kidneys 3-5x daily; ingest 1-3 drops 3-5x daily.

Lemon [T I]
Juniper Berry [T I]
Helichrysum [T I]
Wintergreen [T]
Wild Orange [T I]

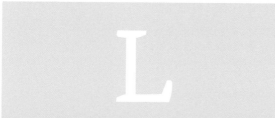

Lactose Intolerance

Ingest 2-4 drops or massage over stomach as needed.

Digestive Blend [T I]
Coriander [T I]
Lemongrass [T I]
Digestive Enzymes [I]
Probiotic Complex [I]

Laryngitis

Diffuse several drops throughout the day; ingest 3-5 drops 3x daily; massage 1-3 drops onto outside of throat.

Protective Blend [A T I]
Melaleuca [A T I]
Pink Pepper [A T I]
Lemon [A T I]
Rosemary [A T I]

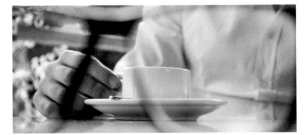

Leaky Gut Syndrome

Combine 3-5 drops in a capsule and take 3x daily after food.

Fennel [I]
Coriander [I]
Helichrysum [I]
Ginger [I]
Melaleuca [I]

Protocol on pg. 223

Leg Cramps

Massage several drops into legs as needed; use carrier oil for improved efficacy.

Soothing Blend [T]
Cypress [T]
Massage Blend [T]
Marjoram [T]
Black Pepper [T]

Leukemia

Ingest 2-4 drops 3x daily; massage 2-4 drops into bottoms of feet and spine 3-5x daily.

Cellular Complex [T I]
Frankincense [T I]
Lemongrass [T I]
Sandalwood [T I]
Myrrh [T I]

Protocol on pg. 186

Libido (low)

Apply 1-3 drops to abdomen, bottoms of feet, and wrists as needed; inhale from cupped hands; diffuse several drops.

Inspiring Blend [A T]
Ylang Ylang [A T]
Jasmine [A T]
Women's Monthly Blend [A T]
Rose [A T]

Protocol on pg. 194

Lice

Apply 3-5 drops with carrier oil to scalp 4x daily.

Melaleuca [T]
Lavender [T]
Cleansing Blend [T]
Clove [T]
Eucalyptus [T]

Lipoma

Massage 3-5 drops to affected area 3x daily.

Grapefruit [T]
Ginger [T]
Patchouli [T]
Frankincense [T]
Melaleuca [T]

Liver Disease

Apply 3-5 drops over the liver 3x daily.

Clove [T]
Grapefruit [T]
Geranium [T]
Rosemary [T]
Frankincense [T]

Lockjaw (Tetanus)

Massage 2-3 drops into jaw joint as needed.

Lavender [T]
Cypress [T]
Frankincense [T]
Copaiba [T]
Massage Blend [T]

Lou Gehrig's Disease

Apply 3-5 drops to spine and back of legs 3x daily.

Frankincense [T]
Myrrh [T]
Lavender [T]
Geranium [T]
Melaleuca [T]

Lumbago

Apply 3-5 drops liberally to affected area as often as needed; use carrier oil for improved efficacy.

Soothing Blend [T]
Wintergreen [T]
Ylang Ylang [T]
Helichrysum [T]
Blue Tansy [T]

Protocol on pg. 154

Lupus

Ingest 2-4 drops 3-5x daily during flare ups; massage 2-4 drops into inflamed areas; diffuse several drops for emotional support.

Frankincense [A T I]
Cellular Complex [A T I]
Soothing Blend [A T]
Copaiba [A T I]
Turmeric [A T I]

Protocol on pg. 194

Lyme Disease

Massage 2-4 drops into lower back 3x daily; take 3-5 drops in a capsule 3x daily.

Melissa [T I]
Thyme [T I]
Oregano [T I]
Geranium [T I]
Vitality Trio [I]

Protocol on pg. 195

Lymphatic Support

Apply 3-5 drops to sides of neck and sides of rib cage 2x daily.

Grapefruit [T]
Lemon [T]
Juniper Berry [T]
Basil [T]
Frankincense [T]

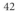

Lymphoma (Non-Hodgkin's)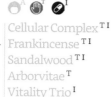

Ingest 3-5 drops 2-4x daily; rub 2-4 drops to sides of throat; supplement for added support

Cellular Complex [TI]
Frankincense [TI]
Sandalwood [TI]
Arborvitae [T]
Vitality Trio [I]

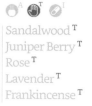

Macular Degeneration

Apply 2-4 drops to lower back and temples.

Sandalwood [T]
Juniper Berry [T]
Rose [T]
Lavender [T]
Frankincense [T]

Malaria

Take 3-5 drops in a capsule 4x daily; rub 2-4 drops onto spine and bottoms of feet.

Ginger [TI]
Grapefruit [TI]
Cinnamon [TI]
Basil [TI]
Thyme [TI]

Measles

Dab a few drops onto spots several times daily; add several drops to bath and soak for at least 30 minutes as needed.

Lavender [T]
Roman Chamomile [T]
Oregano [T]
Eucalyptus [T]
Protective Blend [T]

Melanoma

Apply 2-4 drops to affected areas 3-5x daily; ingest 2-4 drops 3x daily.

Frankincense [T]
Cellular Complex [TI]
Sandalwood [TI]
Rose [T]
Clove [TI]

Memory Loss

Massage 2-4 drops into forehead, temples, back of neck, and chest as needed; inhale from cupped hands.

Rosemary [AT]
Peppermint [AT]
Bergamot [AT]
Lavender [AT]
Frankincense [AT]

Protocol on pg. 195

Meningitis

Ingest 2-4 drops 2x daily; massage 2-4 drops into back of neck with carrier oil daily.

Protective Blend [TI]
Lavender [TI]
Oregano [TI]
Melissa [TI]
Cellular Complex [TI]

Menopause

Apply 2-4 drops topically to abdomen, bottoms of feet, and back of neck daily; ingest 2-4 drops Clary Sage and Siberian Fir as needed.

Clary Sage [TI]
Women's Monthly Blend [TI]
Siberian Fir [TI]
Geranium [TI]
Cellular Complex [TI]

Protocol on pg. 195

Menstrual Bleeding

Massage 2-4 drops into abdomen and lower back; apply to a warm compress over uterus area; ingest 2-4 drops as needed.

Helichrysum [TI]
Geranium [TI]
Clary Sage [TI]
Women's Monthly Blend [TI]
Lavender [TI]

Protocol on pg. 195

Menstrual Cycle (irregular)

Massage 2-4 drops into abdomen and lower back; ingest 2-4 drops 2x daily.

Clary Sage [TI]
Women's Monthly Blend [T]
Ylang Ylang [TI]
Rose [T]
Lavender [TI]

Protocol on pg. 195

Menstrual Pain

Massage 1-3 drops into abdomen, lower back, and shoulders; apply to a warm compress over uterus area; ingest 2-4 drops as needed.

Women's Monthly Blend [T]
Frankincense [ATI]
Peppermint [ATI]
Clary Sage [ATI]
Marjoram [ATI]

Protocol on pg. 195

Mental Fatigue

Massage 1-3 drops into forehead, temples, back of neck, and bottoms of feet; inhale from cupped hands as needed.

Peppermint [AT]
Basil [AT]
Green Mandarin [AT]
Frankincense [AT]
Energy & Stamina Complex [I]

Protocol on pg. 218

Metabolism (low)

Apply 1-3 drops to front of neck. Dilute with carrier oil for easier application. Ingest 2-4 drops 3x daily.

Metabolic Blend [TI]
Clove [TI]
Lemongrass [TI]
Basil [TI]
Frankincense [TI]

Protocol on pg. 205

Migraine

Apply 1-3 drops to forehead, temples, base of skull, back of neck, and bottoms of feet; inhale from cupped hands as needed.

Tension Blend [AT]
Peppermint [AT]
Frankincense [AT]
Soothing Blend [AT]
Copaiba [AT]

Protocol on pg. 196

Milk Supply (Low)

Massage 3-5 drops into breast as often as needed.

Basil ^T
Clary Sage ^T
Geranium ^T
Fennel ^T
Frankincense ^T

Miscarriage

Apply 3-5 drops to lower abdomen and lower back as often as needed.

Clary Sage ^T
Geranium ^T
Frankincense ^T
Myrrh ^T
Bergamot ^T

Mold/Mildew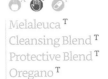

Diffuse several drops where mold is present throughout the day until no longer needed. Mix 20 drops with 4 oz water and apply to area of concern.

Melaleuca ^T
Cleansing Blend ^T
Protective Blend ^T
Oregano ^T
Lemon ^T

Moles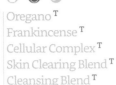

Apply a drop to mole 2-3x daily (avoid surrounding skin with hot oils like Oregano).

Oregano ^T
Frankincense ^T
Cellular Complex ^T
Skin Clearing Blend ^T
Cleansing Blend ^T

Mononucleosis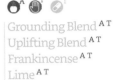

Ingest 3-5 drops 3x daily; apply 2-4 drops to bottoms of feet; diffuse several drops.

Thyme ^{A T I}
Melissa ^{A T I}
Bergamot ^{A T I}
Oregano ^{A T I}
Protective Blend ^{A T I}

Protocol on pg. 196

Mood Swings

Inhale 1-3 drops from cupped hands; apply a few drops to forehead, temples, back of neck, and bottoms of feet; diffuse several drops.

Grounding Blend ^{A T}
Uplifting Blend ^{A T}
Frankincense ^{A T}
Lime ^{A T}
Wild Orange ^{A T}

Protocol on pg. 196

Motion Sickness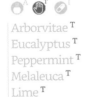

Apply 1-3 drops behind the ears and over navel; inhale from cupped hands; use a drop under the tongue.

Digestive Blend ^{A T I}
Peppermint ^{A T I}
Ginger ^{A T I}
Grounding Blend ^{A T}
Basil ^{A T I}

Mouth Ulcers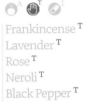

Gargle 1-3 drops mixed with water several times daily; apply a dab to affected area 2-3x daily.

Protective Blend ^{T I}
Clove ^{T I}
Myrrh ^{T I}
Sandalwood ^{T I}
Melaleuca ^{T I}

MRSA

Apply 3-5 drops with carrier oil 3-5x daily to affected areas.

Protective Blend ^T
Detoxification Blend ^T
Patchouli ^T
Geranium ^T
Grapefruit ^T

Mucus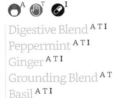

Apply 3-5 drops over the nose and sinuses (avoid the eyes).

Arborvitae ^T
Eucalyptus ^T
Peppermint ^T
Melaleuca ^T
Lime ^T

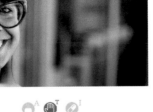

Multiple Sclerosis

Apply 3-5 drops to the bottoms of feet and spine 3x daily.

Frankincense ^T
Lavender ^T
Rose ^T
Neroli ^T
Black Pepper ^T

Protocol on pg. 196

Muscle Cramps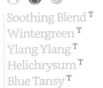

Massage 3-5 drops with carrier oil into affected area as often as desired.

Soothing Blend ^T
Wintergreen ^T
Ylang Ylang ^T
Helichrysum ^T
Blue Tansy ^T

Protocol on pg. 197

Muscle Injury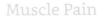

Massage 2-4 drops into affected muscles 3x daily or as needed.

Soothing Blend ^T
Marjoram ^T
Helichrysum ^T
Massage Blend ^T
Yarrow ^T

Muscle Pain

Massage 2-4 drops into affected muscles 3x daily or as needed; use a drop under the tongue for pain relief.

Soothing Blend ^T
Marjoram ^T
Helichrysum ^T
Massage Blend ^T
Copaiba ^{T I}

Protocol on pg. 197

Muscle Spasms

Massage 2-4 drops into affected muscles as needed; use a drop under the tongue.

Black Pepper ᵀ ᴵ
Soothing Blend ᵀ
Copaiba ᵀ ᴵ
Blue Tansy ᵀ
Yarrow ᵀ ᴵ

Muscle Stiffness

Massage 2-4 drops into affected muscles 2-3x daily.

Massage Blend ᵀ
Soothing Blend ᵀ
Cypress ᵀ
Lemongrass ᵀ
Marjoram ᵀ

Muscular Dystrophy

Apply 3-5 drops with carrier oil to spine and back of neck 3x daily.

Frankincense ᵀ
Lavender ᵀ
Rose ᵀ
Neroli ᵀ
Helichrysum ᵀ

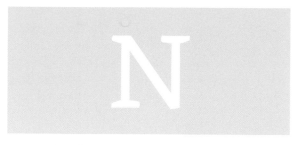

Nails/Nail Beds

Apply 1 drop to nails of concern.

Melaleuca ᵀ
Frankincense ᵀ
Myrrh ᵀ
Eucalyptus ᵀ
Lavender ᵀ

Nasal Congestion

Apply 1-3 drops over bridge of nose, under nose, and rub over sinuses; diffuse several drops.

Respiratory Blend ᴬ ᵀ
Siberian Fir ᴬ ᵀ
Lime ᴬ ᵀ
Eucalyptus ᴬ ᵀ
Peppermint ᴬ ᵀ

Nasal Polyps

Apply 1-3 drops over bridge of nose and under nose.

Frankincense ᵀ
Melaleuca ᵀ
Melissa ᵀ
Respiratory Blend ᵀ
Oregano ᵀ

Nausea

Apply 1-3 drops behind ears and over navel hourly; use a drop under the tongue; inhale from cupped hands.

Digestive Blend ᴬ ᵀ ᴵ
Ginger ᴬ ᵀ ᴵ
Peppermint ᴬ ᵀ ᴵ
Cardamom ᴬ ᵀ ᴵ
Grounding Blend ᴬ ᵀ

Neck Pain

Massage 2-4 drops onto neck several times daily; use carrier oil to improve efficacy; use a drop of Copaiba under the tongue for pain.

Soothing Blend ᴬ ᵀ
Lemongrass ᴬ ᵀ
Copaiba ᴬ ᵀ ᴵ
Wintergreen ᴬ ᵀ
Douglas Fir ᴬ ᵀ

Protocol on pg. 197

Nervous Fatigue

Inhale from cupped hands; apply 1-3 drops to temples, behind ears, and on back of neck as needed; diffuse several drops.

Grounding Blend ᴬ ᵀ
Lemon ᴬ ᵀ
Cedarwood ᴬ ᵀ
Vetiver ᴬ ᵀ
Tangerine ᴬ ᵀ

Nervousness

Apply 1-3 drops over the forehead, back of neck and top of head as needed; diffuse several drops.

Reassuring Blend ᴬ ᵀ
Rose ᴬ ᵀ
Lavender ᴬ ᵀ
Grounding Blend ᴬ ᵀ
Jasmine ᴬ ᵀ

Protocol on pg. 182

Neuromuscular Disorders

Apply 3-5 drops with carrier oil to spine and back of neck 3x daily.

Frankincense ᵀ
Cellular Complex ᵀ
Rose ᵀ
Neroli ᵀ
Helichrysum ᵀ

Protocol on pg. 197

Neuropathy

Apply 2-4 drops to affected areas several times daily; ingest 1-3 drops as needed.

Soothing Blend ᵀ
Frankincense ᵀ ᴵ
Massage Blend ᵀ
Roman Chamomile ᵀ ᴵ
Peppermint ᵀ ᴵ

Protocol on pg. 197

Night Sweats

Apply 2-4 drops to abdomen and back of neck before sleeping.

Detoxification Blend ᵀ
Cellular Complex ᵀ
Peppermint ᵀ
Lavender ᵀ
Lime ᵀ

Nightmares

Apply 2-4 drops to abdomen and back of neck before sleeping; diffuse several drops.

Juniper Berry ᴬ ᵀ
Restful Blend ᴬ ᵀ
Cedarwood ᴬ ᵀ
Lavender ᴬ ᵀ
Reassuring Blend ᴬ ᵀ

Nosebleeds

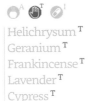

Apply 1-3 drops to the bridge and sides of nose and back of neck as needed.

Helichrysum T
Geranium T
Frankincense T
Lavender T
Cypress T

Obsessive Compulsive Disorder

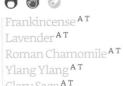

Massage 2-4 drops with carrier oil into spine and neck; inhale from cupped hands; diffuse several drops.

Frankincense A T
Lavender A T
Roman Chamomile A T
Ylang Ylang A T
Clary Sage A T

Protocol on pg. 197

Olfactory Loss

Apply 1-2 drops over nose (avoid eyes) and back of neck 3x daily.

Rose A T
Eucalyptus A T
Lemon A T
Vetiver A T
Bergamot A T

Ovarian Cysts

Blend 1-3 drops with carrier oil and soak tampon to insert overnight; apply 3-5 drops with warm compress over abdomen; take 3-5 drops internally.

Frankincense T I
Clary Sage T I
Cellular Complex T I
Oregano T I
Sandalwood T I

Overeating

Apply 1-3 drops to stomach; take 2-4 drops internally; inhale from cupped hands as needed.

Metabolic Blend A T I
Peppermint A T I
Grapefruit A T I
Renewing Blend A T
Cinnamon A T I

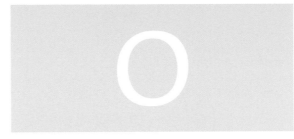

Odors

Diffuse several drops; apply 2-3 drops with a carrier oil to surface odors; ingest 3-5 drops twice daily for body odors.

Cleansing Blend A T
Melaleuca A T I
Cilantro A T I
Lemon A T I
Douglas Fir A T

Osteoarthritis

Massage 2-4 drops into affected areas daily; use carrier oil for improved efficacy.

Soothing Blend T
Frankincense T
Lemongrass T
Copaiba T
Cellular Complex T

Protocol on pg. 183

Overactive Bladder

Take 2-4 drops internally or apply over abdomen as needed.

Peppermint T I
Digestive Blend T I
Ginger T I
Lavender T I
Lemon T I

Overwhelm

Apply 2-4 drops to back of neck and temples; inhale from cupped hands; diffuse several drops.

Cedarwood A T
Spearmint A T
Frankincense A T
Lavender A T
Lemongrass A T

Protocol on pg. 220

Obesity

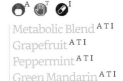

Add 2-5 drops to water to manage cravings and encourage metabolism. Inhale from cupped hands to satisfy cravings.

Metabolic Blend A T I
Grapefruit A T I
Peppermint A T I
Green Mandarin A T I
Lemon A T I

Protocol on pg. 205

Oily Skin

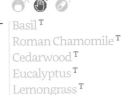

Apply 3-5 drops to affected areas at bedtime.

Basil T
Roman Chamomile T
Cedarwood T
Eucalyptus T
Lemongrass T

Osteoporosis

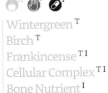

Massage 2-4 drops onto spine and affected areas daily; take 2-4 drops Cellular Complex internally 2x daily.

Wintergreen T
Birch T
Frankincense T I
Cellular Complex T I
Bone Nutrient I

Oxytocin Production

Inhale 1-3 drops from cupped hands 3x daily.

Clary Sage A T
Thyme A T
Sandalwood A T

P

Pain

Combine 3-5 drops with carrier oil and apply liberally to affected area as often as desired; use a drop under the tongue.

Soothing Blend ᴬᵀ
Frankincense ᴬᵀᴵ
Helichrysum ᴬᵀᴵ
Copaiba ᴬᵀᴵ
Turmeric ᴬᵀᴵ

Protocol on pg. 197

Palpitations
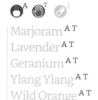
Apply 1-3 drops over heart 3x daily; inhale from cupped hands.

Marjoram ᴬᵀ
Lavender ᴬᵀ
Geranium ᴬᵀ
Ylang Ylang ᴬᵀ
Wild Orange ᴬᵀ

Pancreatitis

Ingest 1-3 drops 3x daily; massage 1-3 drops over abdomen as needed.

Detoxification Blend ᵀᴵ
Marjoram ᵀᴵ
Lemon ᵀᴵ
Coriander ᵀᴵ
Rosemary ᵀᴵ

Panic Attacks

Inhale 1-3 drops from cupped hands; apply to back and front of neck; diffuse several drops.

Cedarwood ᴬᵀ
Spearmint ᴬᵀ
Frankincense ᴬᵀ
Lavender ᴬᵀ
Lemongrass ᴬᵀ

Protocol on pg. 182

Paralysis
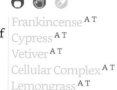
Apply 3-5 drops to back of neck, spine, bottoms of feet, and crown of head 5x daily.

Frankincense ᴬᵀ
Cypress ᴬᵀ
Vetiver ᴬᵀ
Cellular Complex ᴬᵀ
Lemongrass ᴬᵀ

Parasites
Ingest 3-5 drops 3x daily; apply in a warm compress over intestinal area 2-3x daily.

Detoxification Blend ᵀᴵ
Oregano ᵀᴵ
Geranium ᵀᴵ
Clove ᵀᴵ
Thyme ᵀᴵ

Parathyroid Disorder
Apply 1-3 drops to front of neck; dilute with carrier oil for easier application; ingest 1-3 drops a few times daily or as needed.

Frankincense ᵀᴵ
Myrrh ᵀᴵ
Cellular Complex ᵀᴵ
Detoxification Blend ᵀᴵ
Vitality Trio ᴵ

Parkinson's Disease
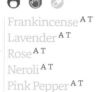
Apply 3-5 drops to spine and back of neck 3x daily; inhale from cupped hands; diffuse several drops throughout the day.

Frankincense ᴬᵀ
Lavender ᴬᵀ
Rose ᴬᵀ
Neroli ᴬᵀ
Pink Pepper ᴬᵀ

Pelvic Pain Syndrome
Apply 3-5 drops to lower abdomen 3x daily.

Clary Sage ᵀ
Eucalyptus ᵀ
Frankincense ᵀ
Ylang Ylang ᵀ
Patchouli ᵀ

Perforated Ear Drum
Apply 1-2 drops behind ear 2-3x daily.

Helichrysum ᵀ
Basil ᵀ
Grounding Blend ᵀ
Rosemary ᵀ
Cypress ᵀ

Perimenopause
Massage 2-4 drops into abdomen, lower back, and shoulders.

Women's Monthly Blend ᴬᵀ
Frankincense ᴬᵀ
Clary Sage ᴬᵀ
Peppermint ᴬᵀ
Marjoram ᴬᵀ

Pernicious Anemia
Take 2-4 drops internally 3x daily; apply to stomach area as needed.

Lemon ᵀᴵ
Lime ᵀᴵ
Helichrysum ᵀᴵ
Cinnamon ᵀᴵ
Cellular Complex ᵀᴵ

Pests

Apply 3-5 drops with carrier oil to skin; add oils to a 20 oz glass spray bottle and spray pest-ridden areas as needed.

Peppermint ᵀ
Eucalyptus ᵀ
Clove ᵀ
Basil ᵀ
Melaleuca ᵀ

Phantom Pains
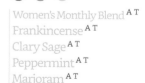
Combine 3-5 drops with carrier oil and apply liberally to affected area as often as desired; inhale from cupped hands.

Wintergreen ᴬᵀ
Ylang Ylang ᴬᵀ
Soothing Blend ᴬᵀ
Helichrysum ᴬᵀ
Blue Tansy ᴬᵀ

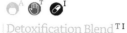

Pineal Gland

Inhale 1-3 drops for 30 seconds from cupped hands 3x daily; apply to pineal gland reflexology point.

Bergamot ᴬᵀ
Clary Sage ᴬᵀ
Lavender ᴬᵀ
Lemon ᴬᵀ
Ginger ᴬᵀ

Pink Eye/ Conjunctivitis

Apply 1-2 drops around (but not in) eyes 3x daily; dilute for sensitive skin.

Melaleuca ᵀ
Rosemary ᵀ
Arborvitae ᵀ
Clary Sage ᵀ
Cleansing Blend ᵀ

Pituitary Gland

Apply 1-3 drops to front of neck; dilute with carrier oil for easier application; ingest 1-3 drops a few times daily or as needed.

Clove ᴬᵀᴵ
Frankincense ᴬᵀᴵ
Sandalwood ᴬᵀᴵ
Lemongrass ᴬᵀᴵ
Basil ᴬᵀᴵ

Plantar Fasciitis

Combine 3-5 drops with carrier oil and apply liberally to affected area 3x daily or as desired.

Soothing Blend ᵀ
Wintergreen ᵀ
Ylang Ylang ᵀ
Helichrysum ᵀ
Blue Tansy ᵀ

Plantar Warts

Apply 1-3 drops to wart several times daily (avoid surrounding skin with hot oils like Oregano.)

Oregano ᵀ
Frankincense ᵀ
Cellular Complex ᵀ
Melissa ᵀ
Rose ᵀ

Pleurisy

Apply 3-5 drops over chest 3x daily; diffuse several drops.

Respiratory Blend ᴬᵀ
Eucalyptus ᴬᵀ
Roman Chamomile ᴬᵀ
Blue Tansy ᴬᵀ
Clove ᴬᵀ

Pneumonia

Apply 2-4 drops to chest, neck, and bottoms of feet 3-5x daily; gargle a drop hourly; inhale from cupped hands as needed; diffuse several drops.

Respiratory Blend ᴬᵀ
Protective Blend ᴬᵀᴵ
Arborvitae ᴬᵀ
Bergamot ᴬᵀᴵ
Roman Chamomile ᴬᵀᴵ

Protocol on pg. 185

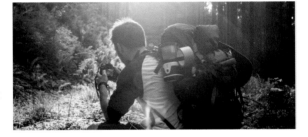

Poison Ivy/Oak

Apply 1-3 drops to affected area with carrier oil a couple times daily or as needed.

Lavender ᵀ
Frankincense ᵀ
Geranium ᵀ
Patchouli ᵀ
Petitgrain ᵀ

Polio

Apply 3-5 drops to spine, back of neck, and bottoms of feet; inhale from cupped hands often.

Frankincense ᴬᵀᴵ
Lavender ᴬᵀᴵ
Rose ᴬᵀᴵ
Neroli ᴬᵀᴵ
Black Pepper ᴬᵀᴵ

Protocol on pg. 198

Polycystic Ovary Syndrome

Apply 3 -5 drops to lower abdomen 3 x daily.

Clary Sage ᵀ
Eucalyptus ᵀ
Frankincense ᵀ
Ylang Ylang ᵀ
Patchouli ᵀ

Polyps

Add 4-6 drops to capsule and take after eating 3x daily.

Frankincense ᵀ
Patchouli ᵀ
Myrrh ᵀ
Oregano ᵀ
Peppermint ᵀ

Post Traumatic Stress Disorder

Apply 2-4 drops to forehead, temples, back of neck, chest, and bottoms of feet; inhale from cupped hands as needed.

Reassuring Blend ᴬᵀ
Sandalwood ᴬᵀ
Frankincense ᴬᵀ
Comforting Blend ᴬᵀ
Renewing Blend ᴬᵀ

Pre-Workout

Massage 2-4 drops with carrier oil into appropriate muscles and joints; apply a drop over the chest; inhale from cupped hands.

Soothing Blend ᴬᵀ
Bergamot ᴬᵀ
Lemon ᴬᵀ
Lime ᴬᵀ
Rosemary ᴬᵀ

Protocol on pg. 212

Preeclampsia

Apply 3-5 drops to lower back and neck.

Lavender ᵀ
Ylang Ylang ᵀ
Roman Chamomile ᵀ
Clary Sage ᵀ
Cedarwood ᵀ

Pregnancy: Delivery

Apply 1-3 drops to hips, lower back, and back of neck; inhale from cupped hands; diffuse several drops.

Lemon ᴬᵀ
Bergamot ᴬᵀ
Lavender ᴬᵀ
Rosemary ᴬᵀ
Jasmine ᴬᵀ

Pregnancy: Hemorrhaging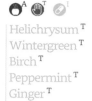

Apply 1-3 drops to spine and abdomen.

Helichrysum ᵀ
Wintergreen ᵀ
Birch ᵀ
Peppermint ᵀ
Ginger ᵀ

Pregnancy: High Blood Pressure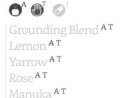

Apply 2-4 drops to bottoms of feet and behind ears 2x daily; inhale from cupped hands.

Grounding Blend ᴬᵀ
Lemon ᴬᵀ
Yarrow ᴬᵀ
Rose ᴬᵀ
Manuka ᴬᵀ

Pregnancy: Labor (during)

Apply 1-3 drops to hips, lower back, and back of neck; inhale from cupped hands; diffuse several drops.

Lemon ᴬᵀ
Bergamot ᴬᵀ
Lavender ᴬᵀ
Rosemary ᴬᵀ
Jasmine ᴬᵀ

Pregnancy: Labor (post)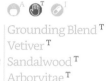

Apply 3-5 drops to lower back 3x daily to stimulate regeneration.

Grounding Blend ᵀ
Vetiver ᵀ
Sandalwood ᵀ
Arborvitae ᵀ
Yarrow ᵀ

Protocol on pg. 199

Pregnancy: Lactation

Massage 1-3 drops with carrier oil over breasts and apply to bottoms of feet; ingest 1-3 drops.

Fennel ᵀ ᴵ
Clary Sage ᵀ ᴵ
Basil ᵀ ᴵ
Vitality Trio ᴵ
Bone Nutrient ᴵ

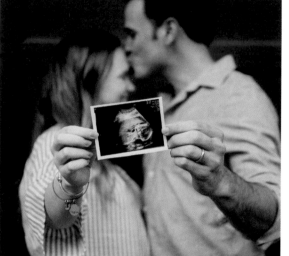

Pregnancy: Low Libido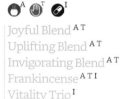

Apply 3-5 drops to inside of thighs and calves 2x daily; diffuse several drops.

Rose ᴬᵀ
Jasmine ᴬᵀ
Ylang Ylang ᴬᵀ
Clary Sage ᴬᵀ
Fennel ᴬᵀ

Pregnancy: Mastitis

Apply 3-5 drops to affected area 3x daily.

Lavender ᵀ
Sandalwood ᵀ
Melaleuca ᵀ
Arborvitae ᵀ
Helichrysum ᵀ

Pregnancy: Morning Sickness

Apply 1-3 drops behind ears and over navel hourly; inhale from cupped hands; ingest 1-3 drops as needed.

Digestive Blend ᴬᵀᴵ
Peppermint ᴬᵀᴵ
Ginger ᴬᵀᴵ
Fennel ᴬᵀᴵ
Coriander ᴬᵀᴵ

Protocol on pg. 199

Pregnancy: Postpartum Depression

Apply 1-3 drops to forehead and temples; use a drop of Frankincense under the tongue; inhale from cupped hands.

Joyful Blend ᴬᵀ
Uplifting Blend ᴬᵀ
Invigorating Blend ᴬᵀ
Frankincense ᴬᵀᴵ
Vitality Trio ᴵ

Protocol on pg. 199

Pregnancy: Sore Nipples

Apply 1-3 drops to affected area 3x daily; dilute for sensitive skin (monitor baby's response and try a different oil if needed).

Lavender ᵀ
Melaleuca ᵀ
Sandalwood ᵀ
Helichrysum ᵀ

Pregnancy: Tender Breasts

Combine 3-5 drops with carrier oil and massage into affected area as often as needed.

Wintergreen ᵀ
Soothing Blend ᵀ
Ylang Ylang ᵀ
Peppermint ᵀ
Yarrow ᵀ

Pregnancy: Uterine Health

Apply 3-5 drops to lower abdomen 3x daily.

Clary Sage ᵀ
Eucalyptus ᵀ
Frankincense ᵀ
Ylang Ylang ᵀ
Patchouli ᵀ

Premenstrual Syndrome (PMS)

Add 3-6 drops to warm bath; apply to abdomen; inhale from cupped hands; ingest 1-3 drops as needed.

Women's Monthly Blend [A T]
Clary Sage [A T I]
Geranium [A T I]
Frankincense [A T I]
Women's Perfume Blend [A T]

Protocol on pg. 195

Prolapsed Mitral Valve

Apply 3-5 drops to inside of arms and chest 3x daily.

Lemon [T]
Lavender [T]
Ylang Ylang [T]
Marjoram [T]
Yarrow [T]

Prostatitis

Apply 3-5 drops to lower abdomen and lower back 3x daily or as needed.

Rosemary [T]
Marjoram [T]
Thyme [T]
Frankincense [T]
Myrrh [T]

Psoriasis

Apply 1-3 drops to affected area a couple times daily with carrier oil; ingest 2-4 drops 2x daily.

Melaleuca [A T I]
Detoxification Blend [A T I]
Thyme [A T I]
Roman Chamomile [A T I]
Probiotic Complex [I]

Protocol on pg. 199

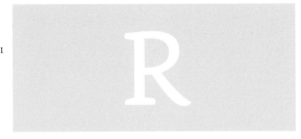

R

Radiation

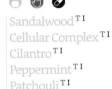

Ingest 2-4 drops 2x daily; apply 1-3 drops to bottoms of feet with carrier oil as desired.

Sandalwood [T I]
Cellular Complex [T I]
Cilantro [T I]
Peppermint [T I]
Patchouli [T I]

Rashes

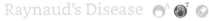

Dilute 1-3 drops with a carrier oil and apply to affected area as needed.

Melaleuca [T]
Roman Chamomile [T]
Lavender [T]
Cedarwood [T]
Magnolia [T]

Protocol on pg. 199

Raynaud's Disease

Apply 3-5 drops to lower back and abdomen and apply a hot compress daily.

Clove [T]
Black Pepper [T]
Geranium [T]
Lavender [T]
Fennel [T]

Reaction Attachment Disorder

Apply 3-5 drops to top of head, forehead and back of neck 3x daily.

Hopeful Blend [A T]
Women's Monthly Blend [A T]
Rose [A T]
Bergamot [A T]
Lavender [A T]

Protocol on pg. 215

Reiter's Arthritis

Massage 1-3 drops into affected areas 3x daily; use a carrier oil for improved efficacy.

Soothing Blend [T]
Frankincense [T]
Cellular Complex [T]
Copaiba [T]
Turmeric [T]

Protocol on pg. 183

Relapse

Apply 2-4 drops as often as needed to back of the neck, temples and ears (not inside ears).

Hopeful Blend [A T]
Encouraging Blend [A T]
Cinnamon [A T]
Rosemary [A T]
Cedarwood [A T]

Protocol on pg. 210

Relaxation

Apply 3-5 drops over the forehead, back of neck and top of head as needed; use 3-6 drops in a hot bath; diffuse several drops.

Reassuring Blend [A T]
Rose [A T]
Lavender [A T]
Grounding Blend [A T]
Blue Tansy [A T]

Protocol on pg. 228

Renal Artery Stenosis

Rub 2-4 drops to bottoms of feet and inner thighs 2x daily; use a carrier oil for improved efficacy.

Cypress [T]
Peppermint [T]
Grounding Blend [T]
Lavender [T]
Douglas Fir [T]

Respiratory Issues

Apply 2-4 drops to chest, neck, under nose, and on bridge of nose; inhale from cupped hands as needed; diffuse several drops.

Respiratory Blend [A T]
Eucalyptus [A T]
Douglas Fir [A T]
Cardamom [A T]
Rosemary [A T]

Respiratory Virus

Apply 3-5 drops 3x daily to chest, outside of arms and nose; diffuse several drops; take 2-4 drops in a capsule 3x daily.

Respiratory Blend [A T]
Protective Blend [A T I]
Eucalyptus [A T]
Lime [A T I]
Arborvitae [A T]

Restless Leg Syndrome

Massage 2-4 drops onto legs and bottoms of feet; diffuse several drops; use 2 drops Yarrow under the tongue.

Soothing Blend ᴬᵀ
Ylang Ylang ᴬᵀ
Cypress ᴬᵀ
Petitgrain ᴬᵀ
Yarrow ᴬᵀᴵ

Restlessness

Inhale 1-3 drops from cupped hands; apply 2-4 drops to bottoms of feet and back of neck as needed.

Grounding Blend ᴬᵀ
Lavender ᴬᵀ
Restful Blend ᴬᵀ
Vetiver ᴬᵀ
Spikenard ᴬᵀ

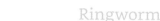
Protocol on pg. 228

Rheumatic Fever
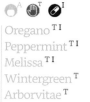

Apply 1-3 drops to bottoms of feet; ingest 1-3 drops twice daily; gargle a few drops mixed with water as needed.

Oregano ᵀᴵ
Peppermint ᵀᴵ
Melissa ᵀᴵ
Wintergreen ᵀ
Arborvitae ᵀ

Rheumatoid Arthritis

Apply 1-3 drops to affected areas daily; dilute for sensitive skin and for easier application.

Soothing Blend ᵀ
Frankincense ᵀ
Oregano ᵀ
Lemongrass ᵀ
Copaiba ᵀ

Protocol on pg. 200

Rhinitis

Inhale 1-3 drops from cupped hands several times daily; apply a couple drops to forehead and bridge of nose; ingest 2-4 drops 3x daily; diffuse several drops.

Respiratory Blend ᴬᵀ
Melaleuca ᴬᵀᴵ
Pink Pepper ᴬᵀᴵ
Siberian Fir ᴬᵀᴵ
Oregano ᴬᵀᴵ

Ringworm

Apply 1-3 drops to affected area 3-4x daily; use with carrier oil for improved efficacy; take 2-4 drops in a capsule 3x daily.

Melaleuca ᵀᴵ
Cleansing Blend ᵀ
Skin Clearing Blend ᵀ
Petitgrain ᵀᴵ
Detoxification Blend ᵀᴵ

Rosacea

Combine 2-3 drops with carrier oil and apply to face at bedtime.

Jasmine ᵀ
Geranium ᵀ
Lavender ᵀ
Patchouli ᵀ
Roman Chamomile ᵀ

Rotator Cuff Issues

Massage 3-5 drops with carrier oil into affected area as often as desired.

Soothing Blend ᵀ
Wintergreen ᵀ
Ylang Ylang ᵀ
Helichrysum ᵀ
Blue Tansy ᵀ

Runner's Knee

Massage 3-5 drops with carrier oil into affected area as often as desired.

Soothing Blend ᵀ
Lemongrass ᵀ
Ylang Ylang ᵀ
Helichrysum ᵀ
Blue Tansy ᵀ

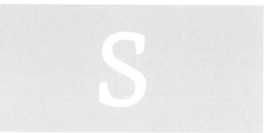

Scabies

Apply 2 drops 2x daily as needed; add 20 drops to glass water bottle and spray furniture as needed.

Peppermint ᵀ
Melaleuca ᵀ
Cedarwood ᵀ
Cleansing Blend ᵀ
Roman Chamomile ᵀ

Scarring

Massage 2-4 drops into scarred area 2x daily.

Anti-Aging Blend ᵀ
Frankincense ᵀ
Helichrysum ᵀ
Sandalwood ᵀ
Neroli ᵀ

Schizophrenia

Apply 3-5 drops to back of neck and spine 3x daily; diffuse several drops throughout the day.

Frankincense ᴬᵀ
Melissa ᴬᵀ
Melaleuca ᴬᵀ
Lavender ᴬᵀ
Grounding Blend ᴬᵀ

Schmidt's Syndrome

Apply 3-5 drops to back of neck, bottoms of feet, and spine 3x daily; ingest 3-5 drops 2x daily; diffuse several drops throughout the day.

Clove ᴬᵀᴵ
Cellular Complex ᴬᵀᴵ
Rosemary ᴬᵀᴵ
Basil ᴬᵀᴵ
Clary Sage ᴬᵀᴵ

Sciatica

Massage 1-3 drops into affected area a couple times daily.

Soothing Blend ᵀ
Frankincense ᵀ
Vetiver ᵀ
Copaiba ᵀ
Helichrysum ᵀ

Protocol on pg. 200

Scleroderma

Apply 1-3 drops to affected areas as needed; use with carrier oil for improved efficacy.

Melaleuca [T]
Skin Clearing Blend [T]
Cedarwood [T]
Detoxification Blend [T]
Frankincense [T]

Scurvy

Take 3-5 drops in a capsule 3x daily after eating; apply 2-3 drops to bottoms of feet.

Lime [T I]
Wild Orange [T I]
Bergamot [T I]
Jasmine [T I]
Lemongrass [T I]

Seizures

Apply 1-3 drops to back of neck and bottoms of feet; inhale from cupped hands as needed; ingest 2-4 drops 2x daily.

Frankincense [A T I]
Grounding Blend [A T]
Spikenard [A T I]
Yarrow [A T I]
Roman Chamomile [A T I]

Protocol on pg. 200

Shin Splints

Massage 3-5 drops with carrier oil into affected area as often as desired.

Soothing Blend [T]
Ylang Ylang [T]
Wintergreen [T]
Helichrysum [T]
Blue Tansy [T]

Shingles

Apply 2-4 drops to affected areas, on back of neck, and along the spine 3x daily; take 2-4 drops 3x daily.

Melaleuca [T I]
Melissa [T I]
Black Pepper [T I]
Yarrow [T I]
Geranium [T I]

Protocol on pg. 201

Shock

Apply 1-3 drops on temples, under nose, and on back of neck as needed; inhale from cupped hands; diffuse several drops.

Grounding Blend [A T]
Frankincense [A T]
Helichrysum [A T]
Uplifting Blend [A T]
Renewing Blend [A T]

Protocol on pg. 233

Sickle Cell Anemia

Combine 3-5 drops of oils on hand (preferably all 5 listed) a capsule and take 3x daily after meals.

Lemon [I]
Rose [I]
Siberian Fir [I]
Rosemary [I]
Geranium [I]

Sinus Infection

Apply 1-3 drops over bridge of nose and sinuses (avoid eyes) 3x daily; diffuse several drops; take 3-5 drops in a capsule 3x daily.

Melaleuca [A T I]
Melissa [A T I]
Oregano [A T I]
Respiratory Blend [A T]
Rosemary [A T I]

Protocol on pg. 201

Skin Tags

Apply a drop to affected areas 3x daily (dilute hot oils like Oregano and avoid surrounding skin).

Frankincense [T]
Oregano [T]
Melaleuca [T]
Rosemary [T]
Basil [T]

Skin Ulcers

Apply 1-3 drops diluted into affected area 2-3x daily.

Lavender [T]
Myrrh [T]
Skin Clearing Blend [T]
Sandalwood [T]
Yarrow [T]

Sleep

Apply 3-5 drops over the forehead, back of neck, and top of head 30 minutes before sleep; diffuse several drops; use a drop under the tongue.

Restful Blend [A T]
Lavender [A T]
Reassuring Blend [A T]
Rose [A T]
Vetiver [A T I]

Protocol on pg. 201

Snoring

Apply 1-3 drops to chest and under nose; diffuse several drops near bedside; gargle Protective Blend with water to open throat.

Respiratory Blend [A T]
Protective Blend [A T I]
Petitgrain [A T]
Eucalyptus [A T]
Douglas Fir [A T]

Protocol on pg. 202

Sore Throat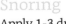

Gargle 1-3 drops with water, then swallow; apply to throat and neck, diluting with carrier oil as needed.

Protective Blend [T I]
Oregano [T I]
Lemon [T I]
Arborvitae [T]
Melissa [T I]

Protocol on pg. 202

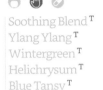

Spasms

Apply 3-5 drops to affected area and bottoms of feet as needed; use a drop under the tongue.

Frankincense ᵀ ᴵ
Black Pepper ᵀ ᴵ
Copaiba ᵀ ᴵ
Ylang Ylang ᵀ ᴵ
Lavender ᵀ ᴵ

Spina Bifida

Apply 3-5 drops to spine and back of neck 3x daily; inhale from cupped hands.

Peppermint ᴬ ᵀ
Roman Chamomile ᴬ ᵀ
Vetiver ᴬ ᵀ
Clove ᴬ ᵀ
Frankincense ᴬ ᵀ

Sprains

Gently apply 2-4 drops to affected area as needed.

Soothing Blend ᵀ
Helichrysum ᵀ
Lemongrass ᵀ
Spikenard ᵀ
Massage Blend ᵀ

Staph Infection

Apply 2-4 drops to the affected 3-5x daily; dilute if necessary.

Detoxification Blend ᵀ
Patchouli ᵀ
Melaleuca ᵀ
Geranium ᵀ
Grapefruit ᵀ

Stenosis (Vessel Narrowing)

Take 1-2 drops of each oil on hand (preferably all 5 listed) in a capsule 3x daily; apply 2-4 drops to bottoms of feet 3x daily.

Frankincense ᵀ ᴵ
Ginger ᵀ ᴵ
Clary Sage ᵀ ᴵ
Cinnamon ᵀ ᴵ
Melaleuca ᵀ ᴵ

Stings

Apply 1-2 drops topically to sting or bite several times daily until symptoms cease.

Lavender ᵀ
Melaleuca ᵀ
Cleansing Blend ᵀ
Roman Chamomile ᵀ
Basil ᵀ

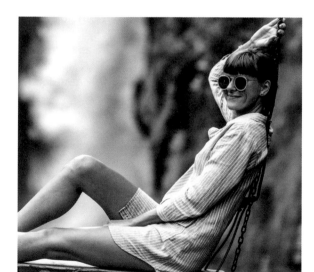

Stomach Ache

Rub 2-4 drops over stomach as needed; ingest 1-3 drops as needed.

Digestive Blend ᵀ ᴵ
Ginger ᵀ ᴵ
Peppermint ᵀ ᴵ
Roman Chamomile ᵀ ᴵ
Wild Orange ᵀ ᴵ

Protocol on pg. 190

Strep Throat

Apply 1-3 drops with a carrier oil to outside of throat 5x daily; ingest 2-5 drops in a capsule; gargle a drop with water.

Arborvitae ᵀ
Oregano ᵀ ᴵ
Thyme ᵀ ᴵ
Protective Blend ᵀ ᴵ
Melaleuca ᵀ ᴵ

Stress

Apply 3-5 drops over the forehead, back of neck, and top of head as needed; inhale from cupped hands; diffuse several drops.

Reassuring Blend ᴬ ᵀ
Grounding Blend ᴬ ᵀ
Lavender ᴬ ᵀ
Frankincense ᴬ ᵀ
Rose ᴬ ᵀ

Protocol on pg. 202

Stretch Marks

Massage 1-3 drops to affected areas 2x daily; use a carrier oil for improved efficacy.

Frankincense ᵀ
Helichrysum ᵀ
Anti-Aging Blend ᵀ
Neroli ᵀ
Yarrow ᵀ

Stroke

Apply 2-4 drops to temples, forehead, behind ears, and back of neck 3-5x daily; ingest 2-4 drops 3x daily; diffuse several drops.

Cypress ᴬ ᵀ
Frankincense ᴬ ᵀ ᴵ
Basil ᴬ ᵀ ᴵ
Fennel ᴬ ᵀ ᴵ
Helichrysum ᴬ ᵀ ᴵ

Sunburn

Apply 1-3 drops to affected area hourly or as needed. Blend 2-3 oils, 2-3 drops each with carrier oil for improved results.

Lavender ᵀ
Helichrysum ᵀ
Peppermint ᵀ
Frankincense ᵀ
Cedarwood ᵀ

Protocol on pg. 203

Swimmer's Ear

Apply 2 drops behind ear 2x daily.

Copaiba ᵀ
Lavender ᵀ
Spearmint ᵀ
Rosemary ᵀ
Wintergreen ᵀ

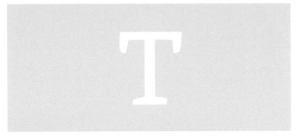

Tachycardia

Apply 3-5 drops to inside of arms and chest 3x daily.

Ylang Ylang ^{T}
Lavender ^{T}
Neroli ^{T}
Vetiver ^{T}
Geranium ^{T}

Taste (loss of)

Apply 1-2 drops directly to tongue 2x daily.

Eucalyptus ^{I}
Lemon ^{I}
Clove ^{I}
Geranium ^{I}
Lime ^{I}

Teeth Grinding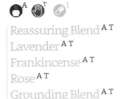

Massage 2-4 drops into jaw joints, back of neck, and top of head as needed.

Reassuring Blend ^{AT}
Lavender ^{AT}
Frankincense ^{AT}
Rose ^{AT}
Grounding Blend ^{AT}

Teething Pain

Dilute with carrier oil and gently massage a drop along baby's jawline, reapplying as needed.

Lavender ^{T}
Clove ^{T}
Magnolia ^{T}
Frankincense ^{T}
Spikenard ^{T}

Tendinitis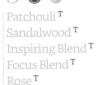

Massage 2-4 drops into affected areas 4-5x daily, or as needed.

Lemongrass ^{T}
Soothing Blend ^{T}
Marjoram ^{T}
Cardamom ^{T}
Siberian Fir ^{T}

Tennis Elbow

Massage 2-4 drops into affected area as needed.

Lemongrass ^{T}
Soothing Blend ^{T}
Siberian Fir ^{T}
Blue Tansy ^{T}
Frankincense ^{T}

Tension

Apply 3-5 drops over the forehead, back of neck and top of head as needed; inhale from cupped hands; diffuse several drops.

Tension Blend ^{AT}
Lavender ^{AT}
Frankincense ^{AT}
Soothing Blend ^{AT}
Rose ^{AT}

Protocol on pg. 202

Testosterone (low)

Apply 2-4 drops to bottoms of feet and inside of thighs 2x daily; inhale from cupped hands as needed.

Patchouli ^{T}
Sandalwood ^{T}
Inspiring Blend ^{T}
Focus Blend ^{T}
Rose ^{T}

Thrombosis, Deep Vein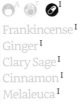

Place 1-2 drops of oils on hand (preferably all 5 listed) in a capsule and take 3x daily.

Frankincense ^{I}
Ginger ^{I}
Clary Sage ^{I}
Cinnamon ^{I}
Melaleuca ^{I}

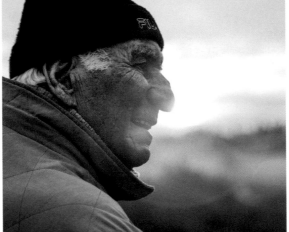

Thrush

Gargle 1-3 drops mixed with water several times daily; apply topically to lower throat and bottoms of feet; ingest 1-3 drops as needed.

Melaleuca ^{TI}
Geranium ^{TI}
Arborvitae ^{TI}
Oregano ^{TI}
Protective Blend ^{TI}

Protocol on pg. 203

Thymus Support

Apply 3-5 drops to throat 2x daily; use carrier oil for improved efficacy.

Frankincense ^{T}
Juniper Berry ^{T}
Rosemary ^{T}
Basil ^{T}
Melaleuca ^{T}

Tick Bites

Apply 1-2 drops to bite frequently for the first hour after carefully removing tick. Dilute Oregano if necessary.

Oregano ^{T}
Melaleuca ^{T}
Cleansing Blend ^{T}
Lavender ^{T}
Outdoor Blend ^{T}

Tingling

Apply 2-4 drops to affected areas several times daily; ingest 1-3 drops as needed.

Peppermint ᵀ ᴵ
Roman Chamomile ᵀ ᴵ
Massage Blend ᵀ ᴵ
Soothing Blend ᵀ ᴵ
Frankincense ᵀ ᴵ

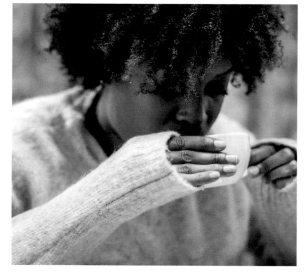

Tinnitus

Apply 1-2 drops behind ear 2-3x daily.

Helichrysum ᵀ
Grounding Blend ᵀ
Basil ᵀ
Frankincense ᵀ
Rosemary ᵀ

Protocol on pg. 204

Tonsillitis

Gargle 1-3 drops mixed with water or ingest 3x daily; apply to outside of throat with carrier oil 3x daily.

Protective Blend ᵀ ᴵ
Oregano ᵀ ᴵ
Arborvitae ᵀ
Melaleuca ᵀ ᴵ
Melissa ᵀ ᴵ

Tourette's Syndrome

Massage 1-3 drops with carrier oil solution into spine and neck; diffuse several drops.

Frankincense ᴬ ᵀ
Lavender ᴬ ᵀ
Roman Chamomile ᴬ ᵀ
Ylang Ylang ᴬ ᵀ
Clary Sage ᴬ ᵀ

Protocol on pg. 204

TMJ (Temporomandibular Joint Dysfunction)

Massage 1-3 drops into jaw joint 3x daily.

Soothing Blend ᵀ
Wintergreen ᵀ
Sandalwood ᵀ
Eucalyptus ᵀ
Rosemary ᵀ

Toothache

Apply a drop to gums and directly onto tooth; swish 1-3 drops with water.

Clove ᵀ ᴵ
Protective Blend ᵀ ᴵ
Helichrysum ᵀ ᴵ
Copaiba ᵀ ᴵ
Wintergreen ᵀ

Toxemia

Gargle a few drops with water several times daily or as needed; take 1-3 drops in a capsule 2x daily; apply 2-4 drops to bottoms of feet 30 minutes before showering.

Cilantro ᵀ ᴵ
Detoxification Blend ᵀ ᴵ
Oregano ᵀ ᴵ
Clove ᵀ ᴵ
Thyme ᵀ ᴵ

Trauma (Emotional)

Apply 2-4 drops to forehead, temples, back of neck, and chest; inhale from cupped hands as needed; diffuse several drops.

Comforting Blend ᴬ ᵀ
Reassuring Blend ᴬ ᵀ
Renewing Blend ᴬ ᵀ
Frankincense ᴬ ᵀ
Rose ᴬ ᵀ

Protocol on pg. 233

Tuberculosis (TB)

Apply 1-3 drops to a carrier solution and massage into spine and neck 3x daily.

Protective Blend ᵀ
Cinnamon ᵀ
Melaleuca ᵀ
Frankincense ᵀ
Arborvitae ᵀ

Tumor

Apply 3-5 drops over the affected area 3-5x daily.

Frankincense ᵀ
Cellular Complex ᵀ
Sandalwood ᵀ
Arborvitae ᵀ
Rosemary ᵀ

Typhoid

Massage 1-3 drops with carrier oil into spine and neck 2-3x daily; ingest 2-4 drops in a capsule.

Protective Blend ᵀ ᴵ
Cinnamon ᵀ ᴵ
Melaleuca ᵀ ᴵ
Frankincense ᵀ ᴵ
Rosemary ᵀ ᴵ

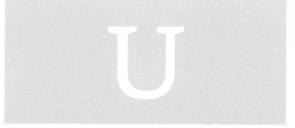

Ulcers (Stomach)

Ingest 1-3 drops at least once daily; massage gently into abdomen as needed.

Lemongrass ᵀ ᴵ
Frankincense ᵀ ᴵ
Myrrh ᵀ ᴵ
Detoxification Blend ᵀ ᴵ
Geranium ᵀ ᴵ

Urinary Support

Massage 1-3 drops over bladder and kidneys before bedtime as needed.

Cypress ^T
Juniper Berry ^T
Ylang Ylang ^T
Lemongrass ^T
Roman Chamomile ^T

Urinary Tract Infection

Massage 1-3 drops over kidneys and on bottoms of the feet; ingest as needed.

Cypress ^T
Basil ^T
Lemongrass ^T
Juniper Berry ^T
Cleansing Blend ^T

Protocol on pg. 204

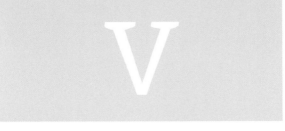

Vaginal Infection

Apply 3-5 drops over lower abdomen and to vaginal area 3x daily.

Lavender ^T
Melaleuca ^T
Rosemary ^T
Frankincense ^T
Arborvitae ^T

Protocol on pg. 205

Vaginitis

Apply 3-5 drops over lower abdomen and to vaginal area 3x daily.

Bergamot ^T
Cedarwood ^T
Melaleuca ^T
Lavender ^T
Myrrh ^T

Protocol on pg. 205

Varicose Veins

Massage 2-4 drops into the affected area several times daily.

Cypress ^T
Helichrysum ^T
Siberian Fir ^T
Detoxification Blend ^T
Cardamom ^T

Vertigo

Apply 2-4 drops to forehead and back of neck as needed.

Ginger ^{A T}
Lavender ^{A T}
Clary Sage ^{A T}
Basil ^{A T}
Rosemary ^{A T}

Viruses

Apply 2-4 drops to bottoms of feet, back of neck, and spine 3-5x daily; ingest 2-5 drops 3x daily.

Protective Blend ^{T I}
Oregano ^{T I}
Melissa ^{T I}
Black Pepper ^{T I}
Lime ^{T I}

Vision Loss

Apply 1-3 drops around eyes (do not get in eyes) and lower back 2x daily.

Clary Sage ^T
Helichrysum ^T
Anti-Aging Blend ^T
Cellular Complex ^T
Yarrow ^T

Vomiting

Apply 1-3 drops over stomach as needed; drink a few drops in water; inhale from cupped hands.

Digestive Blend ^{A T I}
Ginger ^{A T I}
Bergamot ^{A T I}
Peppermint ^{A T I}
Roman Chamomile ^{A T I}

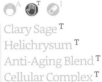

Warts

Apply a drop directly to wart several times daily until the wart disappears. Avoid the surrounding skin with Oregano.

Oregano ^T
Frankincense ^T
Thyme ^T
Skin Clearing Blend ^T
Neroli ^T

Wasp Sting

Apply one drop to sting several times daily or as needed.

Lavender ^T
Roman Chamomile ^T
Cedarwood ^T
Cleansing Blend ^T
Myrrh ^T

Water Retention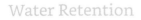

Massage 2-4 drops over bladder and kidneys before bedtime as needed.

Cypress ^T
Black Pepper ^T
Ylang Ylang ^T
Lemongrass ^T
Roman Chamomile ^T

Weight Loss

Add 2-4 drops to water to manage cravings and encourage metabolism; inhale from cupped hands to satisfy cravings.

Metabolic Blend ^{A T I}
Grapefruit ^{A T I}
Peppermint ^{A T I}
Lemon ^{A T I}
Energy & Stamina Complex ^I

Protocol on pg. 205

Wheezing

Rub 2-4 drops over chest with carrier oil; diffuse several drops.

Eucalyptus [A T]
Lavender [A T]
Respiratory Blend [A T]
Frankincense [A T]
Bergamot [A T]

Whiplash

Massage 2-4 drops into affected area 2-3x daily; use with carrier oil to improve efficacy.

Soothing Blend [T]
Siberian Fir [T]
Marjoram [T]
Patchouli [T]
Sandalwood [T]

Whooping Cough
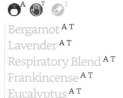
Apply 2-4 drops over chest and on bottoms of feet with carrier oil; diffuse several drops.

Bergamot [A T]
Lavender [A T]
Respiratory Blend [A T]
Frankincense [A T]
Eucalyptus [A T]

Withdrawal Symptoms

Apply 2-4 drops to wrists, chest, and bottoms of feet as often as needed; diffuse several drops.

Detoxification Blend [A T]
Cilantro [A T]
Cinnamon [A T]
Juniper Berry [A T]
Encouraging Blend [A T]

Protocol on pg. 210

Worms

Apply 2-4 drops over abdomen, bottoms of feet, and back of neck; add 2-4 drops to water or take in capsule.

Oregano [T I]
Thyme [T I]
Ginger [T I]
Basil [T I]
Clove [T I]

Wounds

Apply 2-4 drops to affected area; use a carrier oil if needed.

Helichrysum [T]
Melaleuca [T]
Lavender [T]
Roman Chamomile [T]
Myrrh [T]

Wrinkles

Apply 1-3 drops to affected areas as needed 2x daily; add a few drops to facial lotion or use with carrier oil for added benefits.

Anti-Aging Blend [T]
Frankincense [T]
Myrrh [T]
Jasmine [T]
Yarrow [T]

Protocol on pg. 205

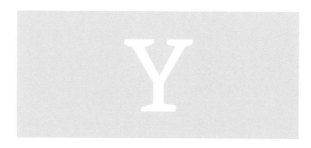

Yeast Infection
Apply 3-5 drops over lower abdomen 3x daily; use with a warm compress; ingest 3-5 drops in a capsule 3x daily.

Melaleuca [T I]
Lavender [T I]
Thyme [T I]
Clove [T I]
Oregano [T I]

Protocol on pg. 205

Section 3

Single *Oils*

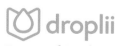

Arborvitae
Thuja Plicata

Application

Main Properties
Antibacterial
Anticancer
Anti-fungal
Astringent
Expectorant

Chemical Constituents
a, B, y-thujaplicin
Methyl thujate
Thujic acid

Other Uses
Colds, Cold Sores, Cysts, Fevers, Intestinal Parasites, Meditation, Respiratory Viruses

Top *Uses*

1 Strep Throat
Rub 2 drops over outside of throat, and gargle 2 drops with water.

2 Bug Repellent
Dilute with several drops of carrier oil, and rub over needed areas.

3 Skin Cancer
Apply diluted to the affected area often and in small amounts.

4 Candida
Rub 2 drops over abdomen and bladder several times a day.

5 Fungal Issues
Apply neat to needed areas.

6 Furniture Polish
Combine 4 drops with 4 drops lemon oil, and rub in using a clean rag.

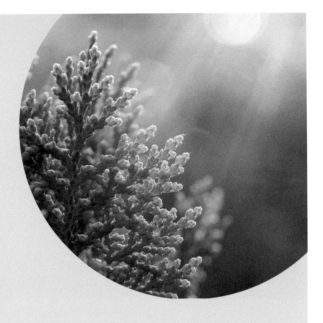

Emotional *Use*

Esters in Arborvitae (Methyl thujate) make it a restorative oil. Use it to restore spiritual balance and to open receptivity to guidance.

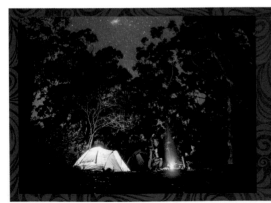

Fireglow Diffuser Blend

1 drop Arborvitae
2 drops Spearmint
2 drops Cinnamon

Arborvitae has a rich, warm, woodsy fragrance. Use less of this oil than you would other tree oils, because a little goes a long way.

Hardwood Floor Cleaner

2 drops Arborvitae
5 drops Lemon
3 drops Juniper Berry
1/2 tsp Murphy's Oil Soap

Mix ingredients with water in a 16 oz. spray bottle for a refreshing floor cleaner that nourishes the wood and your soul!

Basil

Ocimum Basilicum

Application

 A T I

Main Properties
Antibacterial
Anti-infectious
Antispasmodic
Carminative
Nervine

Chemical Constituents
Linalool, 1,8-cineole (eucalyptol), bergamotene, Methyl chavicol

Other Uses
Bee Stings, Bronchitis, Dizziness, Frozen Shoulder, Gout, Greasy Hair, Infertility, Lactation (increase milk supply), Loss of Sense of Smell, Migraines, Nausea, Viral Hepatitis

Top Uses

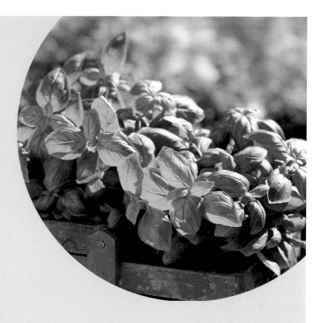

1 Adrenal Fatigue
Apply 1-2 drops directly to the adrenal areas or to the bottoms of the feet.

2 Mental Fatigue
Inhale from cupped hands, or diffuse.

3 Earache
Place a drop on a cotton ball, and rest over the ear for 15 minutes.

4 Muscle Spasms
Massage into muscles with carrier oil.

5 Carpal Tunnel
Massage into wrists & joints.

6 Cramps (abdominal)
Rub a drop clockwise over abdomen.

7 Cooking
Use a toothpick to add to dishes according to taste.

Emotional Use

Alcohols in Basil (Linalool) make it a renewing and calming oil. Use it to feel rejuvenated and renewed in your commitment to a higher life.

Basil Lemonade

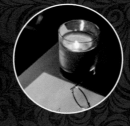

1 drop Basil (or less!)
5 drops Lemon
4-5 fresh-squeezed lemons
Liquid stevia to taste

Combine all ingredients and serve very cold. Adjust ratios to taste.

Insect Repellent Luminaries

1 drop Basil
4 drops Lemon

Add essential oils to a burning tea candle after the wax on the top has melted. For aesthetically pleasing luminaries, place fresh lemon slices and basil leaves in a mason jar with essential oils. Fill with water, and float a tea light candle on the top!

Bergamot
Citrus Bergamia

Application

Main Properties
Antidepressant
Carminative
Neuroprotective
Sedative
Stomachic

Chemical Constituents
d-Limonene, linalyl acetate, linalool, ter-pinene, β-pinene

Other Uses
Brain Injury, Colic, Depression, Fungus Issues, Irritability, Low Energy, Muscle Cramps, Oily Skin, Stress

Safety
Avoid sun for 12 hours after topical application.

Top *Uses*

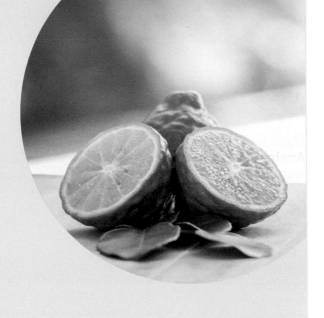

1 Psoriasis
Dilute 1-2 drops heavily with carrier oil, and apply frequently to affected area.

2 Sadness
Inhale from cupped hands or diffuse.

3 Appetite Loss
Drink 1-2 drops in 8 oz. water throughout the day, or diffuse.

4 Addictions
Apply to bottoms of feet, or diffuse.

5 Acne
Apply small amount to affected areas. Avoid sun for 12 hours after.

6 Self-Confidence/Self-Worth
Apply over sacral (belly button).

7 Insomnia
Use 1 drop under tongue or in water.

Emotional Use

Esters like Linalyl Acetate in Bergamot make it a powerful calming oil, perfect for reflecting on and connecting to Self.

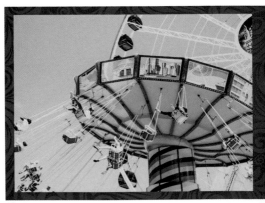

Motion Sickness Relief

2 drops Lime
2 drops Bergamot
2 drops Spearmint or Peppermint

Apply to temples or over stomach, or make a mixture in a roller bottle with a carrier oil and more drops of oil.

Stress Relief Roller

10 drops Lavender
10 drops Wild Orange
5 drops Grounding Blend
5 drops Bergamot

Put all essential oils into a 10 ml roller bottle. Fill remainder with fractionated coconut oil. Rub on your wrists, diffuser bracelet, and back of the neck.

Single Oils

Birch
Betula Lenta

Application

Main Properties
Analgesic
Anti-inflammatory
Antispasmodic
Diuretic
Stimulant

Chemical Constituents
Methyl salicylate
Betulene
Betulinol

Other Uses
Cramps, Gout, Joint Pain, Gallbladder Stones, Kidney Stones, Ulcers

Safety
Avoid during pregnancy. Not for epileptics.

Top *Uses*

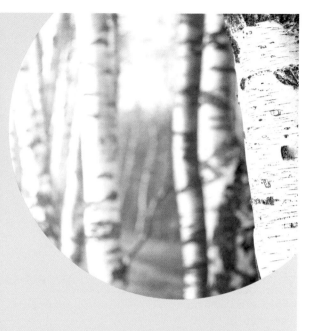

1. Broken bones
Massage 2 drops over and around affected area, avoiding open wounds.

2. Arthritis & Rheumatism
Massage 1-2 drops into affected area.

3. Muscle Aches
Massage 1-2 drops with carrier oil or lotion into muscles.

4. Whiplash
Gently massage with carrier oil. Consider using in Swedish massage.

5. Connective Tissue Injury
Apply neat to affected area.

6. Fever
Apply neat or diluted to back of neck.

7. Bone Spurs
Apply neat to areas of concern.

Emotional *Use*

Esters like Methyl Salicylate make Birch a restorative oil. Use it to achieve feelings of being supported and strengthened.

Stress & Strain Soother

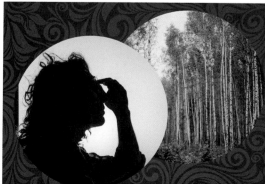

3 drops Birch
3 drops Lavender
3 drops Marjoram
15ml Unscented lotion

Combine ingredients together and store in glass jar. Massage into stressed or strained muscles as needed.

Smoky Skies Diffuser Blend

2 drops Birch
2 drops Arborvitae
2 drops Cedarwood
2 drops Douglas Fir
1 drop Frankincense
1 drop White Fir
1 drop Protective Blend

Enjoy the feeling of a rich autumn evening.

Black Pepper
Piper Nigrum

Application

Main Properties
Analgesic
Anticatarrhal
Anti-microbial
Antiviral
Immunostimulant

Chemical Constituents
β-caryophyllene, l-limonene, sabinene, α-pinene, ß-Pinene, δ-3-carene, caryophyllene oxide

Other Uses
Antioxidant, Anxiety, Cellular Oxygenation, Diarrhea, Digestion, Gas, Emotional Repression, Inflammation, Laxative

Safety
Dilute for use on sensitive skin.

Top *Uses*

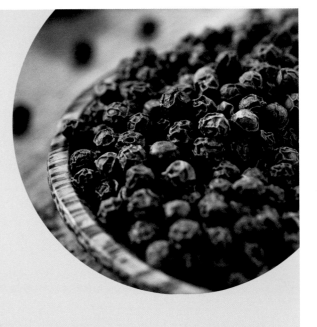

1 Cold & Flu
Take 2 drops in a capsule, or apply to the bottoms of feet.

2 Smoking (quitting)
Apply to bottoms of feet (big toes) several times a day to curb cravings.

3 Circulation
Apply to bottoms of feet.

4 Sprains
Massage into muscles with carrier oil.

5 Congestion
Apply diluted over chest and upper back.

6 Airborne Viruses
Diffuse to cleanse the air.

7 Cooking
Add a drop to soups, sauces, and other dishes.

Emotional Use

Sesquiterpenes like Caryophyllene make Black Pepper a soothing oil that can unmask repressed emotions.

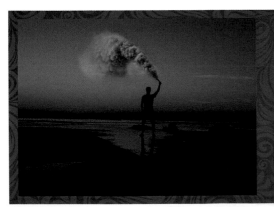

Smoking Stopper
1 drop Black Pepper
1 drop Clove
5 drops FCO

Combine ingredients and use a drop under the tongue to help with cravings and anxiousness. (Be prepared for a numbing sensation from the Clove!)

Fibromyalgia Massage Blend
12 drops Black Pepper
6 drops Marjoram
6 drops Juniper Berry
6 drops Ginger
2 oz. FCO

Combine ingredients in a roller bottle or small jar. Massage small amounts into affected areas as needed.

Blue Tansy

Tanacetum Annuum

Application

Main Properties

Antihistamine
Anti-parasitic
Anti-rheumatic
Hypotensive
Sedative

Chemical Constituents

Sabinene, Chamazulene, p-Cymene, α-Phellandrene, ß-Pinene, Camphor

Other Uses

Bacterial Infection, Constipation, Cramping, Eczema, Fungus, Gas, Gout, Indigestion, Insect Repellent, Psoriasis, Rashes, Rheumatism, Sneezing

Safety

Dilute for use on sensitive skin.

Top Uses

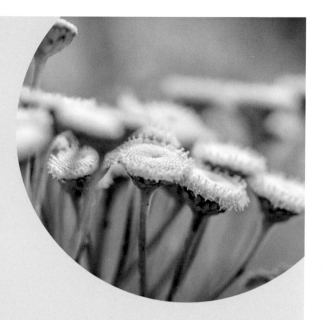

1. **Allergies**
   Put 1-2 drops under the tongue, then swallow with water after 30 seconds.

2. **Arthritis & Muscle Pain**
   Add 5-10 drops to a bath, or massage into affected areas with carrier oil.

3. **Anxiety**
   Apply a drop to pulse points, or diffuse.

4. **Digestive Discomfort**
   Massage 2 drops clockwise onto stomach.

5. **Dry, Itchy, or Inflamed Skin**
   Apply heavily diluted to affected skin.

6. **Headaches**
   Rub a drop into temples and back of skull.

7. **Congestion**
   Rub 2 drops onto chest and mid-back.

Emotional Use

Monoterpenes like Sabinene make Blue Tansy an uplifting oil to conquer procrastination and take inspired action.

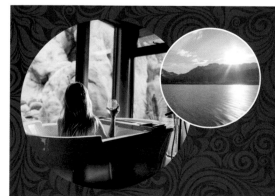

Blue Bath Salt

3 drops Blue Tansy
2 drops Cedarwood
1 drop Ylang Ylang
1 tsp jojoba oil
½ cup Epsom salt

Stir together and add to a full tub for a tranquil and soothing soak.

Positive Morning Diffuser Blend

3 drops Blue Tansy
3 drops Lavender
4 drops Copaiba
2 drops Frankincense

What to notice: This diffuser blend helps encourage a sense of peace and cheer as you start your day.

Cardamom
Elettaria Cardamomum

Application

Main Properties
Anti-infectious
Antispasmodic
Aphrodisiac
Decongestant
Expectorant

Chemical Constituents
a-terpinyl accetate, Linalool, Sabinene, 1,8-cineole

Other Uses
Colitis, Constipation, Headaches, Inflammation, Menstrual Pain, Muscle Aches, Nausea, Pancreatitis, Respiratory Issues, Sore Throat, Stomach Ulcers

Top *Uses*

1 Digestive Discomfort
Drink a drop with a glass of water or in a capsule, or rub over stomach.

2 Congestion
Rub with carrier oil over chest, or diffuse.

3 Indigestion
Drink a drop with water or in a capsule.

4 Cough
Rub with carrier oil over chest.

5 Motion Sickness
Put a drop under the tongue.

6 Asthma, Shortness of Breath
Apply to bottoms of feet or over chest.

7 Cooking
Use a toothpick to add to dishes according to taste.

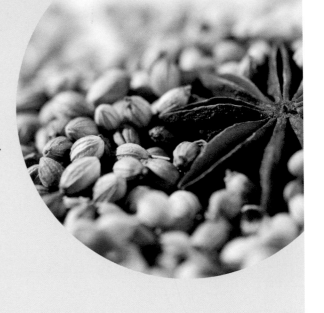

Emotional Use

Ethers like Terpenyl acetate make Cardamom a restoring oil. Use it to replace anger with clear, objective thinking.

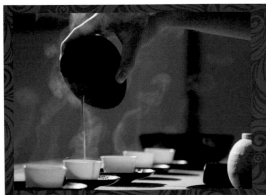

Hot Spiced Tea Diffuser Blend
1 drop Cardamom
3 drops Wild Orange
2 drops Cinnamon
1 drop Clove

This blend is invigorating while keeping your mind focused on the task at hand.

Warm Back Rub
3 drops Cardamom
2 drops Clove
3 drops Ginger
5 drops Marjoram
1 oz. FCO

Stir ingredients together and use in a back massage.

Cassia
Cinnamomum Cassia

Application

Main Properties
Antibacterial
Antiviral
Antispasmodic
Cardiotonic
Decongestant

Chemical Constituents
Trans-cinnamaldehyde, Eugenol , Cinnamyl acetate

Other Uses
Antiseptic, Boils, Circulation, Cold Limbs, Upset Stomach, Typhoid

Safety
Dilute heavily for topical use. Avoid during pregnancy.

Top Uses

1 Vomiting
Take 1-2 drops in a capsule to restore proper digestion.

2 Viruses & Bacteria
Diffuse to cleanse the air, or take 1-2 drops in a capsule to combat internally.

3 Water Retention
Apply to bottoms of feet, take 1-2 drops in a capsule, or add 2 drops to bath.

4 Blood Sugar Balance
Take 1-2 drops in a capsule with food.

5 Sex Drive
Use heavily diluted in massage, or diffuse.

6 Metabolism Boost
Apply to adrenal reflex points.

7 Cooking
Use a toothpick to add to dishes.

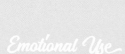

Emotional Use

Aldehydes like Cinnamaldehyde make Cassia ideal for transforming insecurity and shyness into self-assurance.

Gingerbread Diffuser Blend
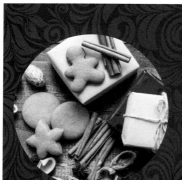
2 drops Cassia
3 drops Ginger
2 drops Clove

This diffuser blend has a warm, inviting feel to it. It's also great for combating airborne pathogens.

Oatmeal Cookie Diffuser Blend
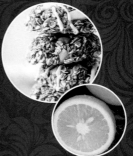
2 drops Cassia
2 drops Cedarwood
3 drops Wild Orange

Who would have thought that Cedarwood, Wild Orange, and Cassia could create a cookie smell? Well, they do!

Cedarwood
Juniperus Virginiana

Application
A T I

Main Properties
Astringent
Decongestant
Depurative
Diuretic
Sedative

Chemical Constituents
a, B, y-thujaplicin, α-cedrene, cedrol, thujo-psene, methyl thujate, thujic acid

Other Uses
Blemishes, Cough, Dandruff, Gums, Insect Repellent, Respiratory Function, Sinusitis, Vaginal Infection, Tension

Safety
Cedarwood is very mild, and safe for even the most sensitive skin.

Top *Uses*

1 Eczema & Psoriasis
Apply neat and often to affected areas.

2 ADD/ADHD
Apply to wrists, temples, and back of neck, or diffuse.

3 Sleep
Rub onto bottoms of feet and back of neck, and diffuse. Blend with Lavender.

4 Anxiety
Apply to wrists and temples.

5 Cuts & Scrapes
Apply around wounded area to promote healing.

6 Urinary & Bladder Infection
Apply over bladder.

7 Seizures & Stroke
Apply to back of neck and bottoms of feet.

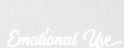

Emotional Use

Alcohols like Cedrol make Cedarwood a Stabilizing oil that takes you from feeling separate to feeling socially connected.

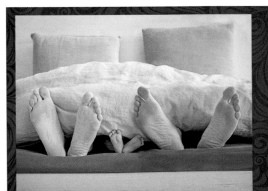

Safe & Sound Sleep Diffuser Blend
2 drops Cedarwood
3 drops Bergamot
1 drop Marjoram

Diffuse this fresh, herbaceous sleep blend to feel comfort and calm at bedtime.

Nighttime Relaxation Blend
2 drops Cedarwood
2 drops Lavender
2 drops Restful Blend

Use this diffuser blend an hour before bedtime to calm things down at home.

Cilantro
Coriandrum Sativum

Application

Main Properties
Antibacterial
Anti-fungal
Antimicrobial
Antioxidant
Detoxifier

Chemical Constituents
Linalool, Methyl chavicol, 1, 8 cineol

Other Uses
Allergies, Antioxidant, Anxiety, Bloating, Gas, Liver Support, Kidney Support

Top *Uses*

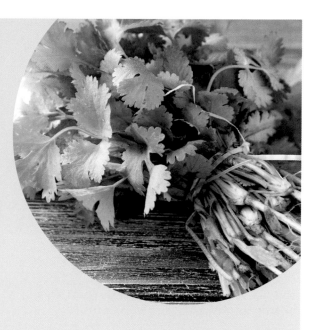

1 Heavy Metal Detox
Apply to the bottoms of feet morning and night.

2 Halitosis
Take 1-2 drops in a capsule.

3 Detox
Apply over liver, kidneys, and bottoms of feet.

4 Fungal Infections
Take 1-2 drops in a capsule for internal issues, or apply topically for external issues.

5 Body Odor
Use small amounts in food, or take 1-2 drops in a capsule to deodorize internally.

6 Cooking
Use a toothpick to add to dishes according to taste.

Emotional *Use*

Alcohols like Linalool make Cilantro a calming oil, perfect for releasing control issues and obsessive compulsive tendencies.

Spring Cleaning Spray

2 drops Cilantro
2 drops Siberian Fir
1 drop Lime
1 Tbs vinegar
16 oz spray bottle with water

Mix together and use on counter tops, trash cans, and other surfaces for a fresh cleaning experience.

Carpet Freshener

5 drops Cilantro
10 drops Siberian Fir
10 drops Melaleuca
10 drops Lime
5 drops Cleansing Blend
2 Cups Baking Soda

Work mixed ingredients into stinky carpet. Vacuum thoroughly after 12-24 hours.

Cinnamon
Cinnamomum Zeylanicum

Application

Main Properties
Antidepressant
Antimicrobial
Antioxidant
Anti-parasitic
Immune stimulant

Chemical Constituents
Transcinnamaldehyde, cinnamyl acetate, eugenol, Linalool

Other Uses
Airborne Bacteria, Cholesterol, Diverticulitis, Fungal Infections, General Tonic, Immune Support, Pancreas Support, Pneumonia, Typhoid, Vaginitis

Safety
Dilute heavily. Avoid during pregnancy. Repeated use can cause sensitivity.

Top *Uses*

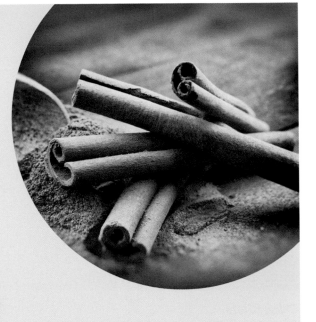

1 High Blood Sugar
Take 1-2 drops in capsule, or drink with large glass of water.

2 Bacterial Infection
Apply heavily diluted for external infection, or take 1-2 drops in a capsule for internal infection.

3 Sex Drive
Use heavily diluted in massage, or diffuse.

4 Cavities
Swish a drop with water as a mouthwash.

5 Diabetes
Take 1-2 drops in a capsule daily.

6 Alkalinity
Drink in water to promote alkalinity.

7 Cooking
Use a toothpick to achieve desired flavor.

Emotional Use

Aldehydes like Cinnamaldehyde make Cinnamon a restoring oil. Use it to restore sexual harmony and expression.

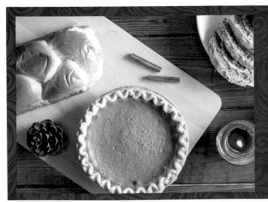

Cinnamint Breath Spray

10 drops Cinnamon
10 drops Peppermint
10ml FCO
Empty oil bottle with spray top

Combine ingredients and shake well. Use as needed for cinnamint fresh breath.

Pumpkin Pie Diffuser Blend

2 drops Cinnamon
4 drops Cardamom
1 drop Clove
1 drop Wild Orange

Enjoy the warmth of the holidays with this nostalgic diffuser blend.

Clary Sage
Salvia Sclarea

Application
 A T I

Main Properties
Anticonvulsant
Antiseptic
Antispasmodic
Nerve tonic
Tonic

Chemical Constituents
Linalyl acetate, Linalool, sclareol

Other Uses
Aneurysm, Breast Enlargement, Cholesterol, Convulsions, Endometriosis, Epilepsy, Fragile Hair, Hot Flashes, Impotence, Lactation, Parkinson's, Premenopause, Seizure

Top Uses

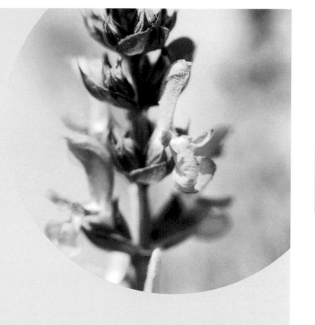

1. **Hormone Balance**
Apply to wrists and behind ears.

2. **PMS**
Apply to bottoms of feet, or take 1-2 drops in capsule.

3. **Postpartum Depression**
Diffuse or apply over heart area.

4. **Abdominal Cramps**
Massage over abdomen.

5. **Pink Eye**
Apply carefully around edge of eye.

6. **Infertility**
Apply to abdomen & uterine reflex points, or take 1-2 drops in capsule.

7. **Breast Cancer**
Apply diluted to breasts, or take 1-2 drops in capsule to regulate estrogen levels.

Emotional Use
Esters like Linalyl Acetate make Clary Sage a calming oil, ideal for calming confusion and bringing about clarified vision.

Epilepsy Diffuser Blend
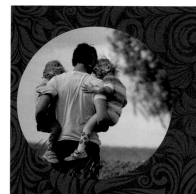

1 drop Clary Sage
1 drop Cedarwood
1 drop Patchouli
1 drop Peppermint
1 drop Grounding Blend
1 drop Frankincense
1 drop Vetiver

Diffuse this throughout the day.

Fresh Start Diffuser Blend
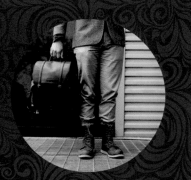

2 drops Clary Sage
2 drops Ylang Ylang
2 drops Sandalwood
2 drops Lavender

Use this blend to begin your week with the right mindset and energy.

Clove

Eugenia Caryophyllata

Application

Main Properties

Analgesic
Anti-infectious
Anti-parasitic
Antiviral
Antioxidant

Chemical Constituents

Eugenol, eugenyl acetate, β-caryophyllene

Other Uses

Addictions, Blood Clots, Candida, Cataracts, Fever, Herpes Simplex, Hodgkin's Disease, Glaucoma, Gingivitis, Lipoma, Lupus, Lyme Disease, Macular Degeneration, Memory Loss, Parasites, Termites

Safety

Can irritate sensitive skin. Use with caution during pregnancy.

Top *Uses*

1 Thyroid (hypo, Hashimoto's)
Apply diluted over thyroid or to thyroid reflex point, or take 1-2 drops in capsule.

2 Toothache
Apply directly to problematic tooth.

3 Smoking Addiction
Rub onto bottom of big toe.

4 Immune Support
Take 1-2 drops in a capsule.

5 Antioxidant
Take 1-2 drops in a capsule, or use in cooking.

6 Liver Detox
Rub over liver or on liver reflex point.

7 Rheumatoid Arthritis
Massage diluted into affected area.

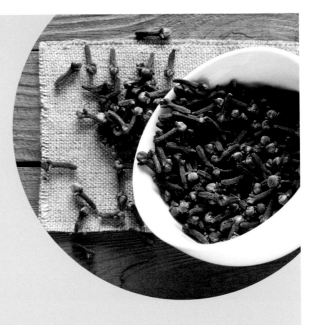

Emotional Use

Phenols like Eugenol make Clove a restoring oil, perfect for defeating victim mentality and holding healthy boundaries.

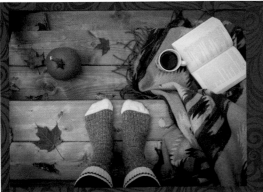

Blood Clot Releaser

3 drops Clove
4 drops Grapefruit
3 drops Lemon
2 drops Helichrysum
Fractionated Coconut Oil

Combine oils in 10ml roller bottle, and top off with FCO. Apply to painful areas as needed.

Immune Booster Diffuser Blend

1 drop Clove
1 drop Rosemary
1 drop Eucalyptus
1 drop Cinnamon
1 drop Wild Orange

Diffuse if you run out of Protective Blend, especially during cold and flu season.

Copaiba
Copaifera Officinalis

Application

Main Properties
Analgesic
Anti-fungal
Anti-inflammatory
Diuretic
Expectorant

Chemical Constituents
β-caryophyllene, d-Limonene, y-terpinene, linalyl acetate

Other Uses
Anxiety, Congestion, Infection, Mood Disorders, Nail Fungus, Skin Strengthening

Top *Uses*

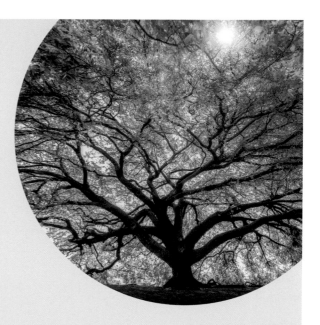

1 Headache & Migraine
Massage gently onto temples, scalp, and the back of the neck.

2 Pain & Inflammation
Inhale or diffuse, or apply topically to affected areas.

3 Wrinkles, Pimples, Blisters
Apply daily with a carrier oil.

4 High Blood Pressure
Apply to the bottoms of feet twice daily.

5 Athlete's Foot
Apply several drops to clean, dry feet.

6 Detox
Apply over bladder to stimulate detox through urination.

Emotional *Use*

Sesquiterpenes like β-caryophyllene make Copaiba a soothing oil, powerful for unveiling the falseness in shame and guilt.

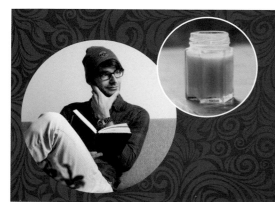

Pain-away Cream
15 drops Copaiba
15 drops Soothing Blend
1/2 cup coconut oil (in solid state)

Beat coconut oil with hand mixer until fluffy. Add essential oils, and stir in slowly. Store in small glass jars in a cool room.

Mind Cleanse Diffuser Blend
5 drops Copaiba
4 drops Rosemary
2 drops Peppermint
2 drops Clary Sage

Enjoy the mental clarity that comes with this diffuser blend. It's the perfect combination of calm and insightful.

Coriander
Coriandrum Sativum

Application

Main Properties
Anti-rheumatic
Carminative
Regenerative
Sedative
Stomachic

Chemical Constituents
Linalool, a-pinene, Geranyl

Other Uses
Alzheimer's, Itchy Skin, Joint Pain, Low Energy, Measles, Muscle Tone, Muscle Spasms, Nausea, Neuropathy, Stiffness, Whiplash

Top *Uses*

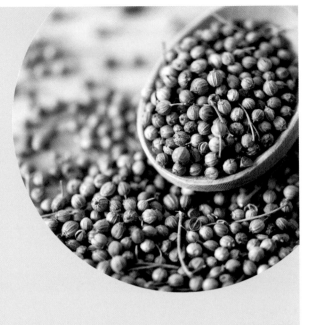

1 Diabetes (high blood sugar)
Combine with 1 drop Cinnamon & Juniper Berry in capsule daily.

2 Food Poisoning
Drink 2 drops in water, or take in capsule.

3 Body Odor
Drink 2 drops in water, or take in a capsule.

4 Cartilage Injury
Massage into affected area with carrier oil.

5 Rashes
Apply diluted to affected area.

6 Muscle Aches
Take a drop in a capsule, or massage with carrier oil onto affected muscles.

7 Cooking
Use a toothpick to add desired flavor.

Emotional *Use*

Alcohols like Linalool make Coriander a calming oil. Use it to turn self-betrayal into integrity.

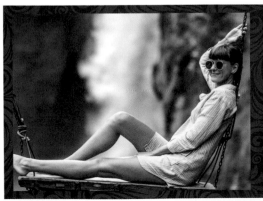

Constipation Relief

5 drops Coriander
2 drops Ginger
4 drops Lemon
4 drops Digestive Blend
7 drops Wild Orange

Combine oils in roller bottle and top with FCO. Rub over stomach 2-3 times daily.

Tummy Calming Bath Salts

3 drops Coriander
10 drops Digestive Blend
1 cup Epsom Salt

Combine ingredients and add to hot bath. Soak for at least 20 minutes to soothe digestive upset.

Cumin

Cuminum Cyminum

Application

Main Properties

Antibacterial
Anti-carcinogentic
Antimicrobial
Antiviral
Sedative

Chemical Constituents

Cuminaldehyde, Beta-pinene, Para-cymene

Other Uses

Skin Warming

Safety

Possible skin sensitivity. Avoid sun for 12 hours after topical application.

Top *Uses*

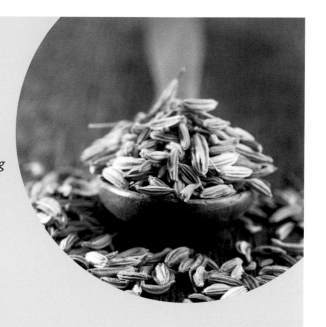

1 Flatulence
Take 1-2 drops in a capsule.

2 Cooking
Use a toothpick to add to dishes according to taste. Especially good for stews, soups, dressings, and sauces.

3 Digestive Discomfort
Take 1-2 drops in a capsule.

4 Organ Detox
Take 1-2 drops in a capsule daily for 3-5 days.

5 Mouth Rinse
Swish a drop with water as a natural mouthwash.

Emotional *Use*

Aldehydes like Cuminal make Cumin a restoring oil, fostering a sense of balanced ambition and non-attachment to success.

Spicy Ribs Rub

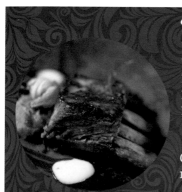

12 drops Cumin
1 drop Cilantro
1 drop Ginger
1 Tbsp cayenne & chili powder
1 tsp white pepper, black pepper, salt, & crushed red pepper

Combine ingredients and rub onto ribs before grilling.

Enchilada Sauce

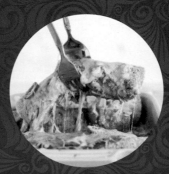

1-2 drops Cumin · 1 tsp sugar
1 Tbsp flour & butter · 1/2 tsp salt
1-3 tsp chili powder · 1 tsp chopped onion
1 cup tomato juice

Heat butter and flour in saucepan. Add other ingredients and bring to a boil. Stir, and simmer for a few minutes.

Cypress
Cupressus Sempervirens

Application

Main Properties
Antibacterial
Anti-infectious
Diuretic
Lymphatic
Vasoconstrictor

Chemical Constituents
a-pinene, cedrol, a-terpinyl acetate

Other Uses
Aneurysm, Bunions, Edema, Hemorrhoids, Flu, Incontinence, Lou Gehrig's Disease, Ovary Issues, Prostate Issues, Raynaud's Disease, Tuberculosis, Varicose Veins, Whooping Cough

Safety
Can irritate sensitive skin. Use with caution during pregnancy.

Top *Uses*

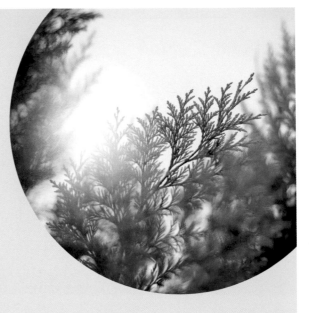

1 **Circulation (poor)**
Apply 2 drops to the bottoms of each foot morning and night.

2 **Bladder/Urinary Tract Infection**
Massage 2 drops with carrier oil over bladder. Repeat every 2 hours as needed.

3 **Bone Spurs**
Apply directly onto affected area.

4 **Concussion**
Massage 2 drops with carrier oil into back of neck, back of skull, and shoulders.

5 **Restless Leg Syndrome**
Massage 2 drops with carrier oil into bottoms of feet, calves, and upper legs.

6 **Bed Wetting**
Apply 2 drops neat over bladder before bed.

Emotional Use

Monoterpenes like a-Pinene make Cypress a restoring oil. It creates motion and flow where energy was once stuck or stagnant.

Laundry Softener

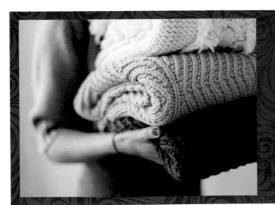

3 drops Cypress
3 drops Siberian Fir
2 drops Wintergreen
1/4 cup baking soda

Combine ingredients and add to laundry before starting the washing machine.

Positive Thinking Diffuser Blend

2 drops Cypress
2 drops Frankincense
2 drops Ylang Ylang

Use this diffuser blend while journaling or during morning meditation.

Dill

Anethum Graveolens

Application

Main Properties
Anti-putrescent
Antispasmodic
Calmative
Cholagogue
Hepatic

Chemical Constituents
δ-limonene, δ-carvone, α & β-phellandrene

Other Uses
Colic, Dyspepsia, Electrolyte Imbalance, Flatulence, Indigestion, Insulin Imbalance, Liver Deficiency, Nervousness, Pancreas Support

Safety
Use with caution when epileptic.

Top *Uses*

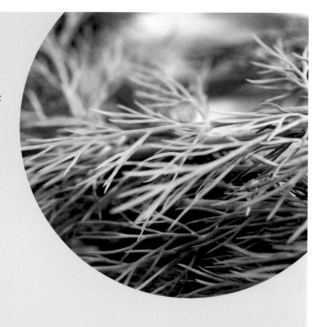

1 Cholesterol
Apply to arches of feet, or take 1-2 drops in a capsule.

2 Flavoring
Use a toothpick to achieve desired flavor in dips and sauces.

3 Constipation
Take 1-2 drops in a capsule.

4 Lactation (increase milk supply)
Take 1-2 drops in a capsule, or massage with carrier oil around breast.

5 Missing Menstrual Cycle
Rub 1 drop with carrier oil over abdomen.

6 Muscle Spasms
Massage with carrier oil over agitated or overactive muscles.

Emotional Use

Ketones like Carvone make Dill an energizing oil, providing mental alertness to incite learning and engagement.

Dill Vinaigrette

2 drops Dill
3/4 cup apple cider vinegar
1/4 cup extra virgin olive oil
1/2 cup Greek yogurt
1/4 tsp onion & garlic powder
Pinch of salt

Blend all ingredients together until smooth.

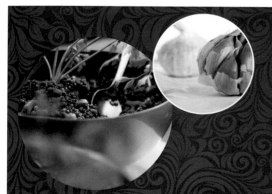

Sunsational Diffuser Blend

1 drop Dill
2 drops Lemon
3 drops Tangerine

This diffuser blend adds a burst of herbaceous and citrusy fun to any day at home.

Douglas Fir
Pseudotsuga Menziesil

Application

Main Properties
Antioxidant
Analgesic
Diuretic
Expectorant
Tonic

Chemical Constituents
β-pinene, α-pinene, δ-3-carene, sabinene

Other Uses
Arthritis, Constipation, Depression, Emotional Congestion, Energy, Generational Patterns, Weight Gain, Sinus Issues

Top *Uses*

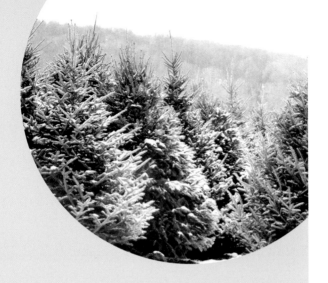

1 Muscle Soreness
Rub 2-4 drops with carrier oil onto sore muscles.

2 Congestion
Rub 1-2 drops over chest, or diffuse.

3 Headache & Migraine
Rub a drop into temples.

4 Focus & Mental Clarity
Inhale from cupped hands, or diffuse.

5 Skin Irritations
Apply heavily diluted to irritated skin.

6 Household Cleansing
Use with Lemon oil for a refreshing household cleaner.

7 Cough
Apply 1-2 drops to chest or lung reflex points.

Emotional Use

Monoterpenes like β-pinene make Douglas Fir an uplifting oil that lifts you from dysfunctional generational patterns.

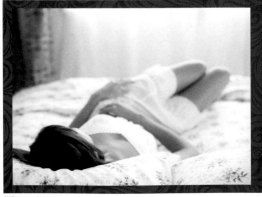

Super Chillax

3 drops Douglas Fir
3 drops Restful Blend
3 drops Grounding Blend

Apply oils to your hands, graze your pillows, rub onto your neck, and brush your hairline. Also diffuse all three oils to fall asleep and stay asleep.

Namaste Breathing

2 drops Douglas Fir
2 drops Juniper Berry
2 drops Grapefruit

Rub oils onto your chest, and take deep breaths from cupped hands.

Eucalyptus
Eucalyptus Radiata

Application

Main Properties
Antiphlogistic
Antispasmodic
Antiussive
Antiviral
Vermifuge

Chemical Constituents
Eucalyptol , 1,8 cineole, a & B-pinenes, a-terpineol

Other Uses
Colds, Fever, Flu, Headache, Earaches, Insect Bites & Stings, Kidney Stones, Muscle Aches, Neuralgia, Rheumatism, Rhinitis

Safety
Not for use topically on newborns.

Top *Uses*

1 Congestion & Cough
Apply 2-4 drops to chest, or diffuse.

2 Bronchitis & Pneumonia
Apply 2-4 drops to chest & mid-back, or diffuse.

3 Sinusitis
Apply heavily diluted to sinuses, carefully avoiding eyes.

4 Asthma
Inhale 2 drops from cupped hands, and apply to lung reflex points.

5 Menstrual Cramps
Rub 1-2 drops with carrier oil over abdomen.

6 Mental Fatigue
Inhale 1-2 drops from cupped hands, or diffuse.

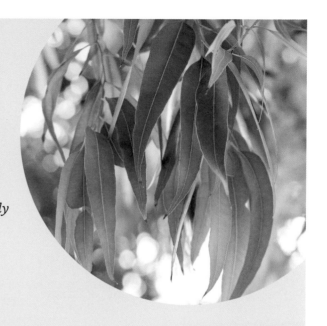

Emotional *Use*

Ethers like 1,8-Cineole make Eucalyptus a restoring oil. It's perfect to release attachment to illness, and to shift into a sense of wellness.

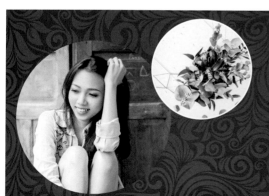

Headache Relief
1 drop Eucalyptus
2 drops Peppermint
2 drops Lavender
1 drop Rosemary

Place oils in palms, and massage onto back of neck and into scalp to relieve headaches.

Freshen Up Diffuser Blend
2 drops Eucalyptus
3 drops Lime
2 drops Thyme

This diffuser blend awakens the senses, stimulates creative thinking, and adds a sense of freshness to the present moment.

Fennel
Foeniculum Vulgare

Application

Main Properties
Carminative
Depurative
Diuretic
Emmenagogue
Stomachic

Chemical Constituents
Trans-anethole, trans-ocimene, fenchone

Other Uses
Blood Sugar Imbalance, Constipation, Digestive Disorders, Edema, Fertility Issues, Fluid Retention, Intestinal Parasites, Menopause, PMS, Spasms, Stroke

Safety
Use with caution if pregnant. Avoid if epileptic.

Top *Uses*

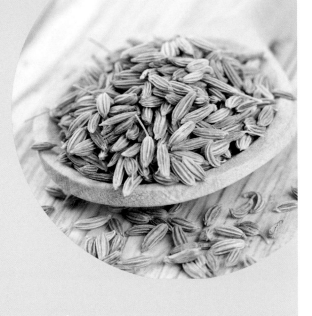

1 **Flatulence**
Rub 1-2 drops over outside of stomach, or drink with water.

2 **Milk Supply (low)**
Massage 1 drop diluted around nipples 2-3 times daily.

3 **Digestive Disorders**
Drink 1-2 drops in water or a capsule.

4 **Nausea**
Rub 1-2 drops over stomach, or drink a drop in water.

5 **Menstrual Discomfort**
Rub a drop over abdomen.

6 **Parasites**
Drink 2-4 drops in a capsule.

7 **Colic**
Rub a drop diluted over stomach.

Emotional Use

Phenylpropenes like Anethole make Fennel an energizer to bring life to sluggish desires and embolden a sense of responsibility.

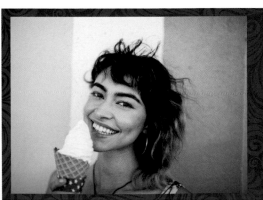

Ease Gut Cramps
3 drops Fennel
1 drop Peppermint
6 drops Rosemary

Add oils to a bowl of hot water, and soak a flannel to make a hot compress. Rest over stomach as needed.

Power Diffuser Blend
3 drops Fennel
3 drops Clary Sage
2 drops Ginger

This blend is invigorates while keeping your mind focused on the task at hand.

Frankincense
Boswellia Frereana

Application

Main Properties
Analgesic
Antidepressant
Antiseptic
Cicatrizing
Cytophylactic

Chemical Constituents
a-phellandrenes, Geranial, Neral, Geraniol, B-elemene, Cis-verbenol

Other Uses
ADHD, Aneurysm, Asthma, Balance, Brain Health, Coma, Concussion, Fibroids, Genital Warts, Immune Support, Lou Gehrig's Disease, Memory, Moles, MRSA, Multiple Sclerosis, Scarring, Sciatica, Warts, Wrinkles

Top Uses

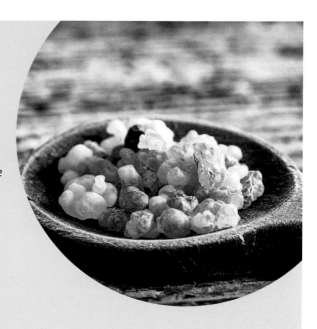

1 Depression & Anxiety
Use a drop under the tongue, apply to pulse points, or diffuse.

2 Alzheimer's & Dementia
Apply 2 drops to bottoms of feet and base of skull twice daily.

3 Cellular Function
Take 1-2 drops in a capsule.

4 Pain & Inflammation
Use a drop under the tongue, or massage into inflamed areas.

5 Parkinson's
Apply 1-2 drops to brain reflex points, and diffuse.

6 Cancer
Take 1-2 drops in a capsule, and apply close to the affected area frequently.

Emotional Use

Monoterpenes like a-Pinene make Frankincense a restoring oil, revealing falseness and restoring awareness of the truth.

Virus Stopper

3 drops Frankincense
5 drops Oregano
5 drops Protective Blend

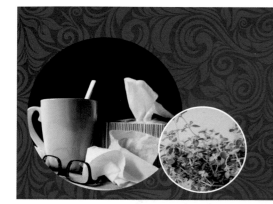

Place all oils in a veggie capsule. Take twice a day to combat viral infections or to boost immune system. Do not take more than 10 days in a row.

Emotion Potion

15 drops Frankincense
15 drops Grounding Blend
15 drops Joyful Blend
FCO

Put ingredients in a 10ml roller bottle and fill the rest with FCO. Apply to pulse points as needed throughout the day.

Geranium
Pelargonium Graveolens

Application

Main Properties
Antidepressant
Carminative
Diaphoretic
Vermifuge
Hypertensive

Chemical Constituents
Citronellol, citronellyl formate, isomenthone, geraniol

Other Uses
Bleeding, Circulation, Depression, Diarrhea, Gastric Ulcers, Hernia, Low Libido, Menstrual Cramps, Menopause, Neuralgia, Raynaud's Disease, Spasms, Vertigo

Safety
Possible skin sensitivity.

Top *Uses*

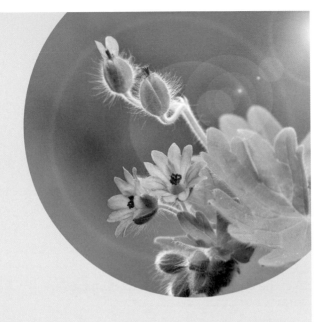

1 Liver & Kidney Support
Rub a drop directly over liver and kidneys.

2 Autism
Apply 1-2 drops to bottoms of feet, or diffuse.

3 Jaundice
Apply 1 drop diluted to bottoms of feet, and diffuse.

4 PMS & Hormone Balance
Apply a drop to pulse points.

5 Hemorrhoids
Apply heavily diluted to affected areas.

6 Reproductive Disorders (female)
Apply 1-2 drops to reproductive reflex points.

7 Varicose Veins
Massage diluted into affected areas.

Emotional Use

Alcohols like Geraniol make Geranium a clarifying oil, reopening the heart to healing, love, and trust.

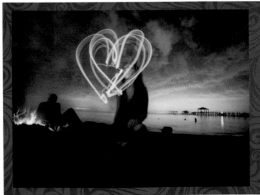

Heart Healing
5 drops Geranium
15 drops Ylang Ylang
12 drops Copaiba
20 drops Cypress
9 drops Litsea
1 oz FCO

Combine in glass spritzer bottle. Apply to chest and heart area, and bottoms of feet.

Fungal Blend
5 drops Geranium
25 drops Melaleuca
15 drops Lavender
5 drops Peppermint
1 oz FCO

Blend all together and apply 2 times a day to the affected areas. This should be dabbed onto lesions with a cotton swab.

Ginger
Zingiber Officinale

Application

Main Properties
Antiseptic
Antispasmodic
Antitussive
Expectorant
Stomachic

Chemical Constituents
α-zingiberene, beta-sesquiphellandrene, zingiberene, camphene, nonanol

Other Uses
Aneurysm, Breast Enlargement, Cholesterol, Convulsions, Endometriosis, Epilepsy, Fragile Hair, Hot Flashes, Impotence, Lactation, Parkinson's, Premenopause, Seizure

Safety
Possible skin sensitivity.

Top *Uses*

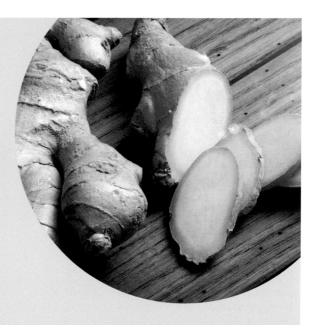

1 Nausea & Stomach Upset
Drink 1-2 drops in a capsule.

2 Vomiting
Rub a drop heavily diluted over stomach.

3 Constipation
Apply 1-2 drops diluted over stomach, or take in a capsule.

4 Immune Support
Apply 1-2 drops to bottoms of feet, or drink in a capsule.

5 Congestion & Cough
Diffuse 3-6 drops.

6 Cold & Flu
Apply 1-2 drops to bottoms of feet, or drink in a capsule.

7 Cooking
Use toothpick to achieve desired taste.

Emotional Use

Sesquiterpenes like Zingiberene make Ginger a calming oil to soothe victim mentality and revitalize a sense of empowerment.

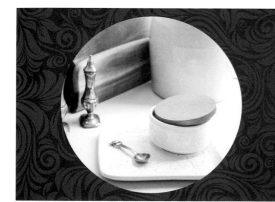

Lactose & Gastritis Aches Blend
10 drops Ginger
4 drops Coriander
10 drops Fennel
4 drops Wild Orange
10 drops Peppermint
FCO

Add oils to a roller bottle and top with FCO. Apply over stomach as needed.

Energizing Sugar Scrub
5 drops Ginger
5 drops Lemongrass
10 drops Lime
1 cup sugar

Combine ingredients in a glass jar. Use in the shower or bath, finishing with an essential oil-infused lotion.

Grapefruit
Citrus X Paradisi

Application

Main Properties
Anti-infectious
Cholagogue
Depurative
Digestive
Tonic

Chemical Constituents
d-Limonene, nonanal, nootketone

Other Uses
Anorexia, Bulimia, Dry Throat, Edema, Energy, Hangovers, Jet Lag, Lymphatic Congestion, Miscarriage Recovery, Obesity, Overeating

Safety
Avoid sun exposure for 12 hours after topical use.

Top Uses

1 Detox
Drink 1-3 drops in water.

2 Weight Loss
Apply 10 drops diluted with carrier oil over cellulite and fatty areas.

3 Smoking Addiction
Drink 1-3 drops in water after meals.

4 Antiviral Support
Apply 1-2 drops to bottoms of feet, or drink in water.

5 Appetite Suppressant
Diffuse several drops, or drink in water.

6 Gallbladder Stones
Drink 1-3 drops in water 3 times daily.

7 Food & Cooking
Use in smoothies, dressings, and sauces.

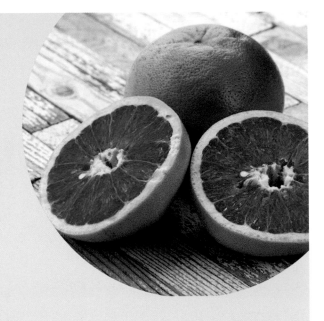

Emotional Use

Monoterpenes like Limonene make Grapefruit an uplifting oil to lift one out of body shame and into honoring the body.

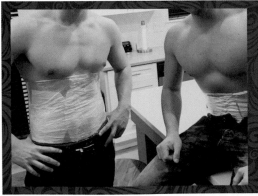

Skinny Wraps
20 drops Grapefruit
20 drops Metabolic Blend
15 drops Cypress
10 drops Lemon
10 drops Detoxification Blend
45 drops FCO

Rub oils over fatty areas and wrap with BPA-free plastic for 1-2 hours.

Spirit-Lifting Spray
15 drops Grapefruit
15 drops Bergamot
10 drops Wild Orange
8 drops Frankincense

Combine oils in a 16 oz. spray bottle with water. Shake before use. Use to brighten a room or as a perfume.

Green Mandarin
Citrus Nobilis

Application

Main Properties
Nervine
Digestive
Sedative
Antiseptic
Immunostimulant

Chemical Constituents
d-limonene, y-terpinene, linalool, myrcene

Other Uses
Antibacterial, Anti-viral, Depression, Numbness, Regenerative, Skin Toner

Safety
Excessive dosing may cause indigestion. Unlike other citrus oil, there is no photo-sensitivity with Green Mandarin.

Top *Uses*

1 Nerve Damage
Apply 2-4 drops to bottoms of feet and along spine.

2 Sensation Loss in Extremities
Massage with carrier oil into affected areas.

3 Pain
Massage 2 drops into affected areas.

4 Simple Antibiotic
Take 2-4 drops in a capsule 3-5x daily as needed.

5 Mood Lift
Diffuse 3-6 drops or inhale from cupped hands as needed.

6 Ageless Skin
Apply 2 drops with carrier oil to fine lines and wrinkles before bed.

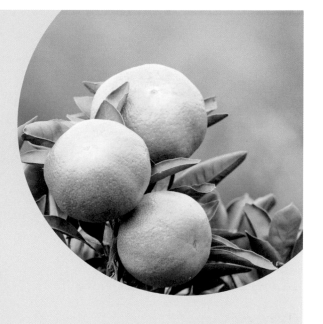

Emotional *Use*

Monoterpenes like y-terpinene make Green Mandarin an uplifting oil. It helps the heart feel light and easy-going.

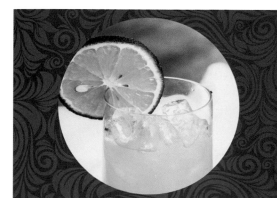

Citrus Pow Water

2 drops Green Mandarin
1 drop Lemon
1 drop Peppermint
Splash of orange juice

Add oils to 44oz of water with a splash of orange juice. Only use stainless steel or glass water bottles (no plastic!).

Skin Tightening Serum

2 drops Green Mandarin
1 drop Melaleuca
1 drop Frankincense
1 drop Hawaiian Sandalwood

Combine oils and massage into face and neck after removing makeup at night.

Helichrysum
Helichrysum Italicum

Application
 A T I

Main Properties
Antibacterial
Anticatarrhal
Anticoagulant
Antispasmodic
Mucolytic

Chemical Constituents
neryl Acetate, alpha pinene, italidione, y-curcumene

Other Uses
AIDS/HIV, Broken Blood Vessels, Bruises, Cuts, Earache, Fibroids, Gallbladder Infection, Hemorrhaging, Hernias, Herpes, Lymphatic Drainage, Nose Bleed, Sciatica, Staph Infection, Stretch Marks, Wrinkles

Top *Uses*

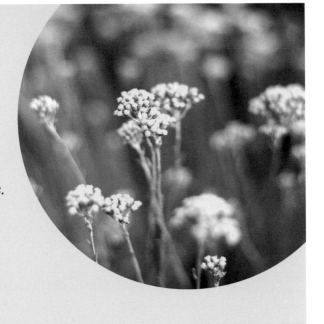

1 Tissue Repair
Apply neat or diluted to wounds.

2 Bleeding
Apply to clean wound to stop bleeding.

3 Eczema & Psoriasis
Apply 1-2 drops diluted to affected areas.

4 Shock
Diffuse 3-6 drops.

5 Tinnitus
Apply a drop behind ear.

6 Viral Infections
Take 1-2 drops in capsule, or diffuse.

7 Cholesterol
Take 1-3 drops in a capsule, and apply to bottoms of feet.

Emotional Use

Esters like Neryl acetate make Helichrysum a restoring oil that ease emotional pain, anguish, and trauma.

Stretch Marks Remover 🌷

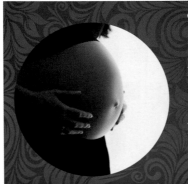

20 drops Helichrysum
20 drops Lavender
FCO

Add oils to a roller bottle and top off with FCO. Apply topically on stretch marks twice daily.

High Blood Pressure Roller 🌷

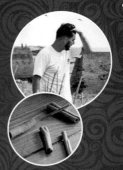

12 drops Helichrysum
12 drops Ylang Ylang
8 drops Cassia
8 drops Frankincense
FCO

Add oils to a roller bottle and top off with FCO. Apply to bottoms of feet, wrists, and over heart twice daily.

Jasmine
Jasminum Grandiflorum

Application

Main Properties
Antidepressant
Antispasmodic
Calmative
Nervine
Sedative

Chemical Constituents
benzyl acetate, benzyl benzoate, phytol, squalene

Other Uses
Apathy, Anxiety, Dry Skin, Insecurity, Labor & Delivery, Low Libido, Menstrual Camps, Nervous Tension, Nervousness, Ovulation, Stress

Top *Uses*

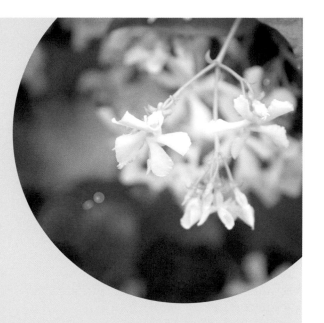

1 **Depression & Self-Esteem Issues**
Inhale 1-2 drops from cupped hands, or apply over heart.

2 **Wrinkles & Fine Lines**
Apply directly to desired areas.

3 **Pink Eye**
Apply carefully around affected eye, avoiding the eye itself.

4 **Infertility**
Apply to pulse points and reproductive reflex points.

5 **Cramps & Spasms**
Apply 1-2 drops to needed areas.

6 **Lethargy & Fatigue**
Inhale from cupped hands, or diffuse.

7 **Sleep & Relaxation**
Apply to bottoms of feet and temples.

Emotional Use

Esters like Benzyl acetate make Jasmine a restoring oil that helps bring back a sense of purity and innocence.

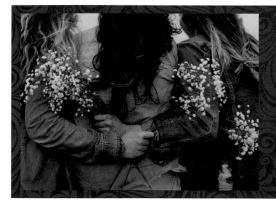

Spring Sunset Perfume

1 drop Jasmine
2 drops Ylang Ylang
2 drops Cedarwood

This floral perfume is soft and bright at the same time. Best of all, it helps keeps hormones in check.

Girly Night Out

6 drops Jasmine
3 drops Patchouli
1 drop Cinnamon
15 ml FCO

Use this blend sparingly on the base of the neck and spine to bring feelings of assertiveness and confidence.

Single Oils

Juniper Berry
Juniperus Communis

Application

Main Properties

Analgesic
Anthelmintic
Antiseptic
Emmenagogue
Nervine

Chemical Constituents

a-pinene, B-caryophyllene, bornyl acetate, sabinene

Other Uses

Acne, Anxiety, Bacteria, Bloating, Cellulite, Cystitis, Detoxifying, Fluid Retention, Heavy Legs, Jaundice, Menstrual Cramps, Mental Exhaustion, Stress, Ulcers, Viruses

Top *Uses*

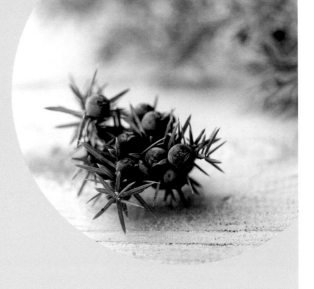

1 Kidney Detox & Infections
Rub 1-2 drops over kidneys, or take in a capsule.

2 Diabetes
Take 1-2 drops in a capsule daily.

3 Kidney Stones
Apply 1-2 drops over kidneys.

4 Urinary Tract Infection
Apply 1-2 drops over bladder.

5 High Cholesterol
Take 1-2 drops in a capsule, or apply to bottoms of feet.

6 Tinnitus
Apply a drop behind affected ear.

7 Chronic Fatigue
Apply 1-2 drops to pulse points, or diffuse.

Emotional Use

Monoterpenes like a-Pinene make Juniper Berry a restoring oil that helps resolve irrational fears and recurring nightmares.

Kidney Support Roll-on

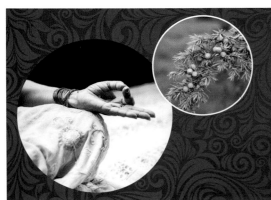

4 drops Juniper Berry
4 drops Geranium
4 drops Lemongrass
4 drops Copaiba
FCO

Mix ingredients in a roller bottle and top with FCO. Apply to kidney area every few hours to support detox and relief.

Mindful Relaxation

4 drops Juniper Berry
3 drops Cedarwood
2 drops Frankincense
3 drops Jasmine
2 Tbsp FCO

Massage onto neck, muscles, and temples. Close your eyes and take several slow, deep breaths to relax.

Kumquat
Fortunella Japonica

Application

Main Properties
Antidepressant
Antioxidant
Cholagogue
Hypotensive
Sedative

Chemical Constituents
Limonene, Myrcene, a-Pinene

Other Uses
Antioxidant, Calming, Detoxification, Mental Stimulation, Revitalization, Shampoo & Conditioner Enhancer, Weight Loss

Top *Uses*

1 **Immune Support**
Drink 1-3 drops in water, or apply to bottoms of feet.

2 **Metabolism Boost**
Drink 1-3 drops in water, or diffuse.

3 **Mood Boost**
Inhale 1-2 drops from cupped hands, or diffuse.

4 **Energy**
Drink 1-3 drops in water, or diffuse.

5 **Household Cleaning**
Use several drops in glass spray bottle with water.

6 **Cardiovascular Health**
Apply 1-2 drops to heart reflex points.

7 **Nervous System Health**
Apply 1-2 drops to bottoms of feet.

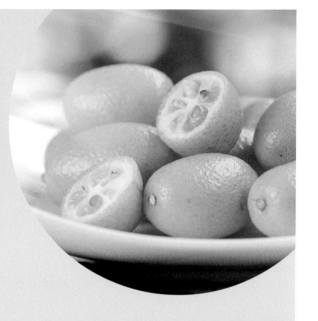

Emotional *Use*

Monoterpenes like Limonene make Kumquat an uplifting oil, perfect for bringing you to a space of authentic presence.

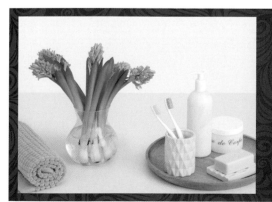

Toothpaste Booster

1 drop Kumquat
Protective Blend enhanced or other fluoride-free toothpaste

Use a drop of Kumquat to enhance the cleansing qualities of your regular toothpaste.

Sunny Forest Diffuser Blend

3 drops Kumquat
2 drop Cedarwood
2 drop Douglas Fir
2 drops Lime

This diffuser blend brings you back to the mountains on a bright, sunny day. Use it to refresh your spirits and to breathe freely.

Lavender
Lavandula Angustifolia

Application
 ^A ^T ^I

Main Properties
Antibacterial
Anti-inflammatory
Anti-venomous
Calmative
Cytophylactic

Chemical Constituents
linalool, linalyl acetate, B-ocimene, ocimene

Other Uses
Allergies, Bee Stings, Bites, Blisters, Chicken Pox, Club Foot, Colic, Convulsions, Crying, Dandruff, Diaper Rash, Gangrene, Giardia, Impetigo, Insomnia, Poison Ivy & Oak, Seizures, Stings, Tachycardia, Teething Pain, Ticks

Top *Uses*

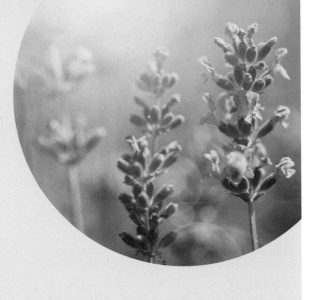

1 Stress & Anxiety
Apply 1-2 drops to temples, or diffuse.

2 Sleep
Apply 2 drops to bottoms of feet and temples, or diffuse near bedside.

3 Skin Irritations & Burns
Apply 1-2 drops with carrier oil.

4 Allergies & Hay Fever
Put a drop under tongue for 30 seconds, then swallow with water.

5 Cuts, Blisters, & Scrapes
Apply diluted to affected areas.

6 Irritability
Apply 1-2 drops to pulse points.

7 Headaches & Migraines
Apply 1-2 drops to temples and base of skull.

Emotional Use

Alcohols like Linalool make Lavender a calming oil. Use it to feel certain and collected through challenging communication.

Soothing Bath Salts

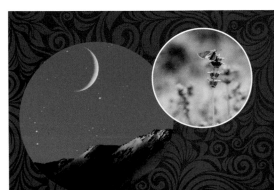

5 drops Lavender
5 drops Melaleuca
1 cup Epsom salt

Combine ingredients in a ceramic bowl. Add to a hot bath and relax!

Rest-Well Diffuser Blend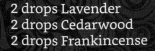

2 drops Lavender
2 drops Cedarwood
2 drops Frankincense

Use this diffuser blend next to your bedside while falling asleep to calm active thoughts.

Lemon
Citrus Limon

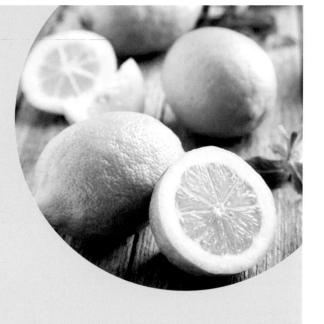

Application

Main Properties
Antimicrobial
Antiseptic
Antiviral
Astringent
Stimulant

Chemical Constituents
d-Limonene, citral, β-pinene, γ-terpinene

Other Uses
Anxiety, Cold Sores, Colds, Concentration, Constipation, Depression, Disinfectant, Dysentery, Flu, Furniture Polish, Greasy Hair, High Blood Pressure, Kidney Stones, MRSA, Pancreatitis, Parasites, Tonsillitis

Safety
Avoid sun exposure for 12 hours after topical use.

Top Uses

1 Energy
Inhale 1-2 drops from cupped hands.

2 Detox
Drink 1-3 drops in water, or apply to bottoms of feet.

3 Permanent Marker
Rub several drops with clean rag.

4 Sore Throat
Take 1-2 drops with a spoonful of honey.

5 Increase Alkalinity
Drink 1-3 drops in water.

6 Household Cleaner
Use several drops with water in glass spray bottle.

7 Food & Cooking
Use in smoothies, juices, and sauces.

Emotional Use

Monoterpenes like Limonene make Lemon an uplifting oil, making it easier to overcome mental fatigue and focus.

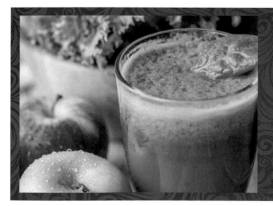

Sunny Green Smoothie
4 drops Lemon
1 cup mixed greens
1/2 cup frozen strawberries
1/2 apple
1 cup almond milk

Blend all ingredients in high speed blender. Add a plant-based protein if desired.

Good Gut Health
1 drop Lemon
2 drops Peppermint
1 drop Protective Blend

Take this blend daily to regulate gut patterns, health, and restore regularity.

Lemon Myrtle
Backhousia Citriodora

Application

Main Properties
Antimicrobial
Antiseptic
Antiviral
Mood lifting
Sedative

Chemical Constituents
Geranial, Neral, Isogeranial, Isoneral,
6-Methyl-5-hepten-2-one

Other Uses
Antiseptic, Antidepressant, Common Cold,
Digestive Issues, Infection, Influenza, Sluggish Digestion

Safety
Avoid during pregnancy. Do not use on broken skin.

Top *Uses*

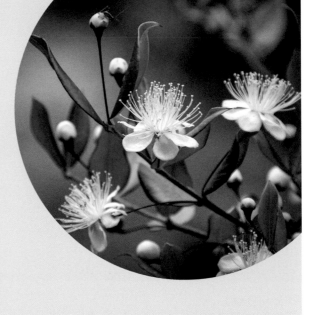

1 Air Purification
Diffuse several drops to help with heavy air pollution.

2 Cold & Flu Prevention
Diffuse several drops during cold & flu season. Apply 2 drops to bottoms of feet.

3 Easy Breathing
Rub 3 drops with carrier oil over chest.

4 Restful Sleep
Diffuse several drops 30 minutes before bedtime. Rub 2 drops on bottoms of feet.

5 Antimicrobial House Cleaning
Add a few drops to a rag while cleaning household surfaces.

6 Air Freshener
Add several drops to a glass spritzer bottle to use in the bathroom or kitchen.

Emotional Use

Aldehydes like Geranial make Lemon Myrtle a restoring oil, useful in bringing a scattered mind back to concentration.

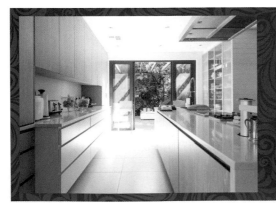

Home Surface Cleaner
5 drops Lemon Myrtle
5 drops Lemon
5 drops Cinnamon
5 drops Lime

Combine oils in a 24 oz glass spray bottle and top with water. Shake before spraying.

Cold & Flu Bomb Diffuser Blend
2 drops Lemon Myrtle
2 drops Cinnamon
2 drops Wild Orange
2 drops Peppermint

Diffuse daily to ward off viruses and airborne pathogens.

Lemongrass
Cymbopogon Flexuosus

Application

Main Properties
Analgesic
Anthelmintic
Antiseptic
Astringent
Tonic

Chemical Constituents
Geranial, neral, Geraniol, a-terpineol

Other Uses
Airborne Bacteria, Bladder Infection, Carpal Tunnel, Charley Horses, Connective Tissue Injury, Constipation, Frozen Shoulder, Lymphatic Drainage, Paralysis, Sprains, Urinary Tract Infection

Safety
Possible skin sensitivity. Do not use internally more than 10 days in a row.

Top *Uses*

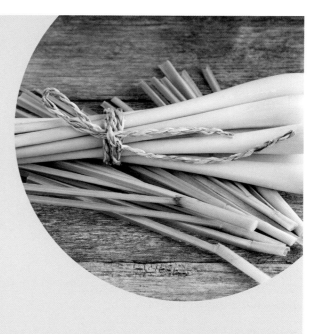

1 Thyroid Support (hypo & hyper)
Apply a drop diluted over thyroid.

2 High Cholesterol
Take 1-2 drops in a capsule.

3 Ligament & Tendon Issues
Apply 1-2 drops diluted to painful areas.

4 Stomach Ulcers
Take 1 drop in a capsule.

5 Immune Support
Apply 1-2 drops to bottoms of feet.

6 Lactose Intolerance
Take 1 drop in a capsule.

7 Cooking
Use toothpick to achieve desired flavor.

Emotional Use
Aldehydes like Geranial make Lemongrass a restoring oil, ideal for cleansing toxic and negative energy.

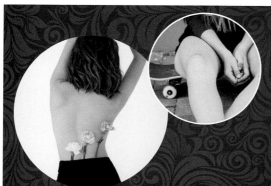

Keloid Scarring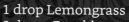
1 drop Lemongrass
1 drop Basil
1 dab protective salve

Combine oils into a dab of protective salve (like a beeswax salve) and rub onto scarring area twice daily.

Pain Killing Bomb
1 drop Lemongrass
2 drops Frankincense
1 drop Marjoram

Take oils in a veggie capsule every 4 hours as needed. Discontinue use after 10 days.

Lime
Citrus Aurantifolia

Application

Main Properties
Anthelmintic
Antimicrobial
Antiviral
Digestive
Restorative

Chemical Constituents
d-Limonene, 1,8 cineol, β-pinene, γ-terpinene, geranial

Other Uses
Antiviral Support, Blood Pressure, Cellulite, Depression, Detox, Energy, Exhaustion, Fever, Gallstones, Gum Removal, Herpes, Memory, Water Purification

Safety
Avoid sun exposure for 12 hours after topical use.

Top *Uses*

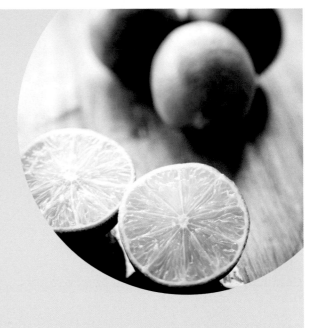

1 Chronic Cough
Apply 2-4 drops over chest, mid-back, and lung reflex points.

2 Colds
Drink 1-3 drops in water, and diffuse.

3 Sore Throat
Gargle 2 drops with water.

4 Cold Sores
Apply 1 drop diluted to affected area.

5 Antioxidant
Drink 1-3 drops in water.

6 Bacterial Infections
Apply 1-2 drops with carrier oil to affected area.

7 Mental Clarity
Diffuse 3-6 drops, or inhale from cupped hands.

Emotional *Use*

Monoterpenes like Limonene make Lime an uplifting oil that dissipates apathy and restores a zest for life.

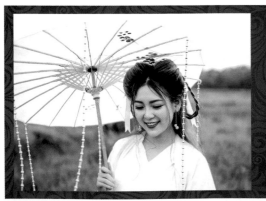

Focus Enhancer
5 drops Lime
5 drops Patchouli
5 drops Frankincense
5 drops Ylang Ylang
5 drops Roman Chamomile
3-5 drops Peppermint

Combine in roller bottle and top with FCO. Apply to back of neck and bottoms of feet.

Don't Worry Diffuser Blend
2 drops Lime
2 drops Peppermint
2 drops Wild Orange
2 drops Frankincense

Use this diffuser blend to go to your happy place.

Litsea
Litsea Cubeba

Application

Main Properties
Antibacterial
Antidepressant
Antiseptic
Antiviral
Hypotensive

Chemical Constituents
Geranial, Neral, Limonene, Methyl heptenone, β-Myrcene

Other Uses
Anxiety, Cold, Cough, Disinfectant, Household Cleaning, Insect Repellent, Odors, Perspiration, Sleep, Stress

Safety
Possible skin sensitivity. Use with caution during pregnancy.

Top *Uses*

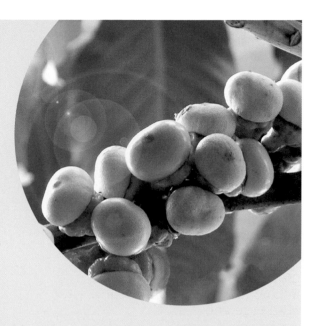

1 **Emotional Balance**
Diffuse several drops, or wear on scarf or sleeve throughout the day.

2 **Mental Rejuvenation**
Inhale 1-2 drops from cupped hands.

3 **Postpartum Depression**
Diffuse, or apply over heart area.

4 **E. Coli**
Apply 1-2 drops diluted to affected areas.

5 **Internal Bacterial Infections**
Drink 2-4 drops in water or in a capsule.

6 **Aging**
Apply 1-2 drops in facial lotion to combat age-promoting free radicals.

7 **Athlete's Foot**
Apply 1-2 drops to clean feet.

Emotional Use

Alcohols like Geranial make Litsea a clarifying oil. Use it to clear self-doubt and fear of rejection, and to expedite manifestations.

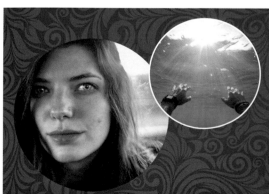

Mermaid Salt Scrub
5 drops Litsea
1 drop Patchouli
1 drop Lavender
1 cup sea salt
1/2 cup coconut oil
Blue food coloring

Mix ingredients in a glass jar and use in the shower.

Zingy Face Scrub
5 drops Litsea
5 drops Lemon
1 Tbsp course sugar
1 Tbsp grape seed oil

Combine all ingredients. Scrub face for 1-2 minutes, then wash. Follow with essential oil-infused skincare products.

Magnolia
Michelia X Alba

Application

Main Properties
Analgesic
Anti-Inflammatory
Calming
Expectorant
Sedative

Chemical Constituents
Linalool, β-caryophyllene, Selinene,
(E)-B-Ocimene

Other Uses
Anger Issues, Bronchitis, Excess Mucus,
Heart Health, Motion Sickness, Nervous
System Support

Top Uses

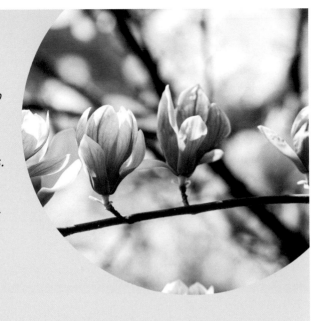

1 Stress & Anxiety
Apply to wrists and temples, taking deep breaths.

2 Menstrual Cramping
Apply over lower abdomen and to wrists.

3 Sore Muscles
Massage onto affected muscles with carrier oil.

4 Depression
Apply over heart in the morning and afternoon.

5 Hives & Rashes
Apply with carrier oil to affected skin.

6 Cough
Apply over chest and mid-back.

7 Chronic Pain
Diffuse 3-6 drops or apply to wrists, spine, and bottoms of feet.

Emotional Use

Alcohols like Linalool make Magnolia a calming oil that enhances the heavenly feeling of genuine connection with others.

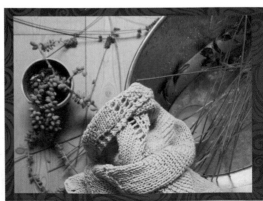

Home Spa Night
4 drops Magnolia
2 drops Lavender
1 tsp pomegranate seed oil

Combine ingredients and stir into hot bath to melt away stress and treat yourself to a little luxury.

Peaceful Surrender Diffuser Blend
3 drops Magnolia
1 drop Tangerine
1 drop Cedarwood
1 drop Geranium

This diffuser blend helps release feelings of upset, grudges, and difficulty forgiving. It helps you surrender to the progression life is calling you to.

Manuka
Leptospermum Scoparium

Application

Main Properties
Cytophylactic
Expectorant
Immunostimulant
Spasmolytic
Vulnerary

Chemical Constituents
eugenol, eugenyl acetate, B-caryophyllene

Other Uses
Athlete's Foot, Bronchitis, Catarrh, Contusions, Cough, Fungal Skin Infections, Head Lice, Influenza, Scabies, Skin Infection, Ulceration

Safety
Possible skin sensitivity. Use with caution when pregnant.

Top *Uses*

1 Blemishes & Complexion
Add a couple drops to skincare products, or apply diluted to affected areas.

2 Hypertension
Apply 1-2 drops to pulse points, or diffuse.

3 Air Purification
Diffuse 4-8 drops.

4 Sleep
Graze pillows with a drop of oil, and diffuse near bedside.

5 Bronchial Infection
Inhale 1-2 drops from cupped hands, or diffuse.

6 Ringworm & Parasites
Apply 1-2 drops diluted to affected areas.

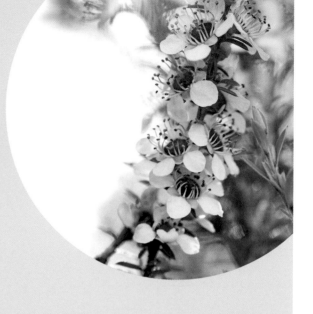

Emotional Use

Phenols like Eugenol make Manuka a restoring oil, providing energetic safety and protection so you never feel abandoned.

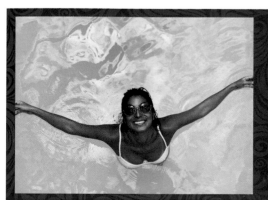

Herbaceous Mouth Wash

3 drops Manuka
3 drops Peppermint
3 drops Melaleuca
1 cup glycerin

Combine ingredients and store in a glass jar or bottle in the bathroom.

Deep Meditation Blend

1 drop Manuka
2 drops Sandalwood
2 drops Jasmine

Use as a perfume or diffuse during meditation to clear the influence of the ego and invite divine support.

Marjoram
Origanum Majorana

Application

(A) (T) (I)

Main Properties
Analgesic
Antibacterial
Antispasmodic
Circulatory
Nervine

Chemical Constituents
a & y-terpinenes, a-terpineol, terpinen-4-ol, trans-sabinene hydrate

Other Uses
Arterial Vasodilator, Bruises, Colic, Constipation, Croup, Headache, Gastrointestinal Disorders, Insomnia, Menstrual Problems, Parkinson's, Prolapsed Mitral Valve, Ringworm, Sprains, Whiplash

Safety
Use with caution during pregnancy.

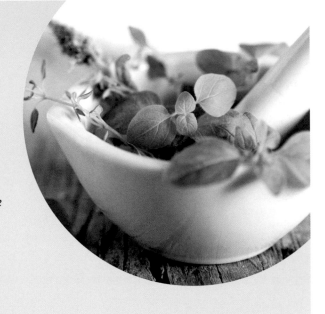

Top *Uses*

1 Muscle Injury
Massage 2 drops with carrier oil into injured muscles.

2 Carpal Tunnel & Arthritis
Apply 1-2 drops neat to affected area.

3 High Blood Pressure
Apply 2 drops to bottoms of feet, or take in a capsule.

4 Irritable Bowel Syndrome
Take 1-2 drops in a capsule, or rub over abdomen.

5 Diverticulitis
Take 1-2 drops in a capsule.

6 Pancreatitis
Apply 1-2 drops neat over pancreas area.

7 Chronic Stress
Rub 1-2 drops onto back of neck.

Emotional Use

Alcohols like Terpinen-4-ol make Marjoram a clarifying oil, bringing closeness and connection where distrust may have been.

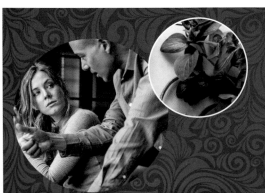

High Blood Pressure Mix
2 drops Marjoram
2 drops Lemon
2 drops Cypress
2 drops Ylang Ylang

Take oils in a veggie capsule twice daily. Also rub a drop of each oil to the bottoms of feet.

Muscle Mend
2 drops Marjoram
1 drop Helichrysum
1 drop Wintergreen

Massage oils into injured muscles 2-3 times daily as needed. Add FCO to use on larger muscle groups.

Single Oils

Melaleuca
Melaleuca Alternifolia

Application

Main Properties
Anthelmintic
Anti-fungal
Antiseptic
Immunostimulant
Vulnerary

Chemical Constituents
a- & y-terpinenes, terpinen-4-ol, a- & o-ca-dinenes

Other Uses
Aneurysm, Bacterial Infections, Cankers, Candida, Cavities, Cold Sores, Cuts, Dermatitis, Ear Infections, Fungal Infections, Hepatitis, Infected Wounds, MRSA, Nail Fungus, Pink Eye, Rubella, Thrush

Safety
Possible skin sensitivity.

Top *Uses*

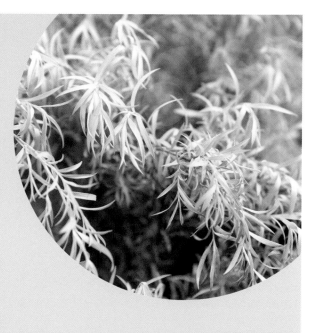

1 Rashes & Eczema
Apply 1-2 drops diluted to affected areas.

2 Dandruff
Add 2 drops to shampoo daily.

3 Athlete's Foot
Apply 1-2 drops neat to clean feet.

4 Acne & Blemishes
Apply a dab to affected areas.

5 Staph Infections
Take 1-2 drops in a capsule.

6 Strep Throat & Tonsillitis
Gargle 2 drops with water, and rub 1-2 drops diluted to outside of throat.

7 Herpes
Apply 1 drop diluted to affected areas.

Emotional Use

Alcohols like Terpen-4-ol make Melaleuca a clarifying oil, powerful for protecting energetic boundaries.

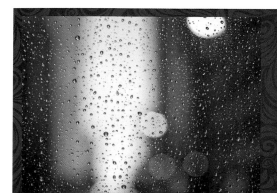

Mold & Mildew Remover

10 drops Melaleuca
10 drops Lemon
2 cups white vinegar

Combine ingredients in a glass spray bottle. Spray and leave for a half hour before scrubbing and rinsing.

Shower Cleaner

20 drops Melaleuca
15 drops Geranium
20 drops Lemon
2 cups white vinegar

Add ingredients to a 16 oz glass spray bottle, filling the remainder with water. Spray shower curtain, walls, and floor liberally to prevent mold and mildew.

Melissa
Melissa Officinalis

Application

A T I

Main Properties
Antibacterial
Antidepressant
Antiviral
Nervine
Soporific

Chemical Constituents
Geranial, Germacrene-D, Neral

Other Uses
Allergies, Anxiety, Blisters, Colds, Dysentery, Erysipelas, Hypertension, Nervousness, Sleep Disorders, Sterility, Viral Outbreak

Safety
Dilute for sensitive skin.

Top *Uses*

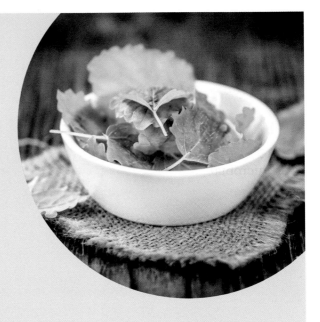

1 Viral Infections
Take 1-2 drops in a capsule.

2 Cold Sores & Herpes
Apply a drop to affected areas.

3 Depression
Use thumb to hold a drop to the roof of the mouth.

4 Bronchitis, Asthma
Apply 1-2 drops diluted over chest.

5 Neurotonic
Apply a drop to the bottoms of feet.

6 Shock
Apply a drop diluted to back of neck, or diffuse.

7 Insomnia
Apply a drop to big toe, or use thumb to hold a drop to the roof of mouth.

Emotional Use

Aldehydes like Neral make Melissa a restoring oil. It sparks enthusiasm and shines light where there was despair or darkness.

Calming Balm

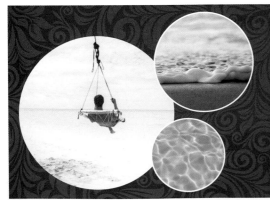

6 drops Melissa
10 drops Geranium
10 drops Lavender
Unscented lotion

Combine oils with lotion according to aroma preference. Massage onto back of neck and lower spine.

Anxiety Relief Diffuser Blend

1 drop Melissa
2 drops Frankincense
2 drops Cedarwood
1 drop Lavender

Use this blend to remedy anxiety - especially anxiety accompanied by despair or fear of moving forward.

Myrrh
Commiphora Myrrha

Application
 A T

Main Properties
Antimicrobial
Antiseptic
Astringent
Cicatrizing
Expectorant

Chemical Constituents
Lindestrene, Methoxyfurogermacrene, Curzenone

Other Uses
Cancer, Chapped Skin, Congestion, Dysentery, Gum Bleeding, Hepatitis, Liver Cirrhosis, Scabies, Stretch Marks

Safety
Use with caution during pregnancy.

Top *Uses*

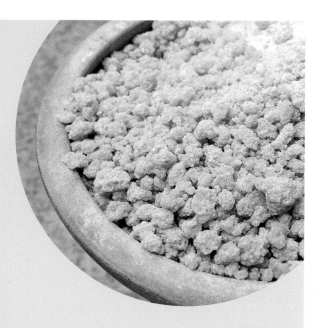

1 Wrinkles & Fine Lines
Massage into needed areas as desired.

2 Gum Disease & Issues
Apply 1-2 drops to gums, or swish with water as mouth rinse.

3 Thyroid Support
Rub 1-2 drops over thyroid.

4 Anxiety & Depression
Inhale 1-2 drops from cupped hands, or diffuse.

5 Mucus & Bronchitis
Apply 1-2 drops to chest, or diffuse.

6 Eczema & Skin Infections
Apply 1-2 drops to affected areas.

7 Nail Fungus
Apply a drop to affected nails.

Emotional Use

Esters like Curzerene make Myrrh a soothing oil, giving it a maternal nurturing quality. It facilitates trust and safety.

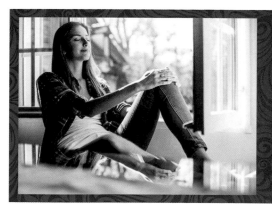

Herbal Mouthwash
5 drops Myrrh
10 drops Peppermint
5 drops Spearmint
5 drops Cinnamon
5 drops Clove
10 oz water
2 Tbsp glycerin

Combine ingredients and store in a glass jar.

Mother's Love Diffuser Blend
2 drops Myrrh
4 drops Wild Orange
1 drop Frankincense
2 drops Lavender

This diffuser blend brings a sense of comfort and safety. Use it when you need the emotional support of a caring world.

Neroli
Citrus Aurantium

Application

 A T I

Main Properties
Antidepressant
Calmative
Circulatory
Cytophylactic
Regenerative

Chemical Constituents
Linalool
Geraniol
Limonene

Other Uses
Convalescence, Indigestion, Insomnia, Intestinal Cramping, Menopausal Anxiety, Sleep Disorders, Tension

Top *Uses*

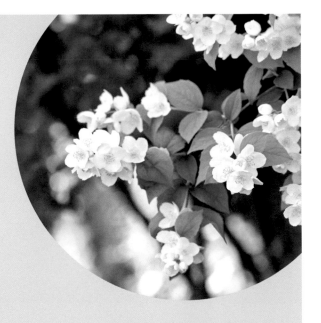

1 Scar Tissue & Stretch Marks
Massage a few drops with carrier oil into needed areas.

2 Perfume
Apply 1-2 drops to pulse points.

3 Cramps & Spasms
Apply neat to affected areas.

4 Emotional Exhaustion
Inhale from cupped hands, or diffuse.

5 Nervousness
Apply a drop to pulse points.

6 Depression
Wear as perfume, inhale from cupped hands, or diffuse.

7 Skin Regeneration
Apply generously to damaged or worn skin.

Emotional Use

Alcohols like Linalool make Neroli a calming oil that brings intimacy, trust, and partnership to relationships.

Scar Smoothing

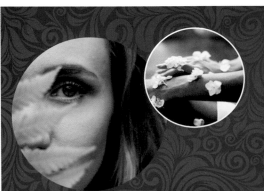

1 drop Neroli
1 drop Lavender
1 drop Basil
2 drops Ylang Ylang

Massage oils into scar tissue 2-3 times daily until scar begins to face.

Peaceful Dreams Diffuser Blend

3 drops Neroli
4 drops Lavender
2 drops Patchouli
1 drop Ylang Ylang

Use this diffuser blend during sleep to enhance the mood and quality of your dreams.

Oregano
Origanum Vulgare

Application

Main Properties
Antibacterial
Anti-fungal
Antiseptic
Antiviral
Rubefacient

Chemical Constituents
carvacrol, B-caryophyllene, rosmaric acid

Other Uses
Athlete's Foot, Calluses, Canker Sores, Carpal Tunnel, Control Issues, Ebola, Fungal Infections, Intestinal Parasites, MRSA, Nasal Polyps, Plague, Ringworm

Safety
Heavily dilute for topical use. Do not use internally for more than 10 days in a row.

Top *Uses*

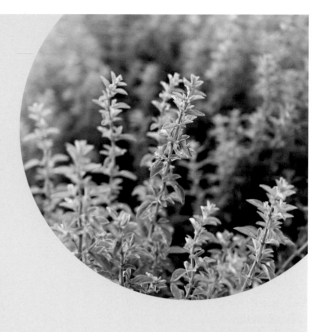

1 Bacterial & Viral Infection
Take 1-3 drops in a capsule for internal issues.

2 Warts
Apply directly to wart with toothpick, avoiding surrounding skin.

3 Candida & Staph Infection
Take 1-3 drops in a capsule.

4 Pneumonia & Whooping Cough
Diffuse 1-3 drops, sitting nearby the diffuser for several minutes. Also rub onto bottoms of feet.

5 Rheumatoid Arthritis
Massage 1 drop heavily diluted into affected area. Also take in a capsule.

6 Strep Throat & Tonsillitis
Gargle a drop in water. Also take 1-3 drops in a capsule.

Emotional Use

Phenols like Carvacrol make Oregano a restoring oil. It brings with it the power of humility and being unattached.

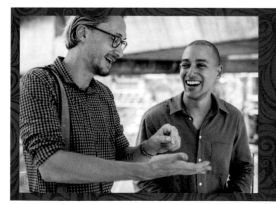

Warts Be Gone

18 drops Oregano
18 drops Clove
13 drops Melaleuca
5 drops Frankincense

Mix oils in an empty oil bottle. Apply to wart with a toothpick 3-5 times a day, avoiding surrounding skin.

Soothing Joints

10 drops Oregano
10 drops Cypress
10 drops Lemongrass
FCO

Combine oils in a 10ml roller bottle, filling the rest with FCO. Roll onto painful joints as needed.

Patchouli
Pogostemon Cablin

Application

Main Properties
Antiseptic
Astringent
Cicatrizing
Cytophylactic
Nervine

Chemical Constituents
a-bulesene, Patchoulol, Pathoulenone

Other Uses
Abscess, Cellulite, Chapped Skin, Depression, Dermatitis, Hemorrhoids, Hives, Irritability, Mastitis, Parasitic Skin Infection, PMS, Weeping Wounds

Top *Uses*

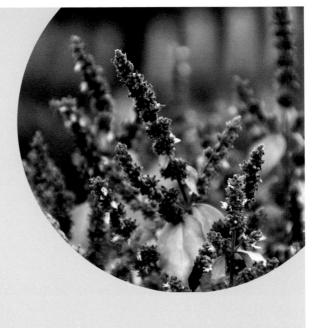

1 Diuretic
Apply 1-2 drops over lower abdomen.

2 Wrinkle Prevention
Add a drop to toner or moisturizer.

3 Shingles
Take 1-2 drops in a capsule, or apply to bottoms of feet.

4 Dopamine Shortage
Diffuse 2-4 drops, or apply to pulse points.

5 Dandruff
Massage 1-2 drops into clean, dry scalp after showering.

6 Weight Loss
Take 1-2 drops with other weight loss essential oils in a capsule.

Emotional Use

Alcohols like Patchoulol make Patchouli a stabilizing oil, which helps with feelings of grounding and body confidence.

Athlete's Foot Soak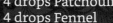

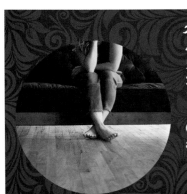

4 drops Patchouli
5 drops Melaleuca
2 drop Myrrh
1 cup Epsom salts

Combine oils with salts, and then add to hot foot bath. Soak feet for 15 minutes.

Appetite Suppressant Tummy Rub

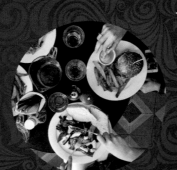

4 drops Patchouli
4 drops Fennel
5 drops Grapefruit
2 oz FCO

Combine ingredients in a glass jar. Rub a small amount over stomach to ease cravings.

Peppermint
Menta Piperita

Application

Main Properties
Analgesic
Anti-inflammatory
Carminative
Stomachic
Tonic

Chemical Constituents
Menthol, a & B-pinenes, germacrene-D

Other Uses
Alertness, Allergies, Autism, Burns, Cravings, Gastritis, Hangover, Hot Flashes, Hypothyroidism, Loss of Sense of Smell, Memory, Milk Supply (Decrease), Osteoporosis, Sciatica, Sinusitis, Typhoid

Safety
Possible skin sensitivity.

Top *Uses*

1 Headache & Migraine
Massage 1-2 drops into temples and base of skull, avoiding the eyes.

2 Digestive Upset
Drink 1-2 drops in water, or massage directly over stomach.

3 Asthma & Cough
Apply 2 drops with carrier oil over chest and lung reflex points, or diffuse.

4 Bad Breath
Lick a dab from your finger.

5 Low Energy & Mental Fog
Drink 1-2 drops in water, or diffuse.

6 Muscle & Joint Pain
Rub a drop diluted into affected areas.

7 Fevers
Apply 1-2 drops to back of neck.

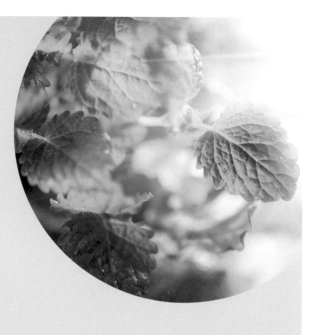

Emotional Use

Alcohols like Menthol make Peppermint an energizing oil. It brings new life to the heart, and reminds you that life can be happy.

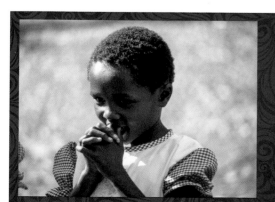

Tender Tummy Roller
4 drops Peppermint
4 drops Copaiba
4 drops Rose
FCO

Combine oils in a 10ml roller bottle. Fill the rest with FCO. Roll over tummy as needed.

Allergy Diffuser Blend
2 drops Peppermint
2 drops Lavender
2 drops Lemon

Diffuse during allergy season to purify the air, reduce histamine response, and support easy breathing.

Single Oils

Petitgrain
Citrus Aurantium

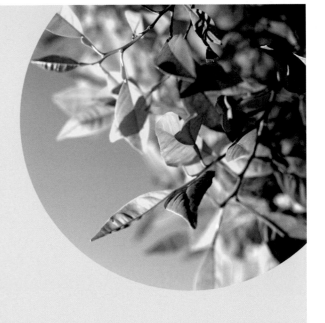

Application

 A   T   I

Main Properties
Antidepressant
Antispasmodic
Cicatrizing
Nervine
Relaxant

Chemical Constituents
linalyl acetate, linalool, alpha-terpineol

Other Uses
Abdominal Cramps/Spasms, Aches, Acne, Convalescence, Depression, Hysteria, Infected Wounds, Nausea, Nervous Asthma, Oily Hair, Shock, Stress-Related Conditions, Tension

Safety
Use with caution during pregnancy.

Top *Uses*

1 Nervous & Muscular Spasms
Apply 1-2 drops to bottoms of feet, or to area of spasm.

2 Seizures
Apply 1-2 drops to bottoms of feet and back of neck.

3 Insomnia
Use a drop under tongue, or on pulse points. Also diffuse.

4 Irritability & Stress
Apply a drop behind ears, or wear as cologne on pulse points.

5 Bacterial Infections
Apply topically to affected area, or take 1-3 drops in a capsule.

6 Spastic Coughing
Apply 1-2 drops with carrier oil over chest and mid-back, or diffuse.

Emotional Use

Esters like Linalyl acetate make Petitgrain a calming oil, providing a space to form new and healthy traditions.

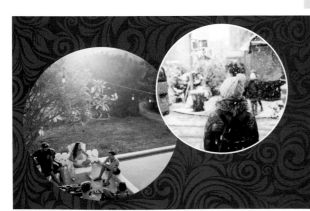

Citrus Blossom Diffuser Blend

3 drops Petitgrain
3 drops Wild Orange
2 drops Bergamot
2 Lime
2 Lavender

This blend is the perfect balance between fresh and calming, right between feminine and masculine.

Winter Blues Diffuser Blend

4 drops Petitgrain
2 Juniper Berry
2 drops Wild Orange

Rejuvenate your spirits during long winter days with this diffuser blend.

Single Oils

Pink Pepper

Schinus Molle

Application

Main Properties

Digestive
Circulatory
Anti-tumoral
Antispasmodic
Antimicrobial

Chemical Constituents

B-Myrcene, a-Phellandrene, p-Cymene, d-Cadinene, Limonene, B-Phellandrene

Other Uses

Arthritis, Bee Stings, Cancer, Chest Pain, Colds, Emotional Upset, Flu, Seizures

Top Uses

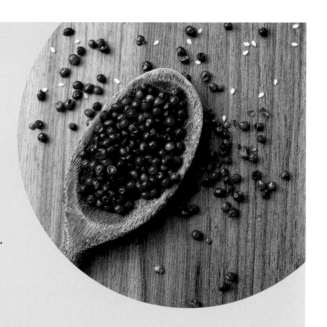

1 Cancer Prevention
Take 2-4 drops in a veggie capsule or massage with carrier oil 2x daily.

2 Muscle Spasms
Massage 2-3 drops with carrier oil into affected areas.

3 Circulatory Disorders
Massage 2 drops with carrier oil into legs.

4 Pain Relief
Take 2 drops in a capsule as needed.

5 Convulsions
Use 2-4 drops on the bottoms of feet, or take 5 drops in a capsule.

6 High Blood Pressure
Apply 3 drops with a carrier oil to chest.

7 Cough Suppressant
Apply 5 drops with carrier oil to chest and upper back.

Emotional Use

Monoterpenes like Myrcene make Pink Pepper an uplifting oil that stimulates capacity to continue giving generously of one's self.

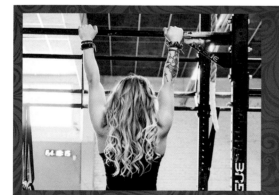

Post-Workout Massage

2 drops Pink Pepper
2 drops Roman Chamomile
2 drops Ginger
2 drops Marjoram
15 drops FCO

Combine oils with FCO and massage into muscles and joints after working out.

Pink Spice Salad Dressing

2 drops Pink Pepper
2 drops Basil
2 drops Lemon Oil
1 cup olive oil
Freshly ground black pepper

Combine ingredients in salad dressing shaker, adding ground black pepper to taste.

Single Oils

Red Mandarin
Citrus Reticulata

Application

Main Properties
Antiseptic
Antispasmodic
Digestive
Stomachic
Tonic

Chemical Constituents
Limonene, Gamma-Terpinene

Other Uses
Household Cleaning, Intestinal Spasm, Irritability, Nervous Spasm, Sleeping Disorders, Stomachache, Stress

Safety
Avoid sun exposure for 12 hours after topical use.

Top *Uses*

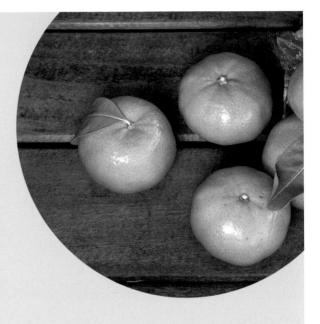

1 Skin Cleansing
Add a drop to facial cleanser.

2 Uplift & Energize
Inhale 1-2 drops from cupped hands, drink in water, or diffuse.

3 Digestive Conditions & IBS
Drink 1-3 drops in water.

4 Cellulite
Massage several drops with carrier oil over cellulite.

5 Antioxidant
Drink 1-3 drops in water, or apply over lymph nodes.

6 Constipation
Rub 2-4 drops clockwise over abdomen.

7 Convalescence
Diffuse and wear on pulse points.

Emotional Use

Monoterpenes like Limonene make Red Mandarin an uplifting oil to bring playfulness and child-like perspective back to life.

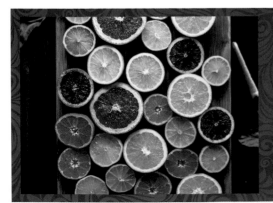

Detox Water
2 drops Red Mandarin
1 drop Lemon
1 drop Lime
1 drop Grapefruit

Add oils to a 20oz glass or stainless steel water bottle and drink throughout the day.

Ignite Diffuser Blend
4 drops Red Mandarin
2 drops Inspiring Blend
2 drops Douglas Fir

This diffuser blend ignites passion and excitement. Use at the beginning of a creative project.

Roman Chamomile
Anthemis Nobilis

Application

Main Properties
Analgesic
Anti-neuralgic
Antispasmodic
Immunostimulant
Sedative

Chemical Constituents
Isobutyl, a- & B-pinene, Pinocarvone

Other Uses
Allergies, Anorexia, Bee/Hornet Stings, Club Foot, Dysentery, Hyperactivity, Menopause, Muscle Spasms, Neuralgia, Rashes, Shock, Sore Nipples

Top Uses

1 Sleep & Insomnia
Apply 1-2 drops to temples and wrists, or diffuse next to bedside.

2 Panic Attacks
Carry on person and breathe a drop deeply from cupped hands as needed.

3 Diaper Rash
Apply 1 drop heavily diluted with carrier oil to baby skin.

4 Crying
Add a drop to front of shirt or sleeve, or diffuse.

5 PMS & Cramps
Apply a drop over abdomen.

6 Parasites & Worms
Apply 1-2 drops over abdomen, and take in a capsule.

Emotional Use

Esters like Methyl-amylangelate make Roman Chamomile a calming oil that beautifully reminds one of spiritual purpose and the greater good.

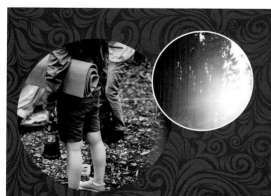

Itchy Bite Remedy

8 drops Roman Chamomile
8 drops Lavender
4 drops Eucalyptus
2 drop Melaleuca
45 drops FCO

Add ingredients to a 10ml roller bottle. Use on itchy bug bites as needed.

Tummy Trouble Capsule

1 drop Roman Chamomile
1 drop Peppermint
1 drop Thyme

Place oils in a veggie cap for a severe stomach upset. Take every 5 hours, not exceeding 5 capsules in a 24-hour period.

Rose
Rosa Damascena

Application

Main Properties
Antidepressant
Astringent
Cytophylactic
Hypnotic
Nervine

Chemical Constituents
Citronellol, Stearoptene, Nonadecane

Other Uses
Anxiety, Astringent, Dysmenorrhea, Endometriosis, Grief, Facial Redness, Impotency, Infertility, Irregular Ovulation, Menstrual Cramping, Phobias

Safety
Use with caution during pregnancy.

Top *Uses*

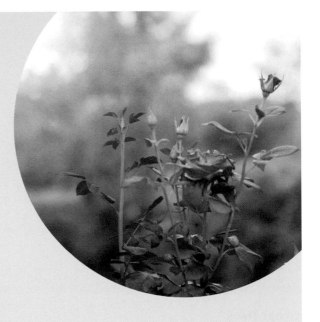

1 Aging Skin
Add a drop to toner or moisturizer, or apply with carrier oil over fine lines, wrinkles, and age spots.

2 Low Libido
Apply 1-2 drops to pulse points, or to reproductive reflex points.

3 Scar Tissue
Massage into scar tissue 3 times daily.

4 Self-Esteem & Depression
Apply 1-2 drops over heart, or diffuse.

5 Aphrodisiac
Diffuse a few drops, or wear on pulse points.

6 Poison Ivy/Oak
Apply 1-2 drops diluted to irritated areas.

Emotional *Use*

Alcohols like Citronellol make Rose a clarifying oil that help connect the mind and soul to divine love and grace.

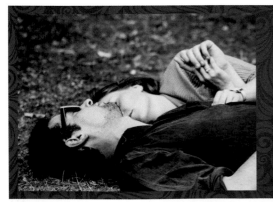

Feel the Romance Salve

5 drops Rose
3 drops Ylang Ylang
2 drops Bergamot
1 drop Sandalwood
Unscented salve (like beeswax salve)

Combine oils with salve and use in sensual massage.

Bloom Diffuser Blend

3 drops Rose
3 drops Wild Orange
3 drops Lavender

This diffuser blend has a graceful aroma that brings a soothing and refreshing air to any day.

Rosemary
Rosmarinus Officinalis

Application

Main Properties
Antimicrobial
Decongestant
Depurative
Restorative
Stimulant

Chemical Constituents
1, 8-cineole, a-pinene, camphor

Other Uses
Alcohol Addiction, Adenitis, Arthritis, Bell's Palsy, Cellulite, Club Foot, Constipation, Headaches, Kidney Infection, Lice, Muscular Dystrophy, Osteoarthritis, Schmidt's Syndrome, Sinusitis

Safety
Avoid during pregnancy, if epileptic, or with high blood pressure.

Top *Uses*

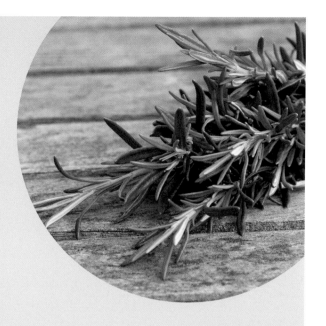

1 Chronic Cough
Apply 2-4 drops to lung reflex points or diluted over chest, or diffuse.

2 Mental & Adrenal Fatigue
Inhale 1-2 drops from cupped hands, or take in a capsule.

3 Focus & Memory Issues
Apply a drop over forehead, or diffuse.

4 Cold & Flu
Apply 1-2 drops diluted over chest.

5 Low Blood Pressure
Massage with carrier oil into legs and on bottoms of feet.

6 Jet Lag
Apply 1-2 drops to temples after flying.

7 Hair Loss.
Work 2 drops into scalp before washing.

Emotional Use
Ethers like 1,8-Cineole make Rosemary a restoring oil that can fortify knowledge and assist in transitioning to new phases of life.

Cellulite & Water Retention Reduction
16 drops Rosemary
20 drops Grapefruit
21 drops Cypress
4 drops Oregano
8 drops Black Pepper
12 drops Geranium
4 oz FCO

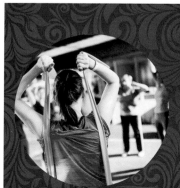

Lather onto tummy, thighs, buns, etc.

Bright-Eyed Diffuser Blend
5 drops Rosemary
4 drops Lemon
2 drops Peppermint
2 drops Wild Orange
1 drop Eucalyptus

This diffuser blend helps with critical thinking and being open to the future.

Sandalwood
Santalum Album

Application

Main Properties
Antidepressant
Antispasmodic
Calmative
Cicatrizing
Tonic

Chemical Constituents
α & ß-santalols, α & ß-santalenes, norticy-cloekasantalic acid, cis-lanceol

Other Uses
Aphrodisiac, Back Pain, Blemishes, Calming, Cartilage Repair, Coma, Dry Skin/Scalp, Exhaustion, Hiccups, Laryngitis, Lou Gehrig's Disease, Moles, Multiple Sclerosis, UV Radiation, Yoga

Top *Uses*

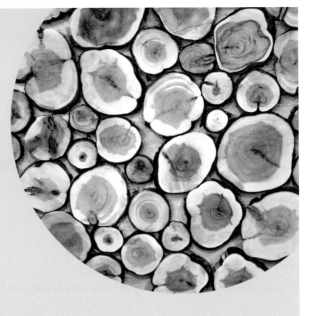

1 Rashes & Skin Conditions
Apply 1-2 drops with carrier oil to affected areas.

2 Cancer & Tumors
Take 1-2 drops in a capsule, apply diluted to affected area, or diffuse.

3 Meditation
Apply a drop to temples during meditation.

4 Low Testosterone
Take 1-2 drops in a capsule, or apply to pulse points and lower abdomen.

5 Scars
Massage 1-2 drops into scars often.

6 Alzheimer's Disease
Apply 1-2 drops to base of skull, or take 1-2 drops in a capsule daily.

Emotional Use

Alcohols like Santalol make Sandalwood a stabilizing oil that grounds one to a higher consciousness and sense of spirituality.

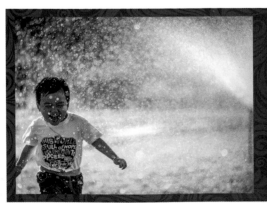

Uplift-Me Spray
12 drops Sandalwood
8 drops Jasmine
8 drops Ylang Ylang
1 tbsp alcohol
4 oz distilled water

Mix oils and alcohol together. Pour into 4 oz spray bottle. Top off with distilled water.

Iron Out Wrinkles
2 drops Sandalwood
3 drops Frankincense
3 Myrrh
2 Tbsp carrier oil

Mix ingredients and massage into face at nighttime to reduce fine lines and wrinkles and even skin tone.

Siberian Fir

Abies Sibirica

Application

Main Properties

Analgesic
Antiseptic
Antitussive
Expectorant
Tonic

Chemical Constituents

Bornyl Acetate, Terpinyl Acetate, δ-3-Carene, α-Pinene, Camphene

Other Uses

Anxiety, Bronchitis, Catarrh, Fever, Sinusitis, Sluggish Nerves, Tension, Urinary Infection

Safety

Use with caution during pregnancy. Possible skin sensitivity.

Top Uses

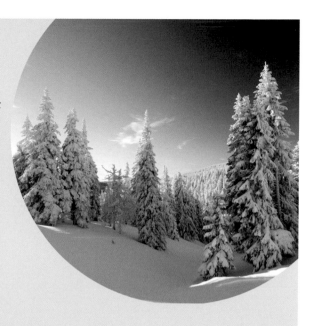

1 Asthma
Apply 1-2 drops with carrier oil over chest or to lung reflex points.

2 Immune Stimulant
Apply 1-2 drops to bottoms of feet.

3 Dry Cough, Cold, & Flu
Inhale 1-2 drops from cupped hands, or apply with carrier oil over chest.

4 Muscle Cramps & Spasms
Massage several drops with carrier oil into affected areas.

5 Emotional Overwhelm
Inhale 1-2 drops from cupped hands.

6 Rheumatism
Apply 1-2 drops neat to affected areas.

7 Mucus
Apply 1-2 drops to throat and chest.

Emotional Use

Esters like Bornyl Acetate make Siberian Fir a restoring oil that illuminates the wisdom and purpose of progressing through life.

Knee Easy Rub

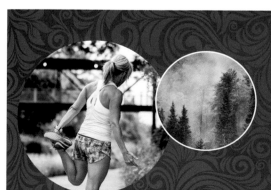

2 drops Siberian Fir
2 drops Copaiba
6 drops FCO

Massage oils with FCO into knees, focusing on connective tissue and muscles around the knee. Repeat as needed.

Seasonal Twist Diffuser Blend

3 drops Siberian Fir
4 drops Protective Blend
2 drops Spearmint

Put an earthy-minty twist on the autumn-like aroma of Protective Blend with this diffuser blend.

Spearmint
Mentha Spicata

Application

 A   T  I

Main Properties
Antiseptic
Decongestant
Digestive
Nervine
Spasmolytic

Chemical Constituents
l-carvone, l-limonene, Carveol, 1, 8-cineole, β-myrcene

Other Uses
Acne, Bronchitis, Headaches, Focus, Migraines, Nervous Fatigue, Respiratory Infection, Sores, Scars

Top *Uses*

1 Indigestion
Drink 1-2 drops in water or in a capsule.

2 Colic
Apply a drop heavily diluted to baby's stomach.

3 Nausea
Inhale 1-2 drops from cupped hands, or rub over stomach.

4 Muscle Aches
Massage 1-2 drops diluted over achy muscles.

5 Bad Breath
Swish 1-2 drops in water as a mouthwash.

6 Heavy Menstruation
Apply 1-2 drops over back of neck and abdomen, or diffuse.

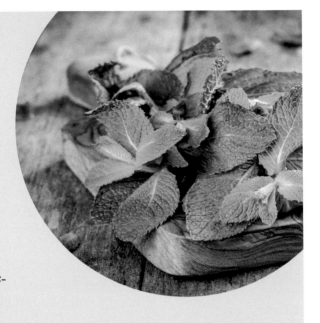

Emotional Use

Ketones like Carvone make Spearmint an energizing oil. Use it to feel energized when public speaking and voicing opinions.

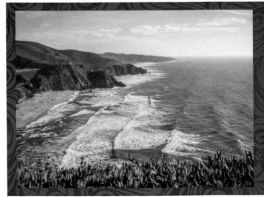

Sea Breeze Diffuser Blend

1 drop Spearmint
3 drops Lavender
3 drops Lime

Return to the seaside with this cool and easy going diffuser blend.

Mint Blast Tongue Scrub

1 drop Spearmint
1 drop Peppermint
1 tsp baking soda

Mix ingredients together. Wet toothbrush and tap into powder. Use to brush tongue (your tongue is where the bad breath is!)

Spikenard
Nardostachys Jatamansi

Application
 A T I

Main Properties
Analgesic
Anti-inflammatory
Nervine
Regenerative
Soporific

Chemical Constituents
Jatamansone, Nardol, a-Selinene

Other Uses
Constipation, Depression, Estrogen Imbalance, Fungal Issues, Mental Fatigue, Pinkeye, PMS Cramping, Progesterone Imbalance, Uterus & Ovaries Detox

Safety
Use with caution during pregnancy.

Top *Uses*

1 **Chronic Fatigue Syndrome**
Apply 1-2 drops to adrenals and pulse points, or take in a capsule.

2 **Insomnia**
Put a drop under the tongue, or take in a capsule.

3 **Toenail Fungus**
Apply neat to affected toenail often.

4 **Digestive Inflammation**
Take 1-2 drops in a capsule.

5 **Pancreatitis**
Apply 1-2 drops neat over pancreas.

6 **Immune Stimulant**
Apply 1-2 drops to bottoms of feet.

7 **Hair Loss**
Add 2 drops to shampoo, and take 1-2 drops in a capsule.

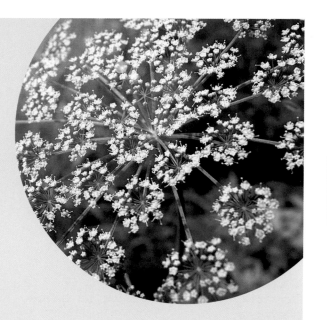

Emotional Use

Ketones like Jatamansone make Spikenard a stabilizing oil that creates a safe space to indulge in deep, luxurious gratitude.

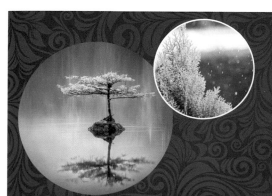

Forest Rain Diffuser Blend
2 drops Spikenard
3 drops Wild Orange
2 drops Juniper Berry

Wake up your senses with this fresh, clean diffuser blend.

Woodland Spice Diffuser Blend
2 drops Spikenard
3 drops Frankincense
4 drops Lavender

This diffuser blend grounds your energy and focus. It's perfect for gratitude journaling.

Star Anise
Illicium Verum

Application

Main Properties
Digestive
Anti-rheumatic
Vermifuge
Sedative
Decongestant

Chemical Constituents
(E)-anethol, Foeniculin, Methyl chavicol, Limonene, Linalool, Nerolidol, Cinnamyl acetate

Other Uses
Arthritis, Cold, Congestion, Cough, Flu, Indigestion, Intestinal Cramps

Safety
Contraindicated in pregnancy and breast-feeding.

Top *Uses*

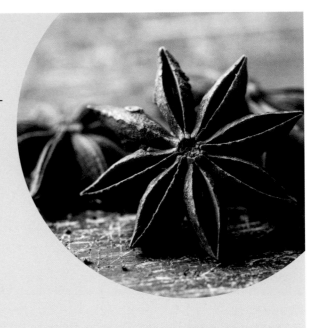

1 Digestive Stimulant
Apply 2 drops to abdomen after an excessive meal.

2 Joint Pain
Apply 2-4 drops to aching joints for pain relief.

3 Intestinal Cramps
Apply 2 drops to abdomen to relieve cramps.

4 Diarrhea
Take 2 drops in a capsule every 30-60 minutes.

5 Gas & Bloating
Massage 4 drops over stomach with carrier oil.

6 Cold (Common)
Apply 2 drops to chest at the earliest signs of cold or flu development.

Emotional Use

Esters like Cinnamyl Acetate make Star Anise a restoring oil. Use it to improve confidence in intimacy and vulnerable connection.

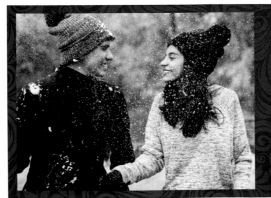

Suave Date Breath Freshener
1 drop Star Anise
1 drop Peppermint
1 drop Lemon Myrtle

Combine oils with 10 drops of FCO and swish for 30 seconds before date night.

Knockout Digestive Roller
3 drops Star Anise
3 drops Coriander
3 drops Ginger
3 drops Basil
3 drops Peppermint
FCO

Combine oils in a 10ml roller bottle and top off with FCO. Use over stomach after meals.

Tangerine
Citrus Reticulata

Application

Main Properties
Antiseptic
Cytophylactic
Depurative
Digestive
Tonic

Chemical Constituents
d-limonene, B-carotene, Linalool

Other Uses
Anxious Feelings, Chronic Fatigue, Circulation, Detox, Digestive Problems, Muscle Aches, Muscle Spasms, Parasites, Water Retention

Safety
Avoid sun exposure for 12 hours after topical use.

Top *Uses*

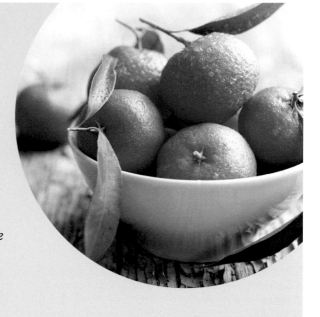

1 Stress-Induced Insomnia
Inhale 1-2 drops during stressful times of the day. Use a drop under the tongue before bedtime.

2 Cellulite
Massage several drops with carrier oil into cellulite areas.

3 Nervous Exhaustion
Diffuse 4-8 drops, or wear a drop on pulse points.

4 Congestion
Rub 2-4 drops over chest and mid-back.

5 Discouragement
Inhale 1-2 drops from cupped hands. Also add 1-3 drops to water.

6 Flatulence & Constipation
Rub 1-2 drops clockwise over stomach, or drink with water.

Emotional *Use*

Monoterpenes like Limonene make Tangerine an uplifting oil. Use it to bring more cheer and creativity to your day.

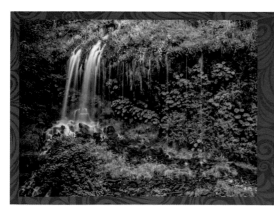

Tropical Shower
2 drops Tangerine
2 drops Eucalyptus

Drop essential oils onto the wall of your hot shower to make an ordinary shower luxurious and invigorating.

Summer Sweet Diffuser Blend
4 drops Tangerine
1 drop Spearmint
1 drop Lime
2 drops Lavender

This diffuser blend brings back the inspiring feel of a cool summer sunset.

Thyme
Thymus Vulgaris

Application

Main Properties
Anthelmintic
Antimicrobial
Antiputrescent
Immunostimulant
Vermifuge

Chemical Constituents
Thymol, p-cymene, Linalool, Paracymene

Other Uses
Antioxidant, Asthma, Bites/Stings, Blood Clots, Croup, Eczema/Dermatitis, Fragile Hair, Fungal Infections, Greasy Hair, Hair Loss, Laryngitis, Mold, Numbness, Parasites, Prostatitis, Tendinitis, Tuberculosis

Safety
Possible skin sensitivity. Use with caution during pregnancy or with high blood pressure.

Top *Uses*

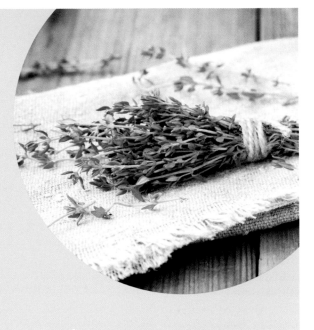

1 Bacterial Infection
Take 1-2 drops in a capsule, or apply to bottoms of feet.

2 Mononucleosis
Take 2 drops in a capsule 3 times daily. Also apply to bottoms of feet.

3 Cough, Cold, & Flu
Diffuse 1-2 drops, and take in a capsule.

4 Bronchitis
Apply 1-2 drops heavily diluted over chest and lung reflex points.

5 Skin Infections
Apply a drop heavily diluted to affected area.

6 Chronic Fatigue
Take 1-2 drops in a capsule, or apply heavily diluted over adrenal glands. Also use one drop in a hot bath.

Emotional Use

Phenols like Thymol make Thyme a restoring oil that can aid in releasing grudges and injured feelings. Use it to release and forgive.

Simple *Foot Powder*

2 drops Thyme
5 drops Rosemary
2 drops Melaleuca
5 oz talc powder

Shake well and let it sit for 24 hours. Shake again and use daily on your feet.

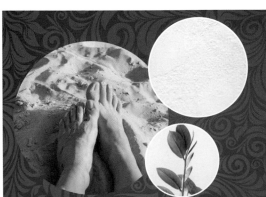

Thyme to Uplift Diffuser Blend

1 drop Thyme
2 drops Eucalyptus
3 drops Lime

This diffuser blend is useful in easing anxious feelings caused by unresolved relationship issues with people or with life in general.

Turmeric
Curcuma Longa

Application

Main Properties
Analgesic
Anti-inflammatory
Antimutagenic
Anti-parasitic
Anti-rheumatic

Chemical Constituents
a-Phellandrene, Terpinolene, 1,8-Cineole, p-Cymene, 2-Octanol

Other Uses
Arthritis, Blood Sugar, Memory Loss, Weight Loss, Wound Healing

Safety
Contraindicated in pregnancy and infants.

Top *Uses*

1 Chronic Pain & Inflammation
Take 2-4 drops under the tongue or in a veggie capsule. Or rub directly onto location.

2 Heart Palpitations
Rub 2-4 drops over chest; ingest 1-3 drops in a capsule.

3 Tumors
Take 5 drops in a capsule for assistance with tumorous conditions.

4 Brain Function
Take 5 drops in a capsule; rub a drop on the bottoms of big toes.

5 Detoxification
Apply 2 drops to lower back and rib cage.

6 Anxiety & Depression
Diffuse 5 drops to improve mood and obsessive thoughts.

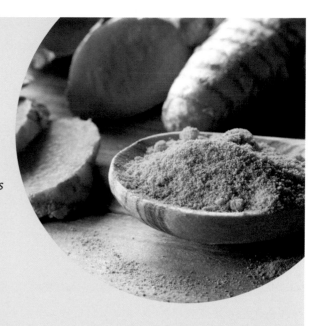

Emotional *Use*

Monoterpenes like a-Phellandrene make Turmeric a restoring oil that helps absorb the seriousness of heavy emotions.

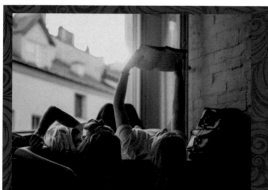

Bright Brain Boost
2 drops Turmeric
2 drops Frankincense
2 drops Rosemary
2 drops Peppermint

Combine in capsule and take two times daily to support healthy brain function.

Cancer Smasher Capsule
2 drops Turmeric
2 drops Frankincense
2 drops Sandalwood
2 drops Lemongrass

Combine in a capsule and take two times daily to assist with inflammation and promote healthy cellular apoptosis while combating cancer.

Vetiver
Vetiveria Zizanioides

Application

Main Properties
Antimicrobial
Astringent
Cytophylactic
Diuretic
Soporific
Stimulant

Chemical Constituents
Isovalencenol, a- & B-vetivones, Vitivene, Khusimol

Other Uses
Breast Enlargement, Depression, Irritability, Learning Difficulties, Memory Retention, Muscular Pain, Nerve Issues, Nervous Tension, PMS, Postpartum Depression, Restlessness, Termites, Workaholism

Top *Uses*

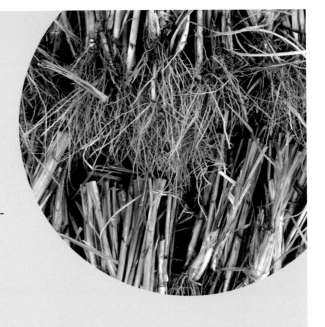

1 ADD/ADHD
Apply 1-2 drops behind ears and on the back of the neck.

2 Sleep & Insomnia
Apply 1-2 drops along spine.

3 Skin Irritation
Apply 1-2 drops with carrier oil to affected area.

4 Neuropathy
Apply 1-2 drops to bottoms of feet, or along spine.

5 Balance Issues
Apply 1-2 drops behind ears.

6 Stress-Related Menstrual Issues
Apply 1-2 drops to lower abdomen.

7 PTSD & Anxiety
Apply 1-2 drops behind ears, or diffuse.

Emotional Use

Alcohols like Isovalencenol make Vetiver a stabilizing oil. It centers the mind and makes space for prioritizing and focus.

Stress Less Roller Bottle

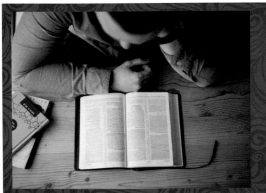

8 drops Vetiver
12 drops Bergamot
8 drops Lavender
8 drops Frankincense
FCO

Combine oils in a 10ml roller bottle and top off with FCO. Apply to wrists and back of neck (be careful of photo-sensitivity).

Focus & Concentrate Diffuser Blend

3 drops Vetiver
3 drops Frankincense
3 drops Cedarwood

This diffuser blend helps the mind stay focused on the task at hand, easily setting aside distractions and non-priorities.

Wild Orange
Citrus Sinensis

Application

Main Properties
Antibacterial
Antiseptic
Depurative
Sedative
Stimulant

Chemical Constituents
d-Limonene, B-carotene, Citral

Other Uses
Cellulite, Colds, Creativity, Depression, Detox, Fear, Fluid Retention, Heart Palpitations, Insomnia, Menopause, Nervousness, Scurvy, Sluggish Digestion, Withdrawal Issues

Safety
Avoid sun exposure for 12 hours after topical use.

Top *Uses*

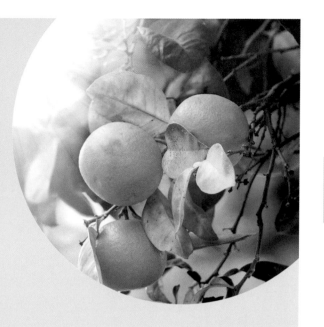

1 Energy
Drink 1-3 drops in water, or inhale from cupped hands.

2 Cheering & Mood Enhancer
Inhale 1-2 drops from cupped hands, or diffuse.

3 Anxiety & Depression
Inhale 1-2 drops from cupped hands, or diffuse 5-10 drops.

4 Immune Support
Gargle 2 drops with water, or apply to bottoms of feet.

5 Sleep Issues
Put a drop under the tongue before bed.

6 Smoothies, Dressings, & Sauces
Add according to taste.

Emotional Use

Monoterpenes like Limonene make Wild Orange an uplifting oil. Use it to lift a scarcity mindset into an abundance mentality.

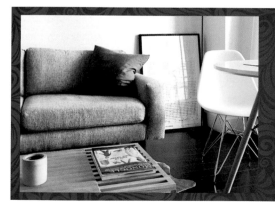

Refreshing Room Spray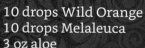
3 drops Wild Orange
2 drops Peppermint
1 drop Rosemary

Add essential oils to a 2 oz spray bottle, then fill with distilled water. Shake well before use.

Orange Tree Hand Sanitizer
10 drops Wild Orange
10 drops Melaleuca
3 oz aloe

Combine ingredients in a 4 oz glass spray bottle. Shake before use.

Wintergreen
Gaultheria Procumbens

Application

Main Properties
Analgesic
Anti-inflammatory
Antirheumatic
Antiseptic
Stimulant

Chemical Constituents
Methyl Salicylate, Salicylic Acid

Other Uses
Bone Spurs, Cartilage Injury, Circulation,
Muscle Development, Rheumatism

Safety
Potential skin sensitivity.

Top *Uses*

1 Muscle Pain & Inflammation
Massage 1-2 drops with carrier oil into affected areas.

2 Arthritis & Gout
Massage 1-2 drops into inflamed joints, diluting if needed.

3 Broken Bones
Apply 1-2 drops gently over injury, avoiding open wounds.

4 Frozen Shoulder & Rotator Cuff
Massage 1-2 drops with carrier oil into affected area.

5 Teeth Whitening
Brush with a drop of oil and baking soda.

6 Dandruff
Add a drop to shampoo, or massage 1-2 drops directly into scalp before shampooing.

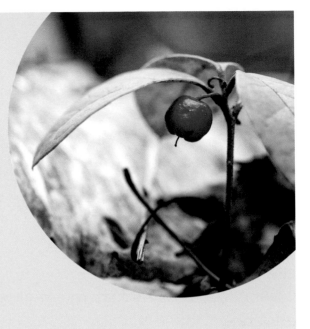

Emotional Use

Esters like Methyl Salicylate make Wintergreen a restoring oil. It transitions control issues and the need to be right into a state of safe surrender.

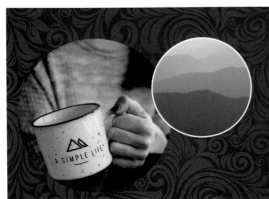

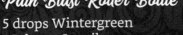

Pain Blast Roller Bottle

5 drops Wintergreen
15 drops Copaiba
10 drops Frankincense
5 drops Clove
FCO

Combine oils in a 10ml roller bottle Top off with FCO. Apply to painful muscles and joints every 3 hours as needed.

Claim Your Truth Diffuser Blend

2 drops Wintergreen
2 drops Spearmint
2 drops Lavender
1 drop Arborvitae
1 drop Helichrysum
1 drop Cardamom

Use this diffuser blend to bring confidence to voicing what you know to be right.

Yarrow
Achillea Millefolium

Application

Main Properties
Antispasmodic
Carminative
Cicatrizing
Circulatory
Expectorant

Chemical Constituents
Azulene, Caryophyllene, Pinene

Other Uses
Congestion, Brain Health, Detox, Excess Sodium, Digestive Discomfort, Flatulence, Gallbladder Pain, Headache, Heart Attack, Inflammation, Metabolism, Muscle Spasms, PMS, Weight Loss

Safety
Contraindicated in pregnancy and with infants.

Top *Uses*

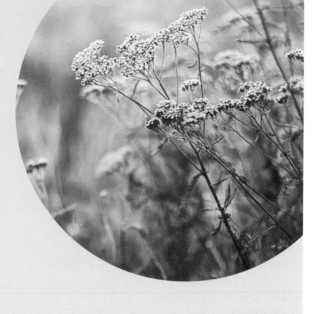

1 High Blood Pressure
Massage 2-4 drops to wrists and bottoms of feet 2x daily.

2 High Cholesterol
Use 2-4 drops under the tongue or in a veggie capsule 2x daily.

3 Heart Health
Rub 2-3 drops over heart and wrists.

4 Insulin Resistance
Rub 2-3 drops onto wrists, and take under tongue or in a veggie capsule.

5 Varicose Veins
Apply 1-2 drops neat to affected areas.

6 Hemorrhoids
Apply 1-2 drops heavily diluted to affected area.

7 Eczema & Skin Irritation
Apply 1-2 drops diluted to affected area.

Emotional Use

Sesquiterpenes like Caryophyllene make Yarrow a soothing oil, granting protection to the courageous warrior.

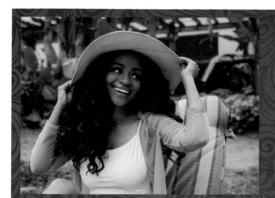

Luxury Body Cream
5 drops Yarrow
5 drops Geranium
3 drops Cedarwood
5 drops Lavender
8 oz unscented cream base

Combine ingredients in a glass jar. Apply liberally to body daily after showering.

Cramp Relief Diffuser Blend
2 drops Yarrow
1 drop Clary Sage
3 drops Bergamot
1 drop Siberian Fir

Breathe in this graceful diffuser blend to help manage pain and cramping.

Ylang Ylang
Cananga Odorata

Application
 A T I

Main Properties
Antidepressant
Antiphlogistic
Antispasmodic
Nervine
Sedative

Chemical Constituents
B-caryophylle, Benzyl Acetate & Benzoate, Linalool

Other Uses
Anxiety, Arterial Hypertension, Balance Issues, Chronic Fatigue, Circulation, Depression, Diabetes, Exhaustion, Hair Loss, Hypertension, Insomnia, Intestinal Spasms, Tachycardia

Safety
Dilute for highly sensitive skin.

Top Uses

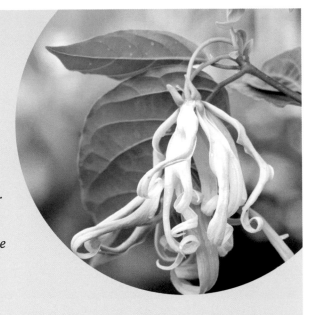

1 Hormone Balance
Apply 1-2 drops to wrists and behind ears.

2 Low Libido
Apply 1-2 drops to pulse points and reproductive reflex points. Diffuse 4-8 drops during intimacy, or use in massage.

3 High Blood Pressure
Apply 2 drops to bottoms of feet, and take in a capsule daily.

4 Infertility
Massage 1-2 drops over abdomen and reproductive reflex points.

5 Heart Palpitations
Apply 1-2 drops over heart, and diffuse.

6 Oily Skin
Add a drop to toner or facial moisturizer, or take 1-2 drops in a capsule daily.

Emotional Use

Sesquiterpenes like Germacrene D make Ylang Ylang a soothing oil that brings out the simplicity and joy of your inner child.

Hair & Scalp Rejuvenation

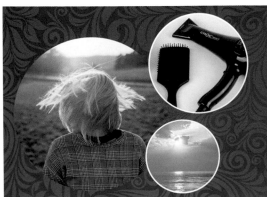

10 drops Ylang Ylang
10 drops Geranium
10 drops Rosemary
10 drops Melaleuca
2 oz Almond Oil

Combine ingredients in a glass bottle with a dropper. Apply a few drops to your hair a few hours before washing.

Migraine Buster

2 drops Ylang Ylang
3 drops Basil
1 drop Marjoram

Apply to the back of the neck, occipital bone and temples. Also use in the diffuser.

Section 4

Oil
Blends

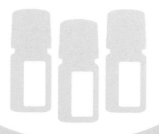

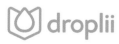

Anti-Aging Blend

place sticker *known name*

Application

A T I

Main Ingredients

Frankincense, Sandalwood, Lavender, Myrrh, Helichrysum, Rose

Other Uses

Aging, Blisters, Chapped Skin, Cuts, Dry Skin, Eczema, Hyper-pigmentation, Psoriasis, Sunburns

"This is my nighttime routine. I swear by this blend! My skin looks more even, and those fine lines are disappearing."
-Emily

"Yeah, guys use this one too. We also like looking young!"
-Marty

Top *Uses*

1 Wrinkles & Fine Lines
Apply to desired areas morning and night.

2 Age Spots
Apply to affected areas 3x daily.

3 Scarring
Massage for 30 seconds into scar tissue 2-3x daily until desired appearance.

4 Skin Cancer
Apply neat to affected area 3x daily.

5 Skin Discoloration
Apply to affected areas 3x daily.

6 Meditation
Apply to pulse points during meditation.

7 Bleeding
Apply neat to stop minor bleeding.

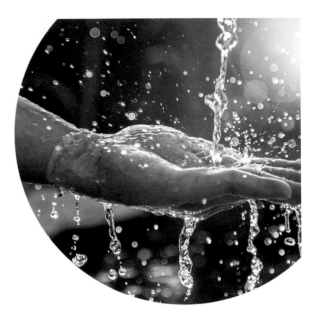

Emotional Use

Sacred trees and woodsy oils in this blend make it ideal for inviting spiritual insight during prayer and meditation.

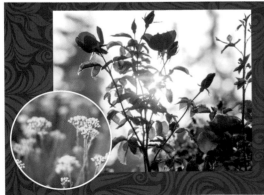

Ageless Serum

20 drops Anti-Aging Blend
10 drops Yarrow
1 tsp jojoba oil
1 tsp coconut oil

Combine ingredients in a glass jar. Massage gently into face using circular motions each night before bed.

Stretch Mark Relief

Anti-Aging Blend
Essential oil body wash
Oscillating facial device

Spread a generous amount of Anti-Aging Blend over stretch marks. Then add a bit of body wash to your oscillating facial device and scrub over stretch marks in the shower. Repeat daily until desired results achieved.

Captivating Blend

place sticker _known name_

Application

 A   T   I

Main Ingredients

Lime, Osmanthus, Bergamot, Frankincense

Other Uses

Addictions behavior, Cold Sores, Cough, Cramps, Depression, Eczema, Herpes, Psoriasis, Scurvy

Safety

Can irritate sensitive skin. Lime may cause photosensitivity. FCF Bergamot does not cause photo sensitivity.

> *"I almost die when I use this blend because I love it so much. It smells like Skittles and rainbows, and it just feels so good."*
> -Tracey

Top *Uses*

1 Self Concept Boost
Roll over wrists and over heart.

2 Energy
Apply to back and sides of neck, wrists, and temples.

3 Viral Infections
Apply generously to bottoms of feet 3-5x daily until symptoms subside.

4 Third Chakra Balance
Apply over naval area.

5 Morning Ritual
Apply to wrists and inhale deeply from cupped hands first thing in the morning while setting intentions for the day.

6 Grief & Trauma Recovery
Apply generously over heart and hip joints while taking deep cleansing breaths.

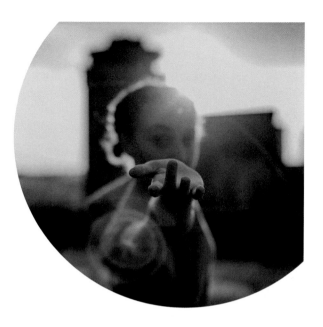

Emotional Use

The balance between bright and grounding aromas in this blend help anchor your perception of self while rising to new levels of self-respect.

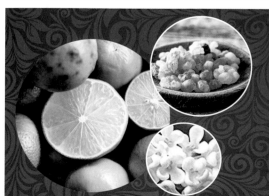

Eczema Be-Gone

Captivating Blend
Colloidal silver
Probiotic Complex

Apply Captivating Blend to eczema 3-5x daily. Use 1 tsp colloidal silver under the tongue 2x daily. Take 1 Probiotic Complex with each meal.

Beautiful Day Diffuser Blend

5 drops Captivating Blend
2 drops Douglas Fir
1 drop Lavender

This diffuser blend sets the emotional temperature of the room to self-care, appreciation, and acceptance. It's also useful when overcoming a virus.

Cellular Complex

place sticker *known name*

Application

 A T I

Main Ingredients
Frankincense, Wild Orange, Lemongrass, Thyme, Summer Savory, Clove, Niaouli

Other Uses
Addictions, Blood Clots, Candida, Cataracts, Fever, Herpes Simplex, Hodgkin's Disease, Glaucoma, Gingivitis, Lipoma, Lupus, Lyme

Safety
Can irritate sensitive skin. Use with caution during pregnancy.

"My Autism Spectrum Disorder/non verbal almost 3-year old son said his first word within 10 minutes after applying this blend over his brain stem. He hasn't stopped talking since!" -Jill

Oil Blends

Top Uses

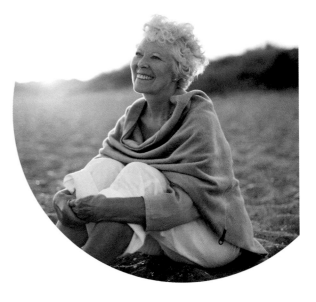

1 Damaged DNA Repair
Apply 2-4 drops to bottoms of feet and spine morning and night.

2 Thyroid (hypo, Hashimoto's)
Apply diluted over thyroid or to thyroid reflex point, or take 1-2 drops in capsule

3 Smoking Addiction
Rub onto bottom of big toe.

4 Immune Support
Take 1-2 drops in a capsule.

5 Antioxidant
Take 1-2 drops in a capsule, or use in cooking.

6 Liver Detox
Rub over liver, or on liver reflex point.

7 Rheumatoid Arthritis
Massage diluted into affected area.

Emotional Use

Just as this blend helps transform health at a cellular and DNA level, it is also useful in emotional transformation. Use it to turn toxicity into a rebirth.

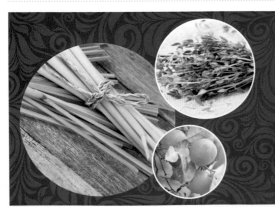

Inflammation Melter

5 drops Cellular Complex
5 drops Copaiba
5 drops Turmeric

Combine oils together. Use a couple drops under the tongue, on the spine, and the bottoms of feet 3x daily to combat inflammation.

Heavy Metal Detox

2 drops Cellular Complex
2 drops Cilantro
1 drop Frankincense

Apply oils to the bottoms of feet 30 minutes before showering. Use a hot shower to allow your body to release toxins through your feet. Repeat daily as needed.

128

Centering Blend

 place sticker *known name*

Application

 A   T   I

Main Ingredients
Bergamot, Coriander, Marjoram, Peppermint, Geranium, Basil, Rose, Jasmine

Other Uses
Body Odors, Dizziness, Mood Disorders, Muscle Injury, Nausea, Neuralgia, Vertigo

Safety
May cause photosensitivity. Use with caution during pregnancy.

> *"I used to get anxious during yoga. I know it's stupid, but I care a lot of what others think of me when I practice. This oil helps me come back to the person my yoga is really for - ME."*
>
> -Jeneay

Top Uses

1. Warrior II, Triangle, & Gate Yoga Pose
Apply 2 drops over heart, turning your attention within. Reach inside for power, identity, and assurance.

2. Completeness, Calmness, Courage
Apply 1-3 drops over heart, pulse points, and naval area.

3. Hyperactivity
Apply a drop to temples; diffuse several drops.

4. Addictions
Apply 2-4 drops to bottoms of feet, focusing on big toes; diffuse several drops.

5. Hormone Balancing
Apply 2-4 drops to wrists and inner thighs 2x daily.

6. Neuropathy
Apply 2-4 drops to bottoms of feet 3x daily.

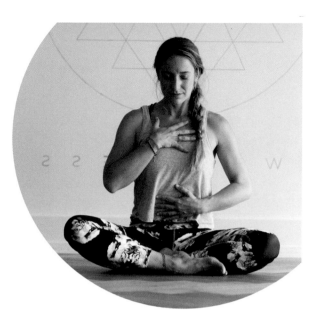

Emotional Use

This yoga blend encourages a sense of harmony and calm progress. Release feelings of hastiness and know that growth happens most often in a subtle, ongoing process.

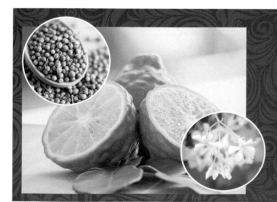

Centering Ritual

2-4 drops Centering Blend
3 affirmation statements
1 journal page

Use Centering Blend on your pulse points as you speak self-affirming statements. Say 3 statements to encourage self-respect. Then spend 5 minutes journaling what you appreciate about yourself.

Embrace Yourself Diffuser Blend

2 drops Centering Blend
2 drops Lime
1 drop Blue Tansy

Find the sweet spot where you can't wait to venture into life's adventures exactly as you are with this deep, meaningful diffuser blend.

Cleansing Blend

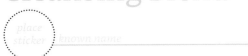

place sticker _known name_ _____

Application

A T I

Main Ingredients
Lime, Lemon, Siberian Fir, Citronella, Melaleuca, Cilantro

Other Uses
Airborne Bacteria & Viruses, Boils, Household Cleaning, Insect Repellent, Mice Repellent, Skin Ulcers

Safety
Can irritate sensitive skin. Avoid direct sun exposure 12 hours after application.

"I love using this blend in my laundry. It's never been fresher, and my grown kids literally fight over my bottle!"
-Debbie

Top Uses

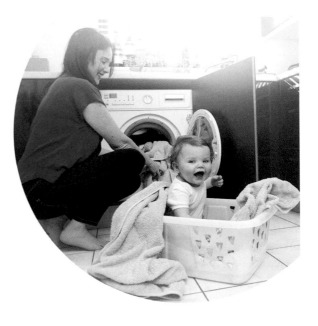

1 Air Freshener
Add 10 drops to glass spray bottle with water. Spray as needed.

2 Foot Odors
Apply neat to feet. Spray inside shoes.

3 Laundry
Add 4-5 drops to detergent.

4 Disinfectant
Add 20 drops to glass spray bottle with water and 1 Tbsp rubbing alcohol.

5 Deodorant
Apply 1-2 drops with carrier oil to armpits.

6 Mildew
Use several drops with a clean sponge.

7 Bites & Stings
Apply 1 drop neat to bite or sting.

Emotional Use

The purifying effects of this blend assist in releasing trapped, unhealthy emotions. It can clear negative energy from a room so that goodness can be noticed and felt.

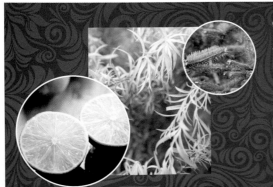

Shoe Deodorant

4 drops Cleansing Blend
8 drops Melaleuca
8 drops Lavender
4 Tbsp baking soda
4 Tbsp corn starch

Mix ingredients and store in airtight container. Sprinkle lightly into shoes and let sit overnight.

No-Energy Vampire Diffuser Blend

4 drops Cleansing Blend
2 drops Melaleuca
1 drop Melissa

Use this diffuser blend to help clear unwanted energy and negative emotions from your space.

Oil Blends

Comforting Blend

place sticker *known name* _____

Application

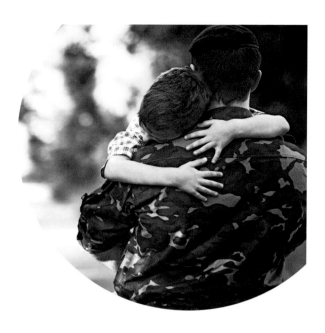

Frankincense, Ylang Ylang, Patchouli, Labdanum, Sandalwood, Rose, Osmanthus

Other Uses

Anger, Brain Health, Bladder Infection, Emotional Processing, Heart Health, Resentment

"I discovered this blend the week after my dad passed away. The timing was incredible. I felt like these oils helped me process my grief in a beautiful way."
                                    -Drew

Top *Uses*

1 Grief, Sorrow, Despair
Apply 1-2 drops over heart, or diffuse.

2 Hormone Balance
Apply 1-3 drops to pulse points before bed.

3 Self-Esteem
Inhale from cupped hands, or diffuse during meditation.

4 Perfume
Wear on pulse points for a floral aroma.

5 Anti-Aging
Apply 1-3 drops with carrier oil to wrinkles, sun spots, and fine lines.

6 Nightmares
Diffuse 3-6 drops next to bedside.

7 Rheumatoid Arthritis
Massage diluted into affected area.

Emotional Use

The soothing qualities of this blend assist in processing grief, loss, and trauma. It facilitates a sense of being whole and knowing that the greater good is unfolding.

Oil Blends

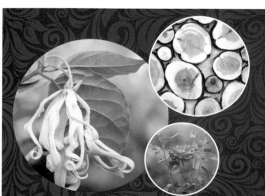

Anti-Anxiety Roller Blend

5 drops Comforting Blend
9 drops Wild Orange
9 drops Peppermint
3 drops Melissa
FCO

Add oils to a 10ml roller bottle and top off with FCO. Apply to pulse points as needed.

Worries Be-Gone Diffuser Blend

3 drops Comforting Blend
3 drops Tangerine
1 drop Douglas Fir

This diffuser blend brings a sense of childlike playfulness where heavy emotions may have been dominant.

131

Detoxification Blend

Oil Blends

Application

 A   T   I

Main Ingredients
Tangerine, Geranium, Rosemary, Juniper Berry, Cilantro

Other Uses
Hangover, Hormone Balance, Gallbladder Detox, Urinary Infection, Weight Loss

Safety
Can irritate sensitive skin. Avoid sun exposure for 12 hours after topical use.

"A lot of detox products are obnoxious to use. I love this blend because you can use it many ways, and you're using the power of essential oils."
　　　　　　　　　　-Tabatha

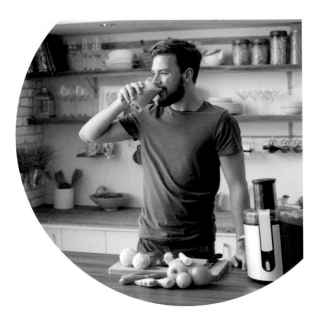

1 Detoxification
Take 2-4 drops in a capsule, or apply to bottoms of feet.

2 Allergies
Apply 2-4 drops to bottoms of feet, or diffuse.

3 Smoking Cravings
Rub onto bottom of big toe, or drink 1-3 drops in water after meals.

4 Liver & Kidney Support
Massage 1-3 drops over liver or kidneys.

5 Antioxidant
Take 1-2 drops in a capsule.

6 Heavy Metal Detox
Apply 2-4 drops to bottoms of feet.

7 Adrenal Fatigue
Massage 1-3 drops over lower back.

Emotional Use

Purging physical toxins also sets the stage for emotional detox. Use this blend to purge self-sabotage and apathy, and transition to vitality.

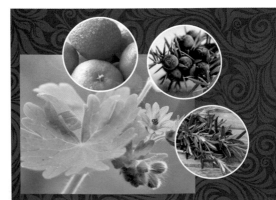

Detox Week

4 drops Detoxification Blend
6 Cellular Complex Softgels

Rub 4 drops of Detoxification Blend onto the bottoms of feet 30 minutes before a hot shower. Take 2 Cellular Complex Softgels 3x daily. Minimize or eliminate dairy, sugars, and GMO grains for 1 week.

Detox Bath

10 drops Detoxification Blend
1 cup coconut milk
2 cups Epsom salt
1 cup baking soda

Pour ingredients into a hot bath and soak for 20 minutes to support hormone balance, liver and kidney function, and toxin discharge. Shower after bath.

Digestive Blend

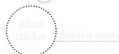

place sticker known name

Application

A T I

Main Ingredients
Peppermint, Ginger, Caraway, Coriander, Anise, Tarragon

Other Uses
Abdominal Cramps, Acid Reflux, Colitis, Crohn's Disease, Gastritis, Heartburn, Morning Sickness, Motion Sickness, Parasites, Sinusitis

Safety
Can irritate sensitive skin. Use with caution during pregnancy.

> "Sometimes I get tummy trouble. Digestive Blend to the rescue! 1-2 drops under the tongue or 3-4 drops right on my stomach...happy tummy in usually 5-7 minutes. So fast!"   -Louise

Top *Uses*

1. **Stomach Upset**
Drink 1-3 drops in water, or take in a capsule.

2. **Gas & Bloating**
Massage 2-4 drops over stomach, or take in a capsule.

3. **Diarrhea & Constipation**
Massage 2-4 drops over stomach, or take in a capsule.

4. **Irritable Bowel Syndrome**
Massage 2-4 drops over stomach, or take in a capsule.

5. **Food Poisoning**
Drink 3-5 drops in water, or take in a capsule.

6. **Nausea**
Put a drop under the tongue, or rub over stomach.

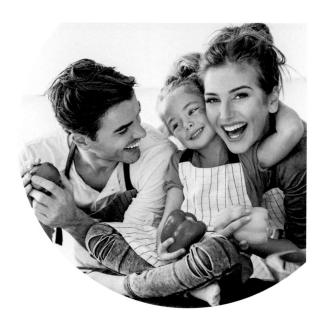

Oil Blends

Emotional Use

The digestion oils in this blend make it useful for digesting difficult emotions, assimilating new information, and achieving a state of feeling nourished.

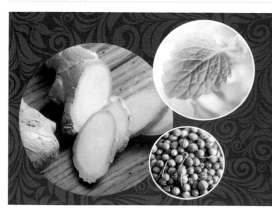

Daily Gut Protocol

2 drops Digestive Blend
2 drops Turmeric
3 Digestive Enzymes
3 Probiotic Complex

Drink Digestive Blend and Turmeric oils in water with heaviest meal of the day. Take 1 Digestive Enzyme and 1 Probiotic Complex with each meal.

Mucus Riddance

3 drops Digestive Blend
Water

Gargle 2 drops of Digestive Blend with water for 30 seconds, then swallow. Rub 1 drop of Digestive Blend over the bridge of nose and sinuses every 30 minutes until mucus lessens.

Encouraging Blend

place sticker known name

Application

Main Ingredients

Clementine, Peppermint, Coriander, Basil, Melissa, Rosemary

Other Uses

Asthma, Confusion, Creativity, Fatigue, Loneliness, Overwhelm, Uncertainty

Safety

Can irritate sensitive skin. Use with caution during pregnancy.

"My son in-law has been struggling with a job he doesn't feel inspired by. We sent a diffuser and Encouraging Blend to his office. It is remarkable how much he felt his attitude shift just from the oils."

-Maryane

Top Uses

1 Discouragement, Low Confidence, Low Motivation
Inhale 1-2 drops from cupped hands, or diffuse.

2 Detox
Apply 1-2 drops to bottoms of feet, or massage over endocrine organs.

3 Adrenal Fatigue
Massage 1-2 drops with carrier oil over lower back.

4 Flatulence
Rub 1-2 drops with carrier oil over stomach.

5 Depression
Diffuse 5-10 drops, or rub 1-2 drops onto temples.

6 Respiratory Issues
Apply 1-2 drops over chest, or diffuse.

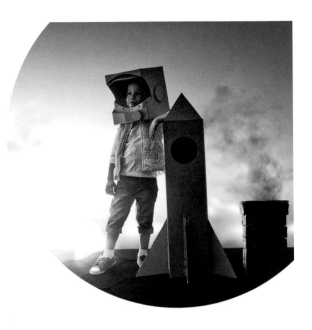

Emotional Use

The combination of citrus and herbs in this blend make it a powerful motivator. It turns lethargic energy into enthusiasm and a sense of "I can do this!"

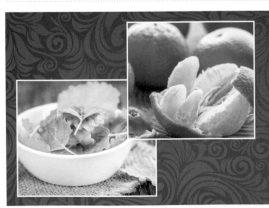

Motivation Monday

5 drops Encouraging Blend
Tart citrus juice (like grapefruit)
Dance music

Most people start their week dreading work. Start your week by dropping a few drops of Encouraging Blend in your shower while waking your senses with a tart fruit juice and dancing to music you love!

Have Courage Diffuser Blend

3 drops Encouraging Blend
3 drops Tangerine
1 drop Spearmint

Add a big splash of aroma-color to your day with this happy, courage-inspiring diffuser blend.

Oil Blends

Enlightening Blend

place sticker *known name*

Application

 A T I

Main Ingredients
Lemon, Grapefruit, Siberian Fir, Osmanthus, Melissa

Other Uses
Depression, Fear, Respiratory Infection, Sinus Infection, Toxicity, Viral Infection

Safety
Avoid sun exposure for 12 hours after topical application.

> "I don't just use this blend for yoga. It's my every-day mood boost. I think it helps me see more opportunities because I feel so inspired by it."
> -Libby

Top *Uses*

1 Standing Arms High, Standing Side Stretch, & Half Moon Yoga Pose
Apply 2-4 drops to inside of arms and wrists. Feel light entering the crown of your head as your own energy rises to meet it.

2 Lacking Motivation
Apply 1-3 drops to temples and back of neck.

3 Mental Clarity & Illumination
Apply 1-3 drops to temples and forehead.

4 Cold & Flu
Massage 2-4 drops into bottoms of feet and spine; diffuse several drops.

5 Overeating
Massage 2-4 drops over stomach; diffuse several drops.

6 Cold Sores
Apply a drop to affected area 5x daily.

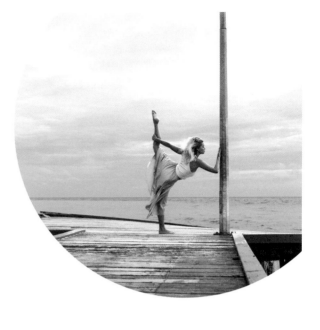

Oil Blends

Emotional *Use*

The Enlightening Blend inspires a sense of freedom. It reminds the user that stability and freedom are the paradoxical duo that allows creativity and inspiration to abound.

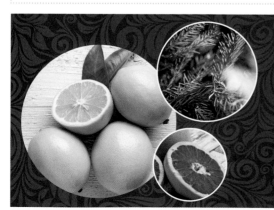

Happy Dish Scrub
10 drops Enlightening Blend
10 drops Lemon
1/4 cup baking soda
5 Tbsp glycerin

Combine ingredients in glass storage container. Wet dish scrub brush and dip into mixture.

Illuminate Diffuser Blend
4 drops Enlightening Blend
2 drops Lemon
1 drop Yarrow

Diffuse this blend to inspire new ideas and to see new possibility.

Focus Blend

Application
 A   T   I

Main Ingredients
Amyris, Patchouli, Frankincense, Lime, Ylang Ylang, Sandalwood, Chamomile

Other Uses
Alzheimer's, Emotional Balance, Hormone Balance, Memory, Parkinson's, Relaxation, Sleep

Safety
Repeated use can irritate highly sensitive skin.

> "My little boy had been struggling in school. His grades suffered, the teacher was frustrated. When we started using this oil, literally nobody could believe how much better he started doing."
>
> -Suzanne D

Top Uses

1 ADD & ADHD
Apply to back of neck and behind ears.

2 Focus & Concentration
Apply to back of neck and behind ears.

3 Anxiety
Apply to pulse points, or inhale from cupped hands.

4 Hyperactivity
Apply to pulse points, or inhale from cupped hands.

5 Seizures
Apply to bottoms of feet and back of neck.

6 Skin Irritations
Apply with carrier oil to affected areas.

7 Sedative
Apply to pulse points or bottoms of feet.

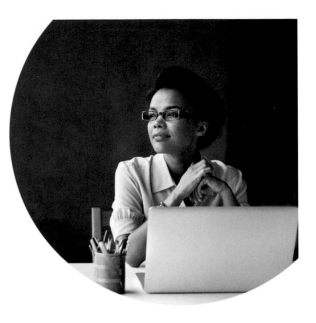

Emotional Use

The bright citrus and deep woodsy fragrance combo in this blend facilitates happily living in the present moment. It promotes indulging in the goodness of the here and now.

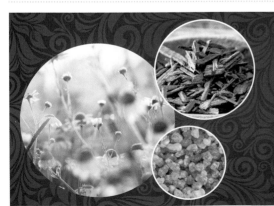

Subtle Focus Rollers
1 bottle of Focus Blend
3 10ml roller bottles
FCO

Make a gentler form of Focus Blend by diluting one bottle into three with FCO. It has the same powerful benefits, but with a softer aroma for places like work where strong scents may be inappropriate.

Reading Hour Diffuser Blend
2 drops Focus Blend
2 drops Ylang Ylang
2 drops Lemon

Use this diffuser blend when diving into a good book or during study time.

Fortifying Blend

place sticker *known name*

Application

Main Ingredients
Buddha Wood, Balsam Canada, Black Pepper, Hinoki, Patchouli, Cocoa

Other Uses
Acne, Anxiety, Dry Skin, Eczema, Fungal Infections, Premature Aging, Rashes

Safety
Use with caution if pregnant or nursing.

"When people talk about their 'soul oil,' this one is mine. I remember who I am and the real purpose I serve in my life when I meditate with this oil, or just use it throughout the day."

-Andrew

Top Uses

1 Deep Meditation
Apply to temples and wrists before beginning meditation. If you slip from a meditative state, focus on the deep aroma.

2 Balding
Massage several drops into scalp every night before bed for at least 4 months.

3 Anxiousness
Apply to pulse points; diffuse several drops.

4 Work Pressure
Take a 30-second reset during intense moments at work; inhale deeply from cupped hands.

5 Spasms and Twitches
Apply generously to bottoms of feet each morning, and to specific affected areas.

6 Aftershave
Apply directly to face after shaving.

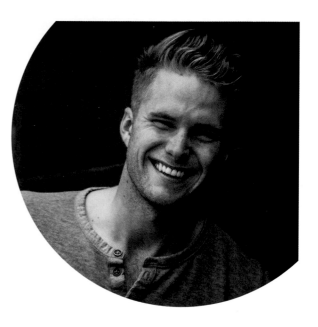

Emotional Use

The spicy aroma of pepper with the intense grounding fragrance of wood oils make this blend ideal for soul-searching. It invites the user to explore the true beauty of one's self in all aspects.

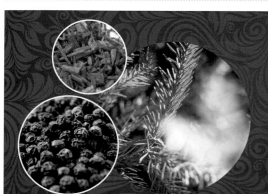

Dream Calibration

Fortifying Blend
List of 3-5 goals & dreams
15 minutes of undisturbed time

Apply Fortifying blend to wrists, temples, and back of neck. Spend 15 minutes vividly visualizing what it looks, feels, sounds, and smells like to experience each goal and dream. Do this exercise daily for 21 days.

Dry Elbow Patch

5 drops Fortifying Blend
2 drops Cedarwood
1 drop Magnolia
Coconut oil or other hydrating salve

Mix essential oils with the coconut oil or salve. Massage into elbows in the morning and before going to bed.

137

Grounding Blend

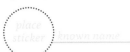

place sticker *known name*

Application

A T ◯ I

Main Ingredients
Spruce, Ho Wood, Frankincense, Blue Tansy, Blue Chamomile

Other Uses
Anger, Back Pain, Brain Integration, Bursitis, Comas, Confusion, Convulsions, Diabetic Sores, Grief, Herniated Discs, Hyperactivity, Lou Gehrig's Disease, Parkinson's Disease, Tranquility

"I use this blend during meditation to really calm down and focus, aligning head and heart to go deep into the meditation practice. It feels so renewing."
                              -Thomas

Top *Uses*

1 Emotional Grounding
Inhale 1-3 drops from cupped hands, or apply to bottoms of feet daily.

2 Focus & Concentration
Apply 1-3 drops to temples and pulse points, or diffuse.

3 Stress & Anxiety
Apply 1-3 drops to pulse points and temples, or to bottoms of feet.

4 Meditation
Apply 1-2 drops to wrists and temples.

5 Neurological Issues
Apply 2-4 drops to bottoms of feet.

6 Stress-Induced Inflammation
Inhale 2-4 drops from cupped hands, apply to bottoms of feet, or diffuse.

7 Balance
Apply 1-2 drops behind ears.

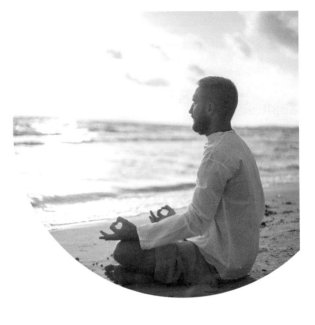

Emotional Use

The earthy character of this blend help bring scattered energy and emotions into a space of stability, consistency, and safety.

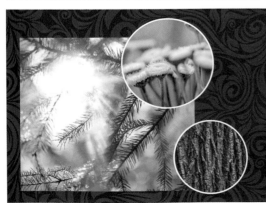

Talua Rising
2 drops Grounding Blend
3 drops Cypress
3 drops Lemon
2 drops Cardamom

Rise out of anger and detach yourself from hyper-focus with Talua (Sanskrit for "rising"). Massage these oils upward and inward from ankles toward pelvic region.

Epilepsy Diffuser Blend
1 drop Grounding Blend
1 drop Cedarwood
1 drop Patchouli
1 drop Clary Sage
1 drop Peppermint
1 drop Frankincense
1 drop Vetiver

Diffuse throughout the day as needed.

Oil Blends

Holiday Joyful Blend

place sticker *unknown name*

Application

 A T I

Main Ingredients

Siberian Fir, Orange, Clove, Cinnamon, Douglas Fir, Vanilla, Nutmeg

Other Uses

Arthritis, Blood Sugar Balance, Muscle Tension, Respiratory Conditions

Safety

Can irritate sensitive skin.

"It literally smells like Christmas. I can't describe it any other way! The fragrance brings that holiday feeling to the air for me, which I associate with joy and happiness."

-Betsy

Top *Uses*

1 Joyful Feelings
Diffuse 5-10 drops, or inhale 1-2 drops from cupped hands.

2 Cover Burnt Food Smell
Diffuse 5-10 drops.

3 Stress & Tension
Apply 1-2 drops with carrier oil to pulse points; inhale from cupped hands.

4 Family Contention
Diffuse 5-10 drops.

5 Cold & Flu
Apply 2-4 drops to bottoms of feet.

6 Airborne Pathogens
Diffuse 5-10 drops.

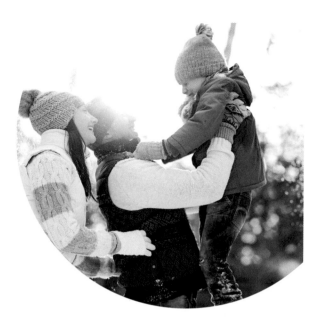

Emotional Use

This warm blend of holiday oils brings with it a reminder to celebrate with love and with healthy boundaries for the people you love.

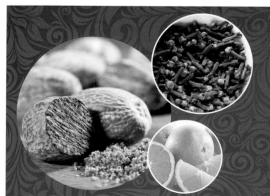

Sanitizing Holiday Soap

15 drops Holiday Joyful Blend
4oz unscented Castile soap
Tap water

Combine oils with unscented soap and water in a foaming hand soap dispenser. The oils in this blend are naturally antibacterial.

Scented Pine Cones

10 drops Holiday Joyful Blend
10 drops FCO
10 pine cones

Mix oils in a small ramekin. Apply to pine cones with a small paint brush. Reapply every couple weeks as needed.

Holiday Peaceful Blend

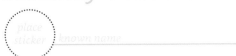

place sticker *known name* _____

Application

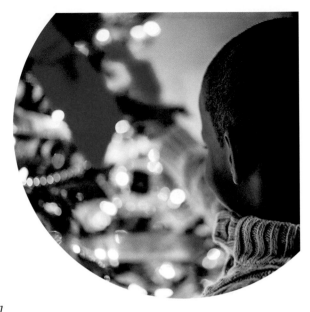

Main Ingredients

Siberian Fir, Grapefruit, Douglas Fir, Himalayan Fir, Frankincense, Vetiver

Other Uses

Arthritis, Bronchitis, Focus, Frozen Shoulder, Joint Pain, Muscle Fatigue, Muscle Pain, Pneumonia, Respiratory Infection, Sprains, Varicose Veins

Did You Know?

The Douglas Fir in this blend is distilled from young trees. It takes an entire tree to make one 5ml bottle, which means there's a lot of holiday tree in your bottle!

Top Uses

1 Peaceful Feelings
Apply 1-2 drops to temples and back of neck; diffuse several drops.

2 Shopping Anxiety
Apply 1-2 drops to pulse points to ease pressure of holiday shopping.

3 Artificial Tree Remedy
Diffuse several drops next to the artificial Christmas tree or add a couple drops to clay ornaments on the tree.

4 Cold Weather Cough
Apply 1-3 drops over chest with carrier oil before venturing into cold weather.

5 Winter Inversion
Diffuse several drops throughout the day to purify the air.

6 Holiday Greed
Inhale 1-2 drops from cupped hands during moments of thanksgiving.

Emotional Use

The many kinds of fir needles in this blend make it an oil for renewing the peace of the holidays. It replaces stress with feelings of freshness to welcome the new year.

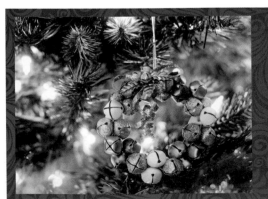

Holiday Peaceful Blend d.i.y.

8 drops Siberian Fir
7 drops Douglas Fir
7 drops Grapefruit
2 drops Frankincense
1 drop Vetiver

Whip up a mock-version of this blend if supplies are scarce and you still need some peace with your holidays.

True Christmas Tree Diffuser Blend

4 drops Holiday Peaceful Blend
4 drops Douglas Fir
1 drop Arborvitae

This diffuser blend has the perfect balance of fresh fir needles and the cool aroma of a freshly cut wooden trunk.

Oil Blends

Hopeful Blend

place sticker / known name

Application

 A T I

Main Ingredients
Bergamot*, Ylang Ylang, Frankincense, Vanilla

Other Uses
Addictions, Alzheimer's, Appetite Loss, Autism, Discouragement, Parkinson's, Self-Worth Issues

Safety
Use with caution during pregnancy.

Did You Know?

FCF Bergamot is distilled with steam distillation, rather than the usual cold pressing of citrus oils. It does not cause photosensitivity.

Top Uses

1 Emotional Trauma
Apply to pulse points, and inhale from cupped hands.

2 Grief & Trust Issues
Apply to pulse points, and inhale from cupped hands.

3 Hormone Balance
Apply to wrists and bottoms of feet.

4 Perfume
Apply 1-2 drops to pulse points.

5 Adrenal Fatigue
Apply to neck and lower back.

6 Stress
Apply to temples, and inhale from cupped hands.

7 Focus & Concentration
Apply to temples.

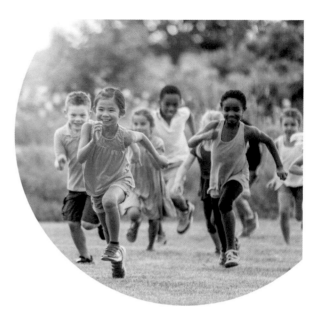

Emotional Use

This blend facilitates renewing trust in people and self after experiencing abuse or trauma. It helps regenerate the ability to connect in safe, healthy, and consensual ways.

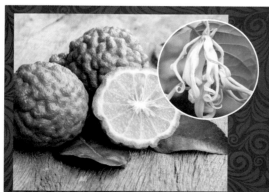

Heart Balancing
Hopeful Blend
Magnolia
Rose

Apply each oil over the heart in turns. Hopeful Blend says it's safe to be you. Magnolia says unseen greater powers have your best interest at heart. Rose says there is genuine love to be given and received.

Cracked Heels Repair
Hopeful Blend
4 drops Cedarwood
Coconut oil
Unscented Lotion

Apply Hopeful Blend and Cedarwood generously with the lotion to heels. Follow with the coconut oil. Cover feet with socks until the oil is absorbed. Repeat nightly.

Inspiring Blend

place sticker *known name*

Application

 A T I

Main Ingredients

Cardamom, Cinnamon, Ginger, Sandalwood, Jasmine, Damiana

Other Uses

Depression, Hormone Balance, Menopause, PMS Discomfort, Slow Bowel Movements

Safety

Can irritate sensitive skin. Avoid topical use during pregnancy.

Did You Know?

Cinnamon, Ginger, Sandalwood, Jasmine, and Damiana are all natural aphrodisiacs. This blend can really turn up the heat.

Top *Uses*

1 Apathy & Boredom
Inhale 1-2 drops from cupped hands, or diffuse.

2 Low Sex Drive
Apply 1-2 drops with carrier oil to pulse points, or use diluted in massage.

3 Digestive Issues
Apply 1-2 drops to stomach reflex points, or apply diluted over stomach.

4 Aphrodisiac
Apply 1-2 drops to pulse points.

5 Slow Digestion
Apply 1-2 drops with carrier oil over stomach.

6 Lack of Creativity
Diffuse 5-10 drops.

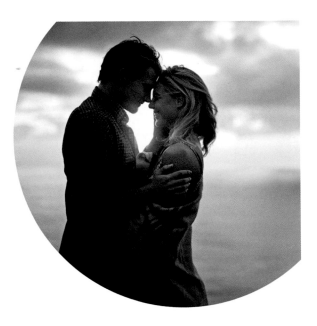

Emotional Use

The passion-inspiring oils in this blend are all about coming out of self-denial and finding the vitality and love of taking risks and being more playful with life.

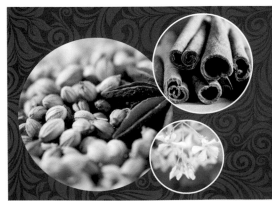

Love Bomb

5 drops Inspiring Blend
3 drops Douglas Fir
FCO

Combine oils with desired amount of FCO and use during intimate massage. Also diffuse several drops of Inspiring Blend with Douglas Fir.

Citrus Summer Remix Diffuser Blend

1 drop Passion
2 drops Bergamot
2 drops Lime
2 drops Green Mandarin

This diffuser blend is filled with both passion and creativity. Use it at parties or at the beginning of a creative project.

Oil Blends

Invigorating Blend

place sticker *known name* _____

Application
 ^A   ^T ^I

Main Ingredients
Orange, Lemon, Grapefruit, Mandarin, Bergamot, Clementine, Vanilla

Other Uses
Air Freshener, Household Cleaning, Eating Disorders, Laundry Freshener, Low Appetite, Mastitis

Safety
Avoid sun exposure for 24 hours after topical use.

Did You Know?

Citrus oils are comprised primarily of d-Limonene, a natural dopaminergic. You feel happy with this oil blend because it stimulates your happy neurotransmitters.

Top Uses

1 **Lack of Creativity & Inspiration**
Inhale 2 drops from cupped hands, or diffuse.

2 **Low Energy**
Apply 2 drops to pulse points, or diffuse.

3 **Morning Moodiness**
Diffuse 5-10 drops next to bedside in the morning, or inhale from cupped hands.

4 **Lymphatic Drainage**
Apply 3-4 drops to bottoms of feet.

5 **Stress & Anxiety**
Inhale 2 drops from cupped hands, or apply to pulse points.

6 **Depression & Gloom**
Inhale 2 drops from cupped hands, or diffuse 5-10 drops.

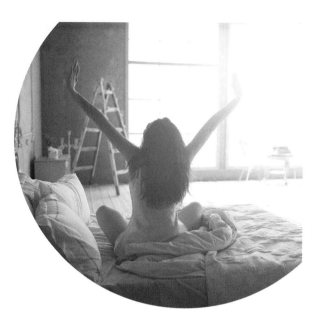

Emotional Use

The blissful aromas of this blend inspire creativity. They help bring out artistic expression and daringness to be bold in what you create.

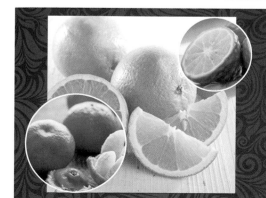

Citrus Grove Bliss Balls

10 drops Invigorating Blend 2 Tbsp coconut oil
1 cup almond meal 2 Tbsp raw honey
1 cup shredded coconut 2 Tbsp lemon juice

Mix ingredients in a bowl, and roll spoonfuls into balls. Roll extra coconut onto balls. Refrigerate for a few hours until firm.

Anthropology Diffuser Blend

4 drops Citrus Bliss
3 drops Grapefruit
2 drops Siberian Fir

Feel like you're treating yourself to a luxurious lifestyle with this blend that smells like everything new and exciting.

Oil Blends

Joyful Blend

place sticker *known name*

Application

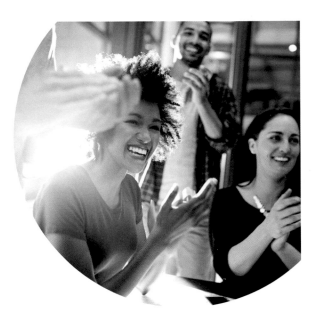

Main Ingredients

Lavandin, Lavender, Sandalwood, Tangerine, Melissa, Ylang Ylang, Osmanthus, Lemon Myrtle

Other Uses

Cushing's Syndrome, Lethargy, Postpartum Depression, Sadness, Shock, Weight Loss

Safety

Can irritate sensitive skin. Avoid sun exposure for 12 hours after topical use.

> "It was love at first sniff! Life was stressful , but after a few inhales, I felt happy again. I felt physically centered and in my heart."
>
> -Louise

Top *Uses*

1 Depression
Carry on your person, and inhale 1-2 drops from cupped hands as needed.

2 Stress & Anxiety
Diffuse 4-8 drops, or inhale 1-2 drops from cupped hands.

3 Abuse Recovery
Apply 1-2 drops to back of neck and over heart.

4 Grief & Sorrow
Apply 1-2 drops to pulse points, or diffuse.

5 Poison Oak/Ivy
Apply 1-2 drops with carrier oil to affected areas.

6 Lupus & Fibromyalgia
Inhale 1-2 drops from cupped hands, and apply diluted to inflamed areas.

Emotional Use

This floral-citrussy aroma brings with it true joy. It elevates the heavy-hearted into an optimistic and care-free state of being.

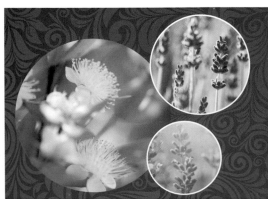

Emotion Potion

10 drops Joyful Blend
10 drops Grounding Blend
8 drops Frankincense
FCO

Combine oils in a 10ml roller bottle and top with FCO. Apply to naval and wrists to experience the healthy paradox of both grounded and elevated emotions.

Spa Elevated Diffuser Blend

1 drop Joyful Blend
2 drops Bergamot
2 drops Wild Orange

Feel like you're in a high-end spa with this bright and classy diffuser blend.

Kids: Courage Blend

place sticker *known name*

Application
 A T I

Main Ingredients
Wild Orange, Amyris, Osmanthus, Cinnamon

Other Uses
Anxiety, Fear, Immune Support, Motivation, Nervousness, Reassurance, Self-Doubt

Safety
Avoid sun exposure for 12 hours after topical use.

"We're using Courage Blend for anything new that might seem hard - like making new friends or potty training!"
-Emily

Top *Uses*

1 **Making New Friends**
Apply to wrists and inhale from cupped hands. Speak out loud a few reasons you make a great friend for others!

2 **Team Sports**
Apply over chest to bring the courage to do your best and be a team player.

3 **Potty Training**
Apply over lower back and back of neck to feel excited about being a big kid.

4 **Electronics Addiction**
Apply to wrists and temples to find ambition to experience new adventures.

5 **Imagination Sparks**
Apply to the back of neck and temples to spur creativity and new ideas.

6 **Trying New Things**
Apply to the naval and chest to feel brave when trying new things.

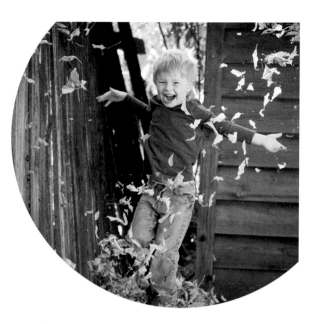

Emotional Use

This blend brings out the bravery in every kid. It reminds kids the value of self-expression, and what it means to be yourself and hold strong to values.

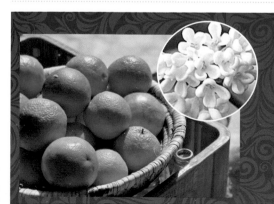

Funny-Again Blend
Kid's Courage Blend
2 drops Tangerine
1 drop Lime

Apply oils over naval and back of neck when things get too serious. This blend helps bring laughter back into the game of life.

Kid-Approved Respiration
Kid's Courage Blend
1 drop Peppermint

Apply Kid's Courage Blend to chest, followed by a drop of Peppermint to open airways and help with things like panic, shortness of breath, or asthma.

Kids: Focus Blend

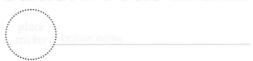

   place sticker known name

Application

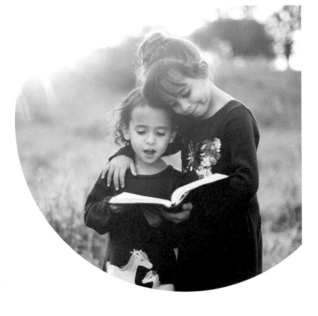

Main Ingredients

Vetiver, Peppermint, Clementine, Rosemary

Other Uses

Autism, Asperger's, Hyperactivity, Mental Handicaps, Nervous Disorders

Safety

Can irritate sensitive skin. Avoid sun exposure for 12 hours after topical use.

Did You Know?

Peppermint and Rosemary enhance memory retention. They make it easier to recall information when they're used first during study time and then during test-taking.

Top Uses

1. **Homework**
Apply to back of neck at the beginning of homework time to boost concentration.

2. **ADD/ADHD**
Apply to the back of neck 3x daily or as needed.

3. **Creative Writing**
Apply to temples to incite new ideas during writing projects.

4. **Household Chores**
Apply to naval and wrists to stay focused during chore time so that playtime can come sooner.

5. **Test Taking**
Apply to temples while studying for a test, and again while taking the test.

6. **Confusion & Distractions**
Apply to temples and inhale from cupped hands to promote mental clarity.

Emotional Use

This blend is the oil for peaceful thoughts. It helps turn agitation and frustration into centered thinking that is both realistic and useful.

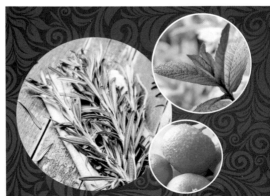

Stressed Thoughts Lifter

Kid's Focus Blend
1 drop Copaiba

Apply Copaiba with Kid's Focus Blend for added stress relief.

Little Rashes Blend

Kid's Focus Blend
1 drop Cedarwood
1 drop Lavender

Apply Kid's Focus Blend, followed by Cedarwood and Lavender to rashes 3x daily. Dilute for sensitive skin.

Oil Blends

Kids: Grounding Blend

Application

 A T I

Main Ingredients

Amyris, Balsam Fir, Coriander, Magnolia

Other Uses

Chronic Pain, Circulation Issues, Cough, Cramps, Depression, Procrastination, Scrapes, Stress

"It took just seconds for the whole family to fall in love with this blend. Everyone feels more steady and confident with it."
-Shilpi

Top Uses

1 Social Anxiety
Apply to wrists and lower back to add a feeling of steadiness to social situations.

2 Frazzled School Mornings
Start the morning right by applying to bottoms of feet and the back of the neck.

3 Useful Time-Outs
Turn time-outs from unhelpful punishment to a time of valuable reflection on the importance of keeping your word and contributing value to the family.

4 Superhero Confidence
Apply over chest and the back of neck.

5 Waaaah-Baby
Apply to temples and wrists to calm temper tantrums.

6 Bad News Buster
Apply over chest to help ease disappointment or discouragement.

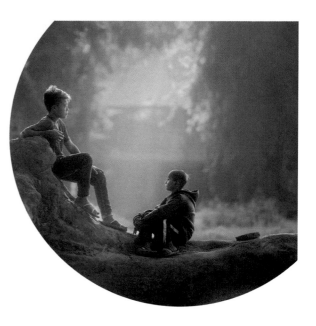

Emotional Use

This blend brings a sense of steadiness to every day. It fosters feelings of safety in the present moment, reminding the user everything can eventually work out.

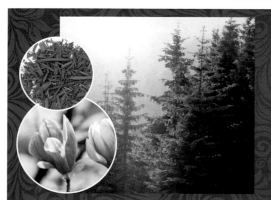

Overwhelm Rescue

Kid's Grounding Blend
1 drop Cedarwood
1 drop Pink Pepper

Apply Kid's Grounding Blend to base of skull, followed by Cedarwood and Pink Pepper. Inhale deeply from cupped hands to manage overwhelm.

Skin Infection Fighter

Kid's Grounding Blend
1 drop Melaleuca
FCO

Apply Kid's Grounding Blend, followed by Melaleuca and a drop of FCO to a rash or skin infection. Repeat 3-5x daily.

Oil Blends

147

Kids: Protective Blend

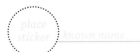 place sticker known name _____

Application
 A   T   I

Main Ingredients
Cedarwood, Litsea, Frankincense, Rose

Other Uses
Athlete's Foot, Dandruff, Fungal Infection, Heartache, Ingrown Toenail

Safety
Can irritate highly sensitive skin.

Did You Know?

Rose is the unanticipated plant with a profound ability to combat serious types of bacteria like MRSA. Yet it's also gentle enough for even the most sensitive skin.

Top Uses

1 Playtime-Ready
Rub on hands, back of neck, and under nose to ward off germs during play with other kids.

2 Cold & Flu
Apply to chest, spine, and bottoms of feet 5x daily.

3 Super Hero Immunity
Apply to bottoms of feet each morning for immune system boost.

4 Zombie Attacks (Bacteria, Virus, Fungus)
Apply 3-5x daily to infected areas.

5 Fatigue
Apply over kidneys and adrenals 2x daily to improve stamina.

6 Inner Circle Friends
Inhale from cupped hands to remember maintaining healthy boundaries and respect in friendships.

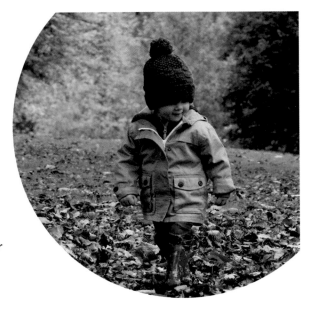

Emotional Use

This blend brings strong heart into social interactions. It helps fortify boundaries of love, promoting a sense of true community.

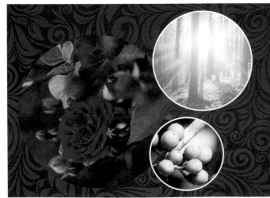

Kiddie Blood Pressure Blend
Kid's Protective Blend
1 drop Lavender

Apply Kid's Protective Blend followed by a drop of Lavender to the bottoms of feet to lower blood pressure, a fast heart rate, and high temperature.

Back to School Immunity
Kid's Protective Blend
1 drop Turmeric

Apply oils to the bottoms of feet before school every day to minimize down-time and stay your strongest.

Kids: Restful Blend

   place sticker *known name*

Application

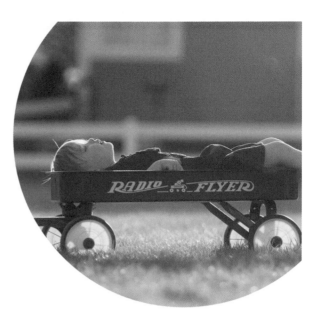

Main Ingredients
Lavender, Cananga, Buddha Wood, Roman Chamomile

Other Uses
Behavioral Disorders, Bee Sting, Crying, Diaper Rash, Hyperactivity, Hyper-pigmentation, Neuralgia, Shock, Spider Bite, Sunburn, Worms

> *"This is my go-to blend when my daughter is fussing. It has a quick soothing effect on her and she enjoys the smell!."*
> -Kaelin

Top *Uses*

1 Easy Sleeping
Apply to bottoms of feet and back of neck 30 minutes before bedtime for an easier time falling asleep.

2 Monsters in the Closet
Apply over chest and wrists to ease nighttime fears.

3 Argument Diffuser
Apply to temples and back of neck to ease contention.

4 Tornado Thoughts
Apply to temples, wrists, and back of neck to soothe runaway and irrational thoughts.

5 Grown-Up Relaxation
Apply liberally to temples and chest before getting into a warm bath to let go of a stressful day of kid's duties.

Emotional Use

The gentle floral aromas of this blend invite purposeful communication. It reminds the wearer to choose words that uplift and edify over words that make you right.

Oil Blends

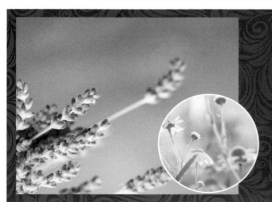

Nightmare Buster

Kid's Restful Blend
1 drop Juniper Berry
1 drop Wild Orange

Apply oils along spine before bed to promote deep, meaningful sleep that's free of nightmares and disturbances.

Chillin' in the Evening

Kid's Restful Blend
1 drop Vetiver

Apply oils to the bottoms of feet after dinner to spend a pleasant and calm evening with the family.

Kids: Soothing Blend

 place sticker _known name_ _____

Application

 A T I

Main Ingredients

Copaiba, Lavender, Spearmint, Zanthoxy-lum

Other Uses

Charley Horse, Growing Pains, Headache, Lethargy, Joint Pain, Muscle Pain, Muscle Tension

Safety

Can irritate sensitive skin. Use with caution during pregnancy.

"I got bumped hard (totally not my fault), and it killed. So we put on the oil. And like by the next morning, I was ready to play hard again. It's awesome."
                                    -Toby

Top *Uses*

1 Battle Wounds
Apply liberally to ease pain and injury that happen with the dangers of being an active kid.

2 Sports Injury
Apply to injured muscles, joints, and connective tissue 5x daily.

3 Bumps & Bruises
Apply every couple hours to reduce the appearance of bruises or bumps.

4 Self-Trust
Apply to the back of neck and temples to remember the power of trusting your good instincts.

5 Stinky Feet
Apply to feet before and after school.

6 Mighty Muscles
Apply to legs, arms, and shoulders as a pre-workout before sports and exercise.

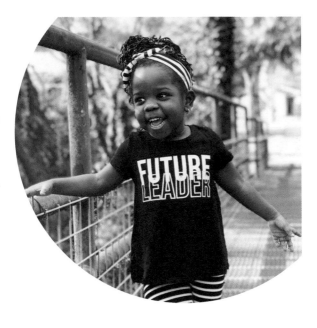

Emotional Use

This blend provides the refresh and reprieve needed for soul-soothing. It turns trouble into a pathway to move forward better and wiser.

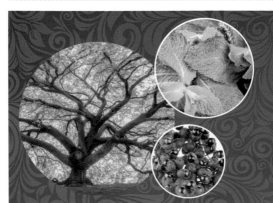

De-Battering Ram

Kid's Soothing Blend
1 drop Helichrysum
Dab of Wintergreen

Apply oils to sore and inflamed muscles after sports or injury. Repeat every few hours until pain is gone.

Crash Remedy

Kid's Soothing Blend
1 drop Marjoram
1 drop Frankincense

Gently apply to severe muscle or tissue injury to promote rapid tissue mend. Repeat every few hours as needed.

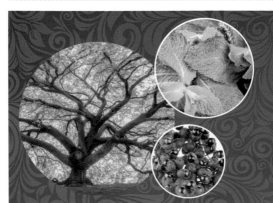

Oil Blends

Massage Blend

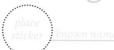

place sticker / known name

Application

A T I

Main Ingredients

Cypress, Peppermint, Marjoram, Basil, Grapefruit, Lavender

Other Uses

Arthritis, Circulation, Ligament Damage, Muscular Dystrophy, Relaxation, Tension

Safety

Can irritate sensitive skin. Use with caution during pregnancy.

Did You Know?

Marjoram and Cypress are a power duo for muscle-mend. They increase circulation and promote faster muscle repair.

Top Uses

1 Muscle Tension & Aches
Massage 2-4 drops with carrier oil into tight muscles.

2 Adrenal Fatigue & Lethargy
Apply 1-2 drops to lower back.

3 Back, Neck, & Shoulder Pain
Massage 2-4 drops with carrier oil into affected muscles, or add to hot bath.

4 Post-Work Stress
Massage 2 drops into back of neck to relieve stress from work.

5 Neuropathy
Apply 1-2 drops to bottoms of feet.

6 High Blood Pressure
Apply 1-2 drops to bottoms of feet.

7 Headache
Apply 1-2 drops to temples, avoiding eyes.

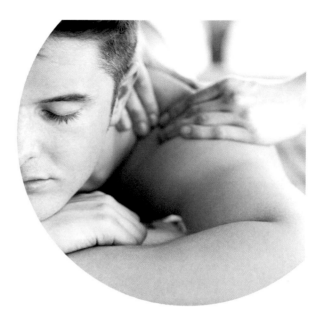

Emotional Use

This blend assists in releasing the tension of the day and shifting into a state of well-deserved relaxation. It opens the mind and heart to the possibility of releasing unnecessary stress.

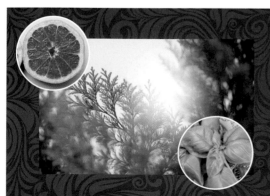

Monday-itis

2 drops Massage Blend
2 drops Lime
2 drops Siberian Fir

Massage oils into neck and shoulders after a long day of work on Mondays to make sure you've got stamina for the remaining week.

Fresh Air Diffuser Blend

3 drops Massage Blend
3 drops Lime
3 drops Grapefruit
1 drop Green Mandarin

Diffuse this blend to clear stale odors from the family area, play room, or anywhere that needs a burst of fresh air.

151

Metabolic Blend

place sticker *known name*

Application

 A   T   I

Main Ingredients
Grapefruit, Lemon, Ginger, Peppermint, Cinnamon

Other Uses
Colds, Congestion, Detox, Energy, Food Addiction, Gallbladder Stones, High Cholesterol, Lymphatic Stimulation, Obesity, Over-Eating

Safety
Can irritate sensitive skin. Use with caution during pregnancy. May cause photosensitivity.

"A new eating plan made me hungry and cranky, and find myself missing chocolate and carbs. After using this blend, I'm now not hungry or cranky, my cravings are gone, and I have even more energy!" -Lou

Top *Uses*

1 Weight Loss
Take 2-4 drops in capsule or drink in water 3-5x daily.

2 Appetite Control
Drink 2-4 drops in water throughout the day, or diffuse.

3 Blood Sugar Regulation
Take 1-2 drops in water or in a capsule.

4 Cellulite & Visceral Fat
Massage several drops with carrier oil into needed areas.

5 Antioxidant
Take 1-2 drops in a capsule.

6 Eating Disorders
Take a drop under the tongue, or diffuse 4-8 drops.

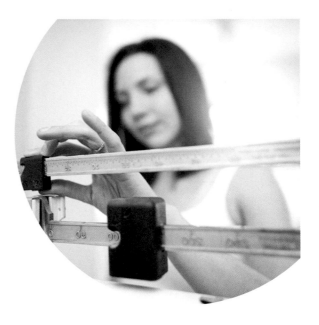

Emotional *Use*

The Metabolic Blend invites the user to release self-criticism, judgment and shame. It turns focus inward where true beauty originates from.

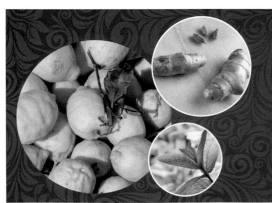

Craving Blaster Smoothie
2-3 drops Metabolic Blend
1 cup mixed greens
1/2 cup frozen strawberries
1 tsp lemon juice
1 cup almond or coconut milk
Pinch of sea salt

Combine ingredients in a high powered blender before lunch time.

Skinny Wrap
10 drops Metabolic Blend
8 drops Cypress
8 drops Grapefruit
5 drops Basil
5 drops Lavender
40 drops FCO

Apply all ingredients to fatty areas and wrap with BPA-free plastic for 60 minutes.

Oil Blends

Outdoor Blend

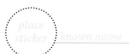

place sticker *known name*

Application

 A   T   I

Main Ingredients

Catnip, Skimmia Laureola, Amyris, Balsam, Orange, White Fir, Eucalyptus, African Sandalwood, Genet, Rose

Other Uses

Ants, Flies, Mites, Mosquitoes, Termites, Tics

"It's that time of year, and this blend is AMAZING! These are the best essential oils for insect and pest repellent."
　　　　　　　　　　　　　　-Jen

"OK. Chemicals are not my favorite, but it's hard to repel mosquitoes without them... Until I found this blend that does it so well! Bye mosquitoes."
　　　　　　　　　　　　　　-Sandy

Top Uses

1 Insect Repellent
Apply directly to exposed skin, and diffuse if possible

2 Fly Infestation
Diffuse 10 drops, or apply lightly over clothing.

3 Energetic Toxicity
Use 1-3 drops during meditation, journaling, or prayer.

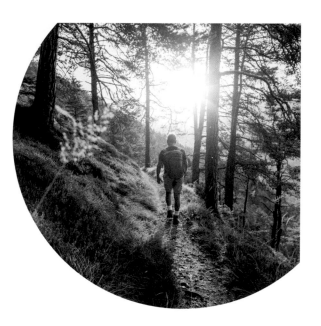

Emotional Use

Just as Outdoor Blend shields you from pests, so can it shield you from relationships or situations where your boundaries may be breached. It lets others be responsible for their energy, and you for yours.

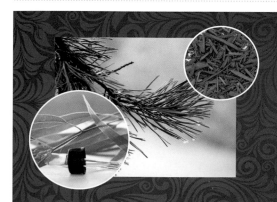

Repellent Booster

4 drops Outdoor Blend
2 drops Arborvitae
2 drops Renewing Blend

Bugs still loving you, even with the Outdoor Blend? Give it a boost with extra Arborvitae and Renewing Blend! Reapply every 5 hours.

Spider Repellent

10 drops Outdoor Blend
10 drops Peppermint
10 drops FCO

Paint bottoms of doorways, ventilation openings, windowsills, and other cracks into the house. Reapply every 1-2 weeks as needed, especially at the beginning of fall.

Protective Blend

Application

A T I

Main Ingredients
Orange, Clove, Cinnamon, Rosemary, Eucalyptus

Other Uses
Autoimmune Disorders, Cough, Germs, Household Cleaning, Hypoglycemia, Laundry Booster, Mold, Pneumonia, Staph Infection, Strep Throat, Warts

Safety
Can irritate sensitive skin. Use with caution during pregnancy.

"My niece uses this blend, along with Melaleuca and Oregano, in a capsule for UTIs. Saves a trip to the doctor."
-Sharon

Top Uses

1 Immune Support
Take 1-2 drops in capsule as daily supplement, or apply to bottoms of feet.

2 Colds & Flu
Apply 1-2 drops to bottoms of feet, and take with water or in a capsule.

3 Airborne Viruses
Diffuse 5-10 drops.

4 Mouthwash
Rinse mouth with 2 drops and water.

5 Cold Sores
Apply a drop with carrier oil to needed areas.

6 MRSA
Apply 1-2 drops diluted to affected areas.

7 Gum Disease & Cavities
Rinse mouth with 2 drops and water.

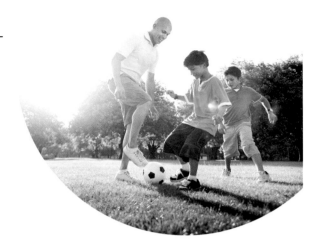

Emotional Use

The protective properties of this blend extend from harmful pathogens to harmful energy. It promotes feelings of being independently capable and strong.

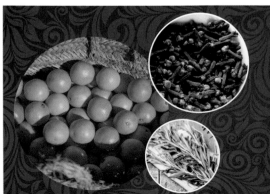

Sanitizing Household Cleaner

10 drops Protective Blend
10 drops Siberian Fir
10 drops Lemon
1 Tbsp white vinegar

Combine oils with white vinegar, then add to 20 oz. glass spray bottle. Shake before use.

Welcome Fall Diffuser Blend

4 drops Protective Blend
2 drops Douglas Fir
2 drops Wild Orange
1 drop Clove

Combine oils in your diffuser for a warm, welcoming aroma that also keeps the family healthy and well.

Oil Blends

Reassuring Blend

place sticker known name

Application

 A T I

Main Ingredients
Vetiver, Lavender, Ylang Ylang, Frankincense, Marjoram, Spearmint, Labdanum

Other Uses
Addictive Personality, Postpartum Recovery, Social Anxiety

Safety
Use with caution during beginning of pregnancy.

"Sometimes I have a lot of stress my life. You never ask for it, but it's there. So I use this blend to calm things down. Just a bit under my nose turns the frenzy into peace and simplicity."

-Cori

Top *Uses*

1 Fear & Insecurity
Apply 1-2 drops over temples or chest.

2 Worry
Inhale 1-2 drops from cupped hands.

3 Restlessness & Irritability
Apply 1-2 drops to temples or bottoms of feet, or diffuse.

4 Sleep Issues
Diffuse 4-8 drops near bedside, or apply 1-2 drops to temples.

5 Focus Issues
Apply 1-2 drops to back of neck or temples.

6 Social Disorders
Inhale 1-2 drops from cupped hands, or rub onto back of neck.

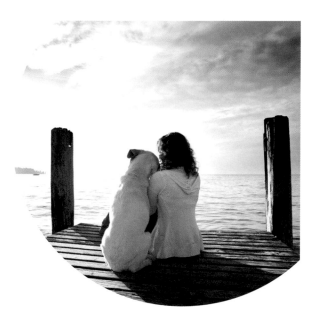

Emotional Use

The peaceful oils in this blend help one move from feeling attacked or controlled by people or life to a place of understanding, lightness, and freedom.

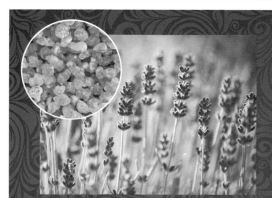

Liquid Anti-Anxiety Roller

10 drops Reassuring Blend
10 drops Grounding Blend
5 drops Vetiver

Combine oils in a 10ml roller bottle and top off with FCO. Apply to pulse points and sides of neck during anxiety attacks.

New Hope Diffuser Blend

3 drops Reassuring Blend
3 drops Grounding Blend
2 drops Bergamot
1 drop Black Pepper

Use this diffuser blend when you need to remember that the best opportunities aren't in the past, but on their way to you.

Renewing Blend

place sticker — known name

Application
 ^A ^T ^I

Main Ingredients
Spruce, Bergamot, Juniper Berry, Myrrh, Arborvitae, Citronella, Thyme, Nootka

Other Uses
Bitterness, Emotional Stagnation, Kidney Stones, Liver Issues, Muscle Pain, Sadness, Shame, Skin Infection

Safety
Can irritate sensitive skin. Avoid sun exposure for 12 hours after topical use.

Did You Know?
Arborvitae and Nootka oils come from sustainable harvesting in British Columbia. The oils are procured from sawdust residue so that not one extra tree is cut down. Even the pulp is recycled into paper.

Top Uses

1 Anger, Resentment, Guilt
Apply 1-2 drops to pulse points, and inhale from cupped hands.

2 Attachment Issues
Apply 1-2 drops to pulse points, and diffuse.

3 Critical Thinking
Apply 1-2 drops to temples and back of neck, and diffuse.

4 Circulation
Apply 2-4 drops to bottoms of feet.

5 Insect Repellent
Apply with carrier oil over exposed skin.

6 Prostate Issues
Apply 1-2 drops over lower abdomen.

7 Irritability
Inhale 1-2 drops from cupped hands.

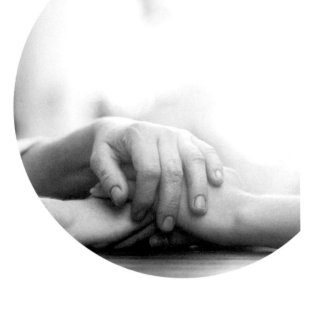

Emotional Use

This oil blend brings the promise of peace that comes with forgiving others and self. It turns resentment and judgment into allowing and acceptance, the two ingredients critical for growth.

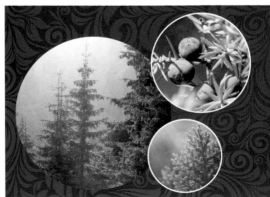

Shame & Guilt Release
2 drops Renewing Blend
2 drops Clary Sage
2 drops Myrrh

Release blockages in your solar plexus by applying these oils to your naval and using the mantra, "I'm sorry. Forgive me. Thank you. I love you."

Raindrop Meadows Diffuser Blend
2 drops Renewing Blend
2 drops Grounding Blend
2 drops Invigorating Blend

This blend brings the feeling of sunshine right after a cleansing rainstorm.

Respiratory Blend

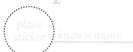

Application

Main Ingredients

Laurel, Eucalyptus, Peppermint, Melaleuca, Lemon, Cardamom, Ravintsara, Ravensara

Other Uses

Constricted Breathing, Emphysema, Exercise-Induced Asthma, Nasal Polyps, Respiratory Infections, Sinusitis, Tuberculosis

Safety

Can irritate sensitive skin. Use with caution during pregnancy.

"I used to suffer from exercise-induced asthma. Now that I have this oil, I can now run more than a mile without an asthma episode!."
                              -Cassi

Top *Uses*

1 Cough, Bronchitis, Pneumonia
Inhale 2-4 drops from cupped hands, and apply diluted over chest.

2 Asthma
Inhale 2-4 drops from cupped hands, and apply to lung reflex points.

3 Cold & Flu
Diffuse 5-10 drops, or apply with carrier oil over chest.

4 Allergies
Apply 1-2 drops over bridge of nose and sinuses, avoiding eyes.

5 Snoring
Apply 1-2 drops over throat and bridge of nose, avoiding eyes.

6 Closed off from Love
Rub a few drops over heart.

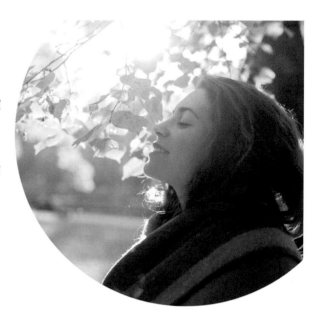

Emotional Use

Rather than being suffocated by sadness or other constricting emotions, this blend helps one exhale that which no longer serves and inhale the support and embrace to make life rich.

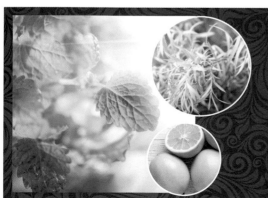

Respiratory Fortifier

2 drops Respiratory Blend
2 drops Protective Blend
2 drops Black Pepper

Combine oils and rub with FCO onto chest and mid back to fight respiratory infections and spastic issues (chronic cough). Use 3-5x daily.

Pollen Relief Diffuser Blend

3 drops Respiratory Blend
3 drops Lavender
2 drops Peppermint
2 drops Lemon

When the trees start blooming and the sneezes start looming, this is the blend to bring relief. Diffuse often.

157

Restful Blend

place sticker / known name

Application

 A T I

Main Ingredients

Lavender, Sweet Marjoram, Chamomile, Ylang Ylang, Sandalwood, Cedarwood, Vetiver, Vanilla

Other Uses

Addictions, Hyperactivity, Insomnia, Lock Jaw, Mental Fatigue, Temporomandibular Joint Disorder (TMJ), Tension

Safety

Use with caution during pregnancy.

"My son with special needs often has a hard time settling down for bed time. A drop on his feet and diffused in his room throughout the night ensures a peaceful and restful sleep for him."

-Thuvan

Top Uses

1 **Sleep Issues**
Apply 1-2 drops to temples and bottoms of feet, and diffuse near bedside.

2 **Stress & Anxiety**
Apply 1-2 drops to pulse points, and inhale from cupped hands.

3 **ADD & ADHD**
Apply 1-2 drops to back of neck, and diffuse.

4 **Itchy Skin**
Apply 1-2 drops with carrier oil to affected areas.

5 **Anger & Restlessness**
Massage 1-2 drops into back of neck.

6 **Hormone Balance & Mood Swings**
Apply 1-2 drops to pulse points, or diffuse.

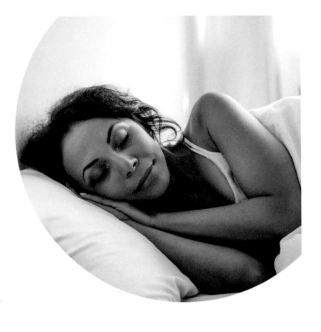

Emotional Use

This oil of tranquility has incredible sedative properties for the mind and heart. It soothes agitation and restlessness to make room for peace, compassion, and connection.

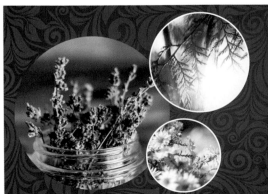

Deep Relief Salt Bath

7 drops Restful Blend
4 drops Soothing Blend
1 cup Epsom Salt
1 cup baking soda

Add ingredients to a hot bath and soak for 20 minutes before bed to soothe fatigued muscles and promote meaningful sleep.

Grounding & Gleeful Diffuser Blend

3 drops Restful Blend
3 drops Lime

When you're not quite ready for bed but also want to ground yourself after a long day, this diffuser blend brings about both serenity and liveliness.

Oil Blends

Skin Clearing Blend

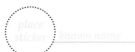

Application

A   T   I

Main Ingredients
Black Cumin, Ho Wood, Melaleuca, Geranium, Eucalyptus, Litsea

Safety
May irritate sensitive skin with continued use.

"I had eczema for about 8 years, and no lotion or steroid helped. It started clearing up within a couple weeks of applying this topical blend to it."

-James

"I love this because it's so easy to put on my face when I have a breakout. It seriously saves me a lot of embarrassment."

-Sophia

Top Uses

1 Acne & Blemishes
Apply directly to areas of concern.

2 Skin Impurities
Rub into skin before washing.

3 Oily Skin
Apply to areas of concern.

4 Eczema & Dermatitis
Apply with carrier oil to affected areas.

5 Bacterial Infection
Apply to affected areas.

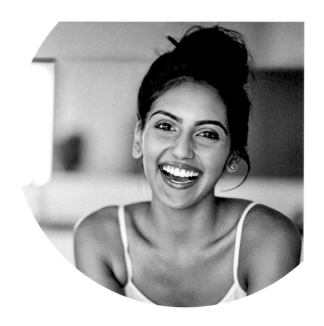

Oil Blends

Emotional Use

This topical blend helps suppressed feelings of anger and blame resolve before they boil to the surface. It's all about understanding the gift of imperfections.

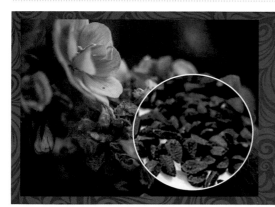

Eczema Salve

10 drops Skin Clearing Blend
10 drops Frankincense
10 drops Melaleuca
15 drops Lavender
5 drops Myrrh
1/2 cup coconut oil
1 Tbsp beeswax pellets
1 Tbsp organic honey

Melt raw ingredients in a double boiler. Let cool slightly, then add the essential oils. Pour into a glass jar.

Breakout Prevention

Skin Clearing Blend
Skin Clearing Face Wash
Skin Clearing Lotion

Wash face first. Then apply a thin layer of Skin Clearing Blend, focusing on blemishes. Wait 5 minutes and then apply lotion.

Soothing Blend

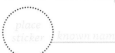
place sticker __known name_____

Application

 A   T   I

Main Ingredients

Wintergreen, Camphor, Peppermint, Blue Tansy, Helichrysum, Blue Chamomile

Other Uses

Back Pain, Bursitis, Frozen Shoulder, Growing Pains, Injured Joints, Tendinitis, Tennis Elbow, Workout (Pre and Post)

Safety

Can irritate sensitive skin. Use with caution during pregnancy.

"After a car accident, my left hip and ribs were very sore and painful. I had no idea essential oils could be anti-inflammatory! I noticed relief within 10 minutes. I'm so grateful!"

-Amy

Top *Uses*

1 Muscle Pain & Inflammation
Massage 2-4 drops with carrier oil or lotion into affected areas.

2 Joint Pain & Arthritis
Apply 1-2 drops to affected areas.

3 Lupus & Fibromyalgia
Apply 1-2 drops with carrier oil when experiencing flare-ups.

4 Whiplash
Apply 2-4 drops to affected areas.

5 Bruises
Gently apply 1-2 drops to bruising.

6 Headache
Apply 1-2 drops to temples and back of neck.

7 Bone Pain
Apply 2-4 drops directly over pain.

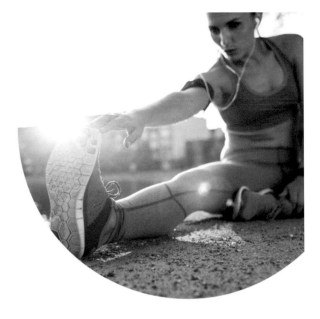

Emotional Use

Sometimes growth is restricted because pain must first be surrendered. This blend encourages the individual to embrace and move through difficulties in order to find the joy that lies beyond pain.

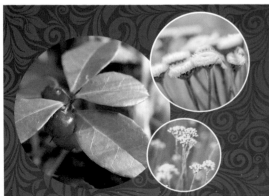

Light Blue Pain Roller

25 drops Soothing Blend
15 drops Frankincense
FCO

Combine oils in a 10ml roller bottle and top off with FCO. Use when straight Soothing Blend is too intense for sensitive tissues.

Pre-Workout Magic

2 drops Soothing Blend
1 drop Lemongrass
2 drops Lime

Apply each oil one at a time and in order to muscle groups before working them out. Massage with carrier oil if needed.

Steadying Blend

Application

 A T I

Main Ingredients

Lavender, Cedarwood, Frankincense, Cinnamon, Sandalwood, Black Pepper, Patchouli

Other Uses

Agitation, Bipolar Disorder, Calming, Courage, Muscle Fatigue, Sleep Issues

Safety

Can irritate sensitive skin. Use with caution during pregnancy.

"As a yoga instructor, you'd think I have it all together all the time. But even yoga instructors need balancing. This blend is so powerful for not only helping with physical balance, but energetic stability too."
— Bernise

Top Uses

1 Seated Meditation, Seated Twist, & Bhu Mudra yoga poses
Apply a couple drops to heels, over ears, and the base of skull.

2 Circulation Issues
Apply 2-4 drops to the bottoms of feet morning and evening.

3 Muscle Spasms
Massage 2-4 drops into the bottoms of feet and into affected muscles.

4 Energetic Focus
Apply a drop to temples and inhale from cupped hands to center your attention.

5 Emotional Numbness
Massage 2-4 drops into sacral area and lower spine.

6 Cracked or Chapped Skin
Massage 2-4 drops with extra FCO into affected areas.

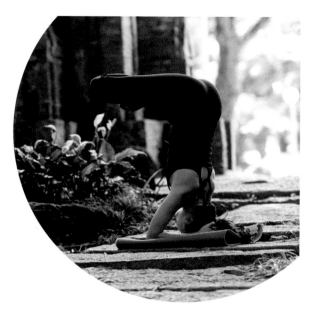

Emotional Use

This is the oil of anchoring to truth. Use this blend to connect to your inner wisdom and what is true to you, independent of social or cultural expectations or changes.

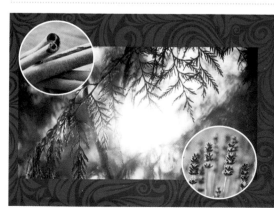

Pranayana Diffuser Blend

2 drops Steadying Blend
2 drops Juniper Berry
2 drops Grapefruit
1 drop Douglas Fir

Use this blend to stabilize upset or agitated emotions while taking deep, intentional breaths.

Anchors Away Diffuser Blend

4 drops Steadying Blend
2 drops Wild Orange
1 drop Yarrow

This diffuser blend encourages steady emotions that still feel fun and playful.

Tension Blend

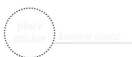

place sticker / known name

Application

Main Ingredients

Wintergreen, Lavender, Peppermint, Frankincense, Cilantro, Marjoram, Chamomile, Rosemary

Other Uses

Alertness, Calming, Inflammation, Muscle Cramps, Swelling

Safety

Can irritate sensitive skin. Use with caution during pregnancy.

"This blend is magic! My daughter and I both suffer from cluster headaches and we both swear by it. As a matter of fact, we don't leave home without it."

-Amy

Top *Uses*

1 Headache & Migraine
Massage into temples and forehead, avoiding eyes.

2 Muscle Tension
Massage into areas of concern.

3 Hot Flashes
Apply to back of neck.

4 Fevers
Apply to back of neck.

5 Bruises
Apply gently over bruises.

6 Hangover
Apply to temples and over stomach.

7 Arthritis
Massage into aching joints.

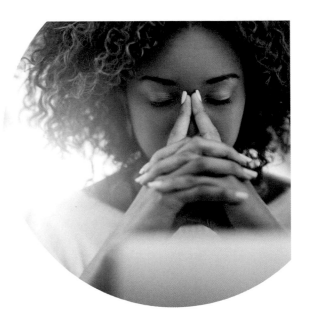

Emotional Use

This blend of relief brings equilibrium and calm where there was nervousness and burnout. It helps relieve stress before it becomes a setback.

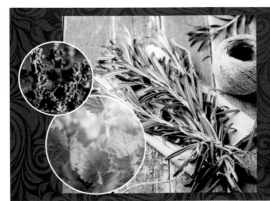

Throbbing Head Relief

Tension Blend
1-3 drops Soothing Blend

Apply tension blend to temples and neck. Then alternate with 1-3 drops of Soothing Blend after 15 minutes. Continue alternating until pain subsides.

Tension in the Past Diffuser Blend

2 drops Tension Blend
2 drops Siberian Fir
1 drop Thyme

This herbaceous diffuser blend helps old patterns of tension and control fall away with ease.

Uplifting Blend

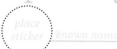

place sticker *known name*

Application

Main Ingredients
Orange, Clove, Star Anise, Lemon Myrtle, Nutmeg, Ginger, Cinnamon, Zdravetz

Other Uses
Digestive Discomfort, Food Addiction, Jaw Pain, Lock Jaw, Low Energy

Safety
Can irritate sensitive skin. Use with caution during pregnancy.

Did You Know?

Spice essential oils are typically high in antioxidants. Application to the bottom of the feet is a great way to eliminate free radicals.

Top *Uses*

1 Gloominess
Inhale 1-2 drops from cupped hands.

2 Self-Sabotage
Apply 1-2 drops over naval, and diffuse.

3 Low Energy
Apply 1-2 drops over adrenals on lower back, and diffuse.

4 Pessimism
Apply 1-2 drops to pulse points, and diffuse.

5 Detoxification
Apply 2-4 drops to bottoms of feet.

6 Emotional Disconnect
Apply 1-2 drops to temples or over heart.

7 Moodiness
Apply 1-2 drops to pulse points, or diffuse.

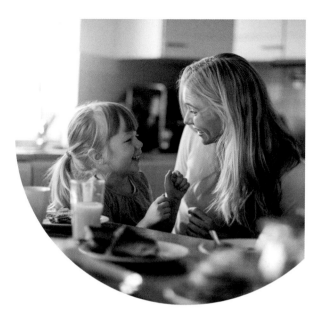

Emotional Use

This oil of cheer and hope is magnetic for optimistic thoughts and laughter. It reminds the soul that fun can happen for no reason other than that life is meant to be cheerful.

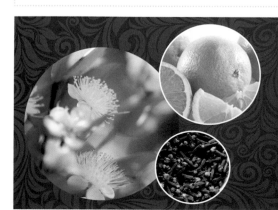

Footprints in the Sand Blend
2 drops Cheer
1 drop Tangerine
1 drop Sandalwood

Use this blend in a diffuser or as a casual cologne/perfume to revisit a happy day at the beach.

Ribbon Candy Diffuser Blend
2 drops Cheer
1 drop Cinnamon
2 drops Cardamom

This blend brings back memories of a favorite childhood treat.

163

Women's Monthly Blend

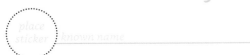

Application

Main Ingredients

Clary Sage, Lavender, Bergamot, Chamomile, Cedarwood, Ylang Ylang, Geranium, Fennel, Carrot Seed, Palmarosa, Vitex

Other Uses

Aphrodisiac, Sedative, Sleep Issues

Safety

Avoid sun exposure for 24 hours after topical use.

> *"I use this on my face every night and it has made the dark circles under my eyes disappear!"*
> -Kimberly

> *"Nothing helps my cramps like this blend."*
> -Lakota

Top *Uses*

1 PMS
Apply to wrists and over lower abdomen.

2 Cramping
Apply to lower abdomen.

3 Hormone Balance
Apply to wrists and over lower abdomen.

4 Hot Flashes
Apply to wrists and back of neck.

5 Mood Swings
Inhale from cupped hands, and apply to pulse points.

6 Self-Confidence
Inhale from cupped hands, and apply to pulse points.

7 Heavy Menstruation
Apply to lower abdomen.

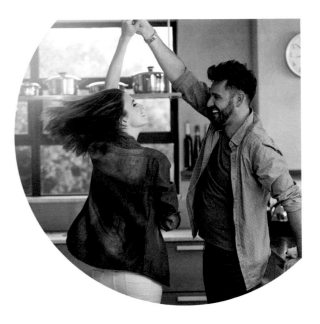

Emotional Use

This oil of vulnerability helps ease fear of rejection and need to constantly meet expectations. It opens a space to feel accepted, nurtured, and enough at any given moment.

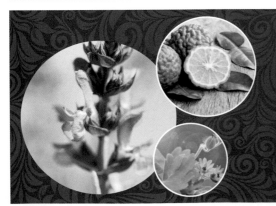

Keep Calm & Clary On Roller

10 drops Women's Monthly Blend
5 drops Tangerine
5 drops Lime
FCO

Combine oils in a 10ml roller bottle and top off with FCO. Use on pulse points to ease emotions during menstruation.

Flirty Purty Diffuser Blend

3 drops Women's Monthly Blend
2 drops Cinnamon
1 drop Melissa

Use this blend to turn an emotionally trying time into something a little fun and sexy.

Oil Blends

Women's Perfume Blend

place sticker *known name*

Application

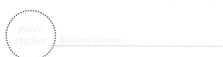

Main Ingredients

Bergamot, Ylang Ylang, Patchouli, Jasmine, Vanilla, Cinnamon, Labdanum, Vetiver, Cocoa, Rose

Other Uses

Loss of Vision, Skin Irritation

Did You Know?

Cocoa absolute oil is a well-known aphrodisiac. Besides being good for feelings of contentment and well-being, it has always been associated with indulgence, love, and sensuality.

Top Uses

1 Perfume
Apply 1-2 drops to pulse points.

2 Hormone Balance
Apply 1-2 drops to pulse points and back of neck.

3 Aphrodisiac
Apply 1-2 drops to neck and wrists.

4 Sedative & Calming
Inhale 1-2 drops from cupped hands.

5 Low Sex Drive
Apply 1-2 drops to pulse points.

6 Menopause
Apply 1-2 drops to pulse points.

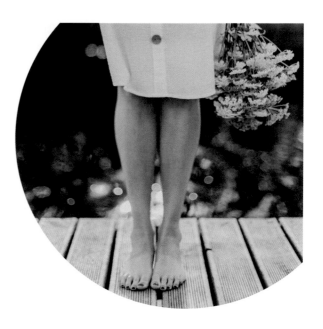

Emotional Use

This blend brings out the best of femininity. Where unexpressed feminine or overtly masculine energy may be a pattern, this blend brings balance to embracing your sexuality.

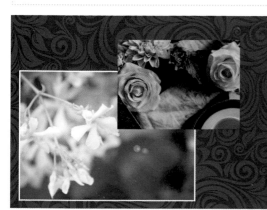

Ladies Night Out Perfume

2 drops Women's Perfume Blend
2 drops Inspiring Blend
1 drop Tangerine

Combine oils and apply to pulse points before a fun night out with the girls.

Woodland Whispers Diffuser Blend

2 drops Women's Perfume Blend
2 drops Siberian Fir
2 drops Invigorating Blend

Indulge yourself with a meditative visit to the woods through this cool and collected blend.

Oil Blends

Section 5

Supplements
& Softgels

Vitality Supplement *Trio*

place sticker *known name* _____

Components
- Cellular Vitality Complex
- Essential Oil + Omegas
- Food Nutrient Complex

Key Uses
- Vitality & Wellness
- Immune System Support
- Pain & Inflammation
- Sleep
- Mood, Depression, Anxiety
- Energy
- Hormone Balance
- Provides bioavailable crucial nutrients to cells for building healthy organs, tissues, and body systems.

Every protocol starts with the trio!

Every ailment and disease has roots in inflammation, and every real solution happens at the cellular level. Essential oil protocols should always include the vitality trio.

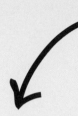

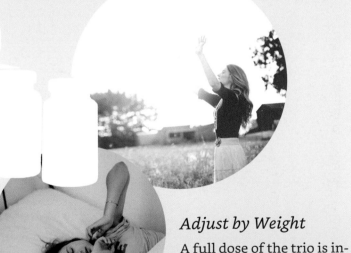

Adjust by Weight

A full dose of the trio is intended for an average-size adult. Try increasing or decreasing dosage for bigger or small body sizes!

Bone Nutrient

place sticker *known name*

Main Ingredients
Calcium (coral calcium), Vitamin C, Vitamin D-2, Biotin, Magnesium, Zinc, Copper, Manganese, Boron

Key Uses
- Promotes Bone Health
- Prevents age-related calcium loss
- Maintains bone mineralization
- Maximizes calcium utilization

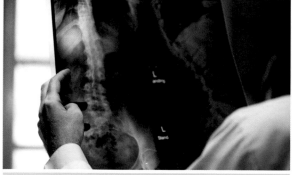

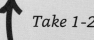 *Take 1-2 capsules twice daily for:*

- Osteoporosis
- Weak bones
- Fragile hips
- Aggressive sports

Cellular Complex Softgel

place sticker *known name*

Main Ingredients
Frankincense, Orange, Lemongrass, Thyme, Summer Savory, Niaouli, Clove

Key Uses
- Aids in elimination of unhealthy cells
- Facilitates DNA repair
- Promotes healthy cellular function
- Useful for cancer, tumors, inflammation, infections, nervous system issues, immune system issues

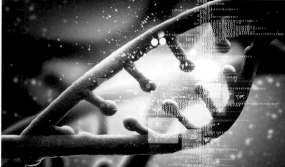

Take 1 softgel 1-3x/day for:

- Cancer prevention
- Lupus & Fibromyalgia
- Genetic disorders
- Damaged DNA repair
- Other auto-immune issues

Cellular Vitality Complex

place sticker *known name*

Main Ingredients
Boswellia Serrata, Scuttelaria Root, Milk Thistle, Pineapple Extract, Polygonum Capsudatum, Turmeric Root, Red Raspberry, Grape Seed, Marigold Flower, Tomato Fruit

Key Uses
- Protects body against free radicals
- Maintains proper cellular function
- Improves cellular vitality & energy
- Reduces inflammation

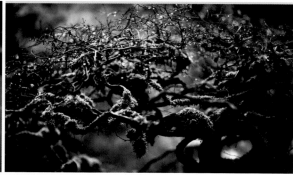

Take 2 twice daily for:

- Food-based nutrition
- Supplementing imperfect diet
- Cellular fuel
- Low energy

Supplements

169

Children's Chewable

place sticker *known name*

Main Ingredients
Vitamins A, C, D, E, B1, B2, B3, B6, B12, B5, Folic Acid, Biotin, Calcium, Iron, Iodine, Magnesium, Zinc, Copper, Manganese, Superfood Blend, Cellular Vitality Blend

Key Uses
• Complete daily nutrient for children
• Food-derived nutrients
• Easy to ingest
• Pairs perfectly with other supplements

Children's Omega-3

place sticker *known name*

Main Ingredients
Fish Oil (EPA, DHA), Vitamin D, Vitamin E, Vitamin C, Orange Essential Oil

Key Uses
• Provides benefits of fish oil without fishy taste
• Easy to take plain, or add to juice
• Supports brain, joint, and cardiovascular development

Children's Probiotic

place sticker *known name*

Main Ingredients
Lactobacillus Rhamnosus, Lactobacillus Salivarius, Lactobaccilus Plantarum LP01 & LP02, Bifidobacterium Breve, Bifidobacterium Lactis

Key Uses
• 5 billion live cells of 6 strains of flora
• Supports healthy digestive, neurological, immune, and brain function
• Shelf-stable unique delivery process
• Special micro-encapsulation protects probiotics until they reach the gut

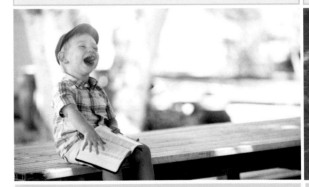

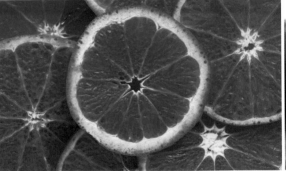

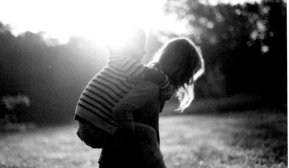

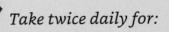

Take twice daily for:
• Supplementing imperfect diet
• Supporting proper development

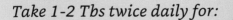

Take 1-2 Tbs twice daily for:
• Heart support
• Brain support & development
• Joint support
• Healthy skin
• Use extra for ADD/ADHD, Autism, and developmental issues

Take twice daily for:
• Healthy immune system
• Proper digestive function
• Healthy mood balance

Supplements

Daily Supplement (Duo)

 place sticker *known name* _____

Main Ingredients
Food Nutrient Complex, Essential Oil + Omegas

Key Uses
- Provides complete daily nutrients derived from whole foods
- Complex omegas without standard preservatives, combined with essential oils
- Bioavailable nutrients to support body systems, organs, and cellular health

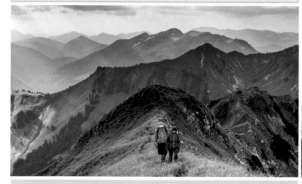

 Take 2 of each bottle twice daily for:
- Cellular fuel & support
- Providing omegas for brain, heart, joint, and integumentary support
- Starting point for other regimens

Detox Herbal Complex

 place sticker *known name* _____

Main Ingredients
Psyllium Seed Husk, Barberry Leaf, Turkish Rhubarb, Kelp, Milk Thistle, Osha Root, Safflower, Acacia Gum, Burdoc Root, Clove, Enzyme Assimilation Complex

Key Uses
- Natural detoxification herbal blend
- Promotes healthy endocrine system
- Promotes toxin filtration
- Complements Detoxification Oil Blend

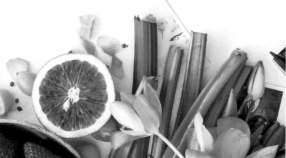

Take 1-3x daily for:
- Liver & kidney issues
- Fatigue
- Toxicity-related acne & skin issues
- Toxicity from medications
- Toxicity from food, air, or other environmental factors

Detoxification Softgels

 place sticker *known name* _____

Main Ingredients
Tangerine, Rosemary, Geranium, Juniper Berry, Cilantro

Key Uses
- Endocrine Support
- Promotes release of toxins
- Hormone Balance
- Antioxidant
- Stimulates adrenals
- Cleanses filtration organs

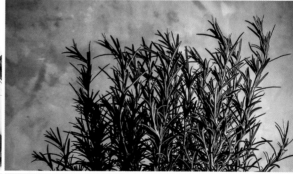

Take 1-3x daily for:
- Complementing the Detox Herbal Complex
- Adrenal fatigue
- Parasites

Digestion Comfort Tablets

place sticker *known name* _____

Main Ingredients
Calcium Carbonate, Ginger, Fennel, Coriander, Peppermint, Tarragon, Anise, Caraway

Key Uses
• Soothes GI discomfort
• Relieves heartburn and indigestion
• Relieves sour stomach
• Reduces belching and bloating

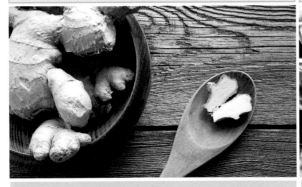

Take 1-2 as needed for:
• Excessive gas
• Stinky gas
• Diarrhea
• Gurgling stomach
• Acid reflux

Digestive Enzymes

place sticker *known name* _____

Main Ingredients
Protease, Amylase, Lipase, Alpha Galactosidase, Cellulase, Maltase, Sucrase, Tummy Taming Blend, Enzyme Assimilation Blend

Key Uses
• Facilitates breakdown of food
• Increases nutrient absorption
• Promotes comfortable digestion
• Increases usability of nutrients
• Facilitates proper gut function

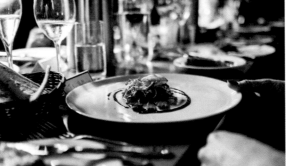

Take 1-3x daily with meals for:
• Digestive comfort after eating out
• Increasing nutrient absorption
• Gluten sensitivities
• Lactose sensitivities
• Restoring proper digestive function

Digestive Blend Softgels

place sticker *known name* _____

Main Ingredients
Ginger, Peppermint, Tarragon, Fennel, Caraway, Coriander, Anise

Key Uses
• Soothes digestive discomfort
• Reduces gas and flatulence
• Reduces nausea
• Reduces diarrhea and constipation

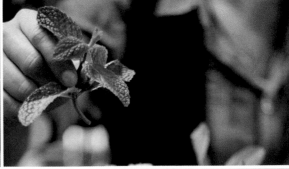

Take 1-3 as needed (up to 5-8 daily) for:
• Queasiness
• Motion sickness
• Stomach upset
• Diarrhea & constipation
• Heartburn

Energy & Stamina Complex

place sticker *known name*

Main Ingredients
Acetyl-L-Carnitine, Alpha-Lipolic Acid, Co-enzyme Q10, Lychee Fruit, Green Tea Leaf, Quercetine Dihydrate, Cordyceps Mycelium, Ginseng, Ashwagandha

Key Uses
- Increases cellular energy
- Improves micro-circulation
- Stimulates mitochondria
- Improves stamina

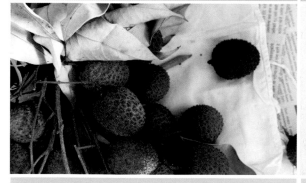

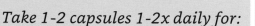
Take 1-2 capsules 1-2x daily for:
- Low energy
- Pre-workout
- Exhaustion
- Cold extremities
- Endurance

Essential Oil + Omegas

place sticker *known name*

Main Ingredients
Fish Oil (EPA DHA), Astaxanthin, Flaxseed Oil, Borage Seed Oil, Cranberry Seed Oil, Pomegranate Seed Oil, Vitamin D

Key Uses
- Promotes heart, brain, joint, eye, skin, and circulatory health
- Protects against lipid oxidation
- Molecularly filtered fish oil combined with internal dose of 9 essential oils

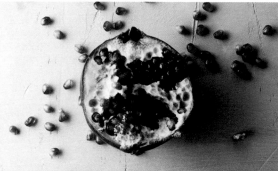

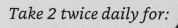
Take 2 twice daily for:
- Brain support
- Depression, Anxiety, & ADD/ADHD
- Heart support
- Joint support
- Healthier skin

Food Nutrient Complex

place sticker *known name*

Main Ingredients
Vitamins A, C, D, E, K, B6, B12, Thiamin, Riboflavin, Niacin, Folate, Biotin, Pantothenic Acid, Calcium, Iron, Iodine, Magnesium, Zinc, Selenium, Copper, Manganese

Key Uses
- Whole-food comprehensive vitamin and mineral nutrient
- Provides bioavailable crucial nutrients to body systems, organs, and cells

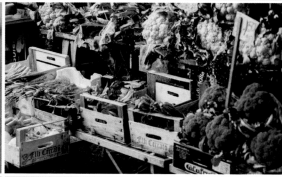

Take 2 twice daily for:
- Sustainable energy
- Fuel for your cells & body systems
- Supplementing more veggies & fruits into your diet

Supplements

Fruit & Veggie Drink Mix

place sticker *known name* _____

Main Ingredients
Kale, Dandelion, Collard Greens, Wheat Grass, Alfalfa, Barley Grass, Goji Berry, Mangosteen, Lemon & Ginger Oil

Key Uses
- Provides essential nutrients
- Supports Immune Health
- Supports Digestive Health
- Supports Weight Loss
- All natural ingredients

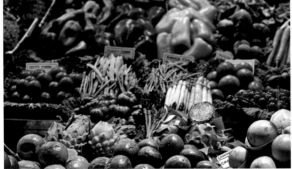

Use 1-2 servings daily for:
- Supplementing low produce consumption
- Higher energy
- Enhancing smoothies & juices
- Better nutrition while traveling

GI Cleansing Complex

place sticker *known name* _____

Main Ingredients
Caprylic Acid; Oregano, Melaleuca, Lemon, Lemongrass, and Thyme Oils

Key Uses
- Helps rid gut of parasites, Candida, and other harmful agents
- Supports healthy digestive environment
- Helps improve microbial balance

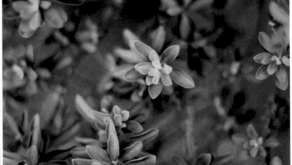

Take 1 capsule with each meal (no more than 10 days*) for:

- Candida & parasite cleanse
- Removing biofilm in gut

* Begin with 1 capsule/day. Work your way up to 3.

Phytoestrogen Complex

place sticker *known name* _____

Main Ingredients
Soy Extract (64% isoflavones, 50% Genistein), Flaxseed Extract (40% Lignan), Pomegranate Extract (40% Ellagic Acid)

Key Uses
- Promotes hormone balance by blocking estrogen binding to cells
- Manages harmful metabolite byproducts of hormone metabolism

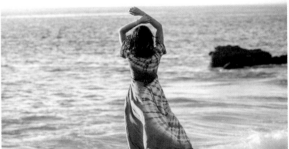

Take 1-2 capsules daily for:
- Pre-menopausal hormone balance (take 1-2)
- Post-menopausal hormone balance (take 2)

Polyphenol Complex

place sticker *known name*

Main Ingredients
Frankincense Extract, Turmeric, Ginger, Green Tea Extract, Pomegranate Extract, Grape Seed Extract, Resveratrol

Key Uses
- Reduces inflammation and pain
- Provides relief to tension headaches, as well as back, neck, and shoulder pain
- Antioxidant support
- Internal complement to Soothing Blend

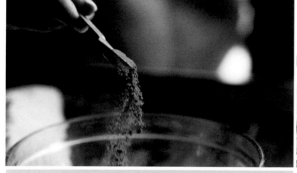

Take 1-3 daily for:
- Chronic pain (take 2 twice daily)
- Headaches & migraines (take 3)
- Lupus, Fibromyalgia, and other inflammatory issues (take 2 twice daily)
- Post-workout recovery

Probiotic Complex

place sticker *known name*

Main Ingredients
L. acidophilus, B. lactis, L. salivarius, L. casei, B. longum, B. bifidum

Key Uses
- 6 billion CFUs
- Supports digestive & immune systems
- Unique double-encapsulated delivery
- Shelf stable with prebiotics to sustain probiotics
- Helps digestion of food nutrients

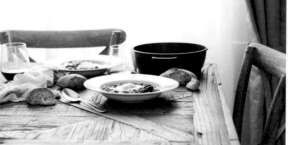

 Take 1-3x daily for:
- Healthy immune system
- Replenishing flora after antibiotics
- Hormone balance
- Proper digestive functions
- Higher absorption rates than other probiotic delivery forms

Protective Blend Softgels +

place sticker *known name*

Main Ingredients
Clove, Wild Orange, Black Pepper, Cinnamon, Eucalyptus, Oregano, Rosemary, Melissa

Key Uses
- Supercharged Protective Blend
- Combats viral and bacterial infections
- Supports immune system

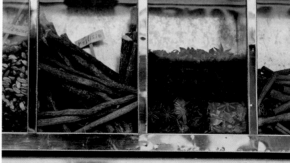

Take 1-2 softgels as needed for:
- Combating cold & flu
- Preventing illness
- Immune system boost
- Antioxidant support

Restful Complex

place sticker *known name* _____

Main Ingredients
Lavender, L-theanine, Lemonbalm, Passion Flower, Chamomile

Key Uses
- Promotes falling asleep faster
- Supports more meaningful sleep
- Promotes waking up feeling refreshed

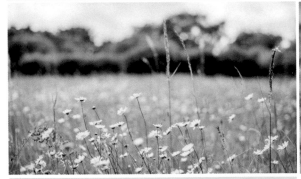

↑ *Take 2 30 minutes before bed for:*

- Falling asleep more easily
- Waking feeling more refreshed
- Use in addition to Restful essential oil blend (diffuse & rub 2 drops on bottoms of feet)

Seasonal Blend Softgels

place sticker *known name* _____

Main Ingredients
Lemon, Lavender, & Peppermint Essential Oils

Key Uses
- Reduces histamine response
- Opens airways
- Relieves itchiness
- Eases sinus congestion
- Useful for seasonal and pet allergies

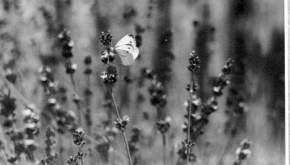

↑ *Take 1-2 as needed:*

- Hayfever
- Pet allergies
- Constricted airways

* *Let 1 softgel dissolve under the tongue for faster results.*

Trim Shake

place sticker *known name* _____

Main Ingredients
Whey & Egg White Protein, Fiber Blend, Stevia, Annatto, Ashwagandha, Potato Protein, Trim Complex

Key Uses
- Meal replacement shake
- Reduces cortisol levels to reduce fat retention
- Manages appetite and cravings
- Healthy protein-carb-fat ratio

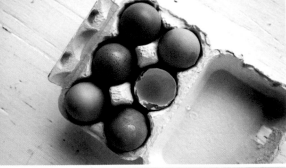

↑ *Use 1-2 servings daily for:*

- Enhanced appetite control
- Weight loss program support
- Smoothie & shake enhancement
- Added protein for diets

Section 6

Ailment
Protocols

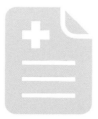

How to Use *Ailment Protocols*

While using plant-based medicine to remedy a health challenge is very much an individual process, this chapter offers protocols that provide more specific direction.

Each protocol gives detailed instructions on which essential oils and supplements to use, including dosage, frequency, and duration.

It is recommended that you use the protocols as they are written in order to achieve the best results. Consistency creates greatest impact.

How to Stay Consistent

- Set recurring reminders in your phone
- Place your oils and supplements where you'll see them
- Take products you need when you leave the house
- Commit to fully experiencing the protocol

Safety & Dosage

These protocols are not intended to replace instruction or care from your physician. Consult your physician before changing medications or other prescribed routines.

If the recommended dosage of oils or supplements feels off to you, adjust how much you're using. Certain protocols suggest using oils internally. The maximum recommended daily limit is *12-24 drops* for adults, and *3-12 drops* for children. Listen to your body.

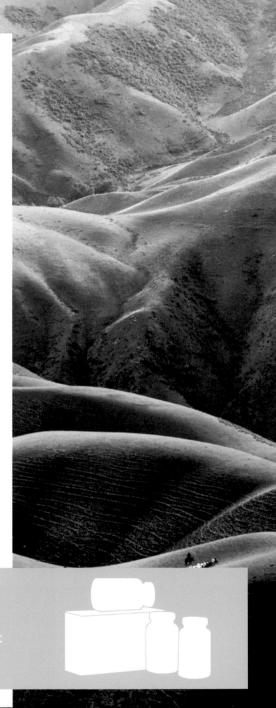

Build from the *Trio*

The Vitality Supplement Trio is recommended as the basis for all protocols. Every health challenge will involve at least one of the main focuses of the Trio: *Inflammation, Immune Response, Energy, and Hormones.*

Protocols

Acid Reflux

Condition in which acidic gastric fluid is regurgitated into the esophagus.

Description
Improves the integrity of gut cell junctions and repairs the intestinal mucosa. Doing so will reduce the symptoms of acid reflux.

Suggested Duration
3-6 months

Digestive Blend (1), **Turmeric** (1), **Yarrow** (2)
Combine oils in an empty capsule and take 3x daily on an empty stomach.

Apply a drop of each to upper abdomen 3x daily at the same time the capsule is taken.

Digestive Blend Softgels
Take 2 capsules with food.

Notes
Additional Support
- Probiotic Complex (take 2 capsules 2x daily on an empty stomach)
- Digestive Enzymes (take 1 capsule with each meal)

Acne (bacteria)

Inflamed sebaceous glands and pimples due to bacteria trapped in pores.

Description
Combats bacterial overgrowth that becomes trapped in pores.

Suggested Duration
Ongoing

Skin Clearing Blend
Apply a small amount evenly over clean skin after showering daily.

Melaleuca & Lavender
Apply a dab to blemishes.

Frankincense
Apply a dab to healing blemishes to prevent scarring.

Notes
Additional Support
- Anti-Aging Blend
- Helichrysum

Acne (hormones)

Inflamed sebaceous glands and pimples due to hormonal imbalance.

Description
Balances hormone production and maintenance throughout the body, including the gut.

Suggested Duration
Until desired appearance is achieved, then as needed

Vitality Supplement Trio
Take 2 of each supplement twice daily.

Phytoestrogen Complex
Take 1 capsule with each dose of Vitality Supplements (for men and women).

Clary Sage
Rub 1 drop on pulse points before bed.

Skin Clearing Blend
Apply a small amount to blemishes daily as needed.

Notes
Additional Support
- Melaleuca
- Helichrysum

Acne (toxicity)

Outbreak occurring when the skin is used to eliminate toxins from the body.

Description
Alleviates toxicity overload by detoxing organs and skin.

Suggested Duration
3-5 weeks

Detoxification Softgels
Take 1 softgel with each meal.

Detox Herbal Complex
Take 1 capsule with breakfast and dinner.

Cellular Complex Softgels
Take 1 softgel with each meal.

Skin Clearing Blend
Apply small amount to blemishes daily as needed.

Notes
Additional Support
- GI Cleansing Complex
- Helichrysum
- Detoxification Blend (use on bottoms of feet)

ADD/ADHD

Behavioral disorder with symptoms of poor concentration and hyperactivity.

Description

Designed to activate the parasympathetic nervous system and induce a more calm and focused mental state.

Suggested Duration

6 months, then as needed

Vetiver, Frankincense, Rose

Apply 1-2 drops of each oil to back of neck, spine and bottoms of feet 2x daily.

Focus Blend

Carry in your pocket, and roll a small amount on back of neck as needed for focus.

Probiotic Complex

Take 2 capsules in the morning on an empty stomach.

Notes

Additional Support
- Ylang Ylang
- Sandalwood
- Siberian Fir
- Roman Chamomile

Adrenal Fatigue

Stress-related deterioration of adrenal glands' ability to produce hormones.

Description

Supports healthy adrenal function.

Suggested Duration

4-8 weeks

Lemon (8), **Basil** (3), **Rosemary** (3), **Frankincense** (3)

Combine in roller bottle. Fill the rest with carrier oil. Massage into neck and kidneys daily as often as needed.

Rosemary & Peppermint

Breathe a drop of each from cupped hands, or diffuse for energy as needed.

Vitality Supplement Trio

Take 2 of each bottle 2x daily.

Energy & Stamina Complex

Take 2 capsules 2x daily.

Notes

Additional Support
- Invigorating Blend
- Detoxification Blend

AIDS/HIV

Sexually transmitted retrovirus that can become autoimmune dysfunction.

Description

Provides emotional support, promotes a properly functioning immune system.

Suggested Duration

6 months, then as needed

Cellular Complex Blend

Rub 3-5 drops onto spine morning & night.

Cellular Complex Softgels

Take 2 softgels 3x daily.

Vitality Supplement Trio

Take 2 of each bottle 2x daily.

Protective Blend & Melissa

Rub 2 drops each on bottoms of feet 2x daily.

Joyful Blend

Carry with you, and inhale from hands for emotional support throughout the day.

Notes

Additional Support
- Helichrysum
- Pink Pepper
- Detoxification Blend

Allergies (food)

Abnormal immune response to certain foods.

Description

Lowers histamine response triggered by food allergies and creates calm in the gut.

Suggested Duration

4 weeks to begin, then as needed

Lavender

Put 1 drop under tongue. Drink water after 30 seconds.

Probiotic Complex

Take 1 capsule 3x daily on an empty stomach.

Polyphenol Complex

Take 1 capsule 3x daily.

Digestive Enzyme Complex

Take 1 with each meal.

Notes

Additional Support
- Do a 14-day bone broth cleanse
- Detox Herbal Complex
- Detoxification Blend

Protocols

Allergies (seasonal/pet) *Overreaction of the immune system to ordinarily harmless substances.*

Description
Reduces histamine response and boosts immune response.

Suggested Duration
4-8 weeks, then as needed

Lemon, Lavender, Peppermint
Put 1 drop each under tongue. Drink water after 30 seconds.

Respiratory Blend
Inhale from cupped hands when experiencing attack.

Probiotic Complex
Take 1 capsule 3x daily on an empty stomach.

Protective Blend
Gargle 2 drops with water nightly, then swallow.

Notes
Additional Support
• Seasonal Blend Softgels
• Siberian Fir
• Vitality Supplement Trio

Allergies (skin) *Hypersensitivity to typically harmless substances that come in contact with skin.*

Description
Calms irritation due to skin contact with allergens.

Suggested Duration
As needed

Lavender, Helichrysum, Frankincense, Lemon
Combine 10 drops of each in a roller bottle. Fill the rest with carrier oil. Roll onto affected area often.

Lavender
Put a drop under tongue. Drink water after 30 seconds.

Probiotic Complex
Take 1 capsule 3x daily on an empty stomach.

Notes
Additional Support
• Detox Herbal Complex
• Detoxification Blend

Alzheimer's *Progressive mental deterioration due to degeneration of the brain.*

Description
Supports healthy mental activity, boosts alertness.

Suggested Duration
Ongoing

Vitality Supplement Trio
Take 2 of each bottle 2x daily.

Cellular Complex Blend
Rub 3-5 drops along spine and bottoms of feet 3x daily.

Cellular Complex Softgels
Take 1 softgel 3x daily.

Peppermint & Rosemary
Massage a drop each into scalp and diffuse several drops daily to increase alertness & memory.

Notes
Additional Support
• Cilantro
• Frankincense
• Extra Omega Complex
• Grounding Blend

Anxiety *Condition of worry, nervousness, or unease.*

Description
Increases a general calming state due to the interaction of oils with neurotransmitters.

Suggested Duration
3 months, then as needed

Roman Chamomile, Lavender, Vetiver
Apply a drop of each to back of neck, spine, and bottoms of feet 3x daily.

Focus Blend
Apply to temples and sides of neck 3x daily.

Probiotic Complex
Take 2 capsules in the morning on an empty stomach.

Magnolia
Roll over back of neck 3x daily and as needed.

Notes
Additional Support
• Frankincense
• Rose
• Sandalwood

Arthritis

Painful inflammation and stiffness of the joints.

Description
Decreases the inflammatory response within the joint tissues.

Suggested Duration
6 months, then as needed

Copaiba, Turmeric, Frankincense
Apply a drop of each to affected areas 3x daily.

Soothing Blend
Massage lotion into affected areas after above oils 3x daily.

Polyphenol Complex
Take 2 capsules in the evening with food.

Notes

Additional Support
• Marjoram
• Lemongrass
• Wintergreen
• Myrrh

Asperger's

Developmental disorder impacting social interactions and communication.

Description
Increases the integrity of the gut lining and promote brain health.

Suggested Duration
1 to 3 years

Frankincense, Vetiver, Turmeric, Clary Sage
Apply a drop of each to back of neck and bottoms of feet 3x daily.

Cellular Complex
Apply 2 drops to spine 3x daily.

Focus Blend
Apply roller blend to temples and sides of neck 3x daily.

Probiotic Complex
Take 2 capsules in the morning on an empty stomach.

Notes

Additional Support
• Digestive Softgels (2x daily)
• Restful Complex (2 at bedtime)
• Yarrow (under the tongue)
• Lavender
• Sandalwood

Asthma

Respiratory condition marked by spasms in the bronchi of the lungs.

Description
Promotes open airways and easy breathing.

Suggested Duration
As needed

Respiratory Blend
Inhale 2 drops from cupped hands during attacks.

Lavender
Massage a drop behind and over ears to promote calm.

Cardamom
Gargle a drop for 30 seconds, then swallow as needed.

Probiotic Complex
Take 1 capsule 2x daily.

Notes

Additional Support
• Rosemary
• Siberian Fir
• Eucalyptus

Autism

Developmental disorder impacting social interactions and communication.

Description
Increases the integrity of the gut lining and promotes brain health.

Suggested Duration
1 to 3 years

Frankincense, Vetiver, Turmeric, Clary Sage
Apply a drop of each diluted to back of neck and bottoms of feet 3x daily.

Cellular Complex & Rose
Apply 2 drops each diluted to spine 2x daily.

Probiotic Complex
Take 2 capsules in the morning on an empty stomach.

Lavender, Melaleuca, Frankincense, Digestive Blend, Copaiba
Roll diluted clockwise over stomach 2x daily.

Digestive Enzymes
Take 1 capsule with each meal.

Notes

Additional Support
Digestive Softgels (2x daily)
• Restful Complex (2 at bedtime)
• Yarrow (under the tongue)

Auto-Immune

Condition in which the immune system turns on healthy cells.

Description

Induces the parasympathetic nervous system, eliminates antigens and latent infections, and reduces the immune response.

Suggested Duration

1 to 3 years

Frankincense, Yarrow, Turmeric, Clary Sage
Apply a drop of each to back of neck and bottoms of feet 2x daily.

Cellular Complex
Apply 2-4 drops to spine 2x daily. Also take 2 softgels 2x daily.

Detoxification Blend
Apply 2 drops to sides of neck 2x daily.

Probiotic Complex
Take 2 capsules in the morning on an empty stomach.

Notes

Additional Support
• Vitality Supplement Trio
• Copaiba
• Sandalwood
• Detox Herbal Complex
• Restful Complex

Back Pain

Inflammation and pain in the back due to injury, aging, or other issues.

Description

Increases circulation, reduces scar tissue, promotes healing.

Suggested Duration
6-12 months

Frankincense, Turmeric, Copaiba
Take a drop of each in a capsule or under the tongue 3x daily.

Polyphenol Complex
Take 2 capsules 2x daily on an empty stomach.

Marjoram, Frankincense, Lemongrass, Siberian Fir, Soothing Blend (lotion)
Apply a drop of each onto spine and painful areas 3x daily.

Notes

Additional Support
• Yarrow
• Sandalwood
• Wintergreen
• Fennel

Bipolar Disorder

Mood disorder resulting in mania, depression, and psychotic issues.

Description

Normalizes brain activity and regulates nervous system.

Suggested Duration
12 months

Frankincense, Vetiver, Turmeric, Clary Sage
Apply a drop of each to back of neck and bottoms of feet 2x daily.

Cellular Complex
Apply 2-4 drops to spine 2x daily.

Probiotic Complex
Take 2 capsules in the morning on an empty stomach.

Grounding Blend
Carry throughout the day and apply to temples as needed.

Notes

Additional Support
• Siberian Fir
• Rosemary
• Cedarwood
• Sandalwood
• Lavender

Blood Pressure (high)

Hypertension resulting unhealthy pressure on artery walls.

Description

Regulates blood pressure by dilation of blood vessels and reducing the viscosity of the blood.

Suggested Duration
6-12 months

Cypress, Marjoram, Ylang Ylang, Lemon
Apply a drop of each over the chest and bottom of feet 2x daily.

Marjoram, Ylang Ylang, Lemon, Yarrow
Take 2 drops each in a capsule 2x daily.

Notes

Additional Support
• Clary Sage
• Lavender
• Cellular Complex

Bone Spurs

New bone material that develops along the edges of existing bones.

Description
Alleviates agitation of surrounding tissue and decreased functionality by decreasing pain and inflammation.

Suggested Duration
2-3 months

Frankincense & Turmeric
Massage a drop of each into affected area 3x daily.

Soothing Blend
Massage lotion into affected areas after above oils 3x daily.

Cellular Complex Softgels
Take 2 softgels or apply 2 drops oil onto spine 3x daily.

Notes

Additional Support
• Rosemary
• Yarrow
• Wintergreen
• Eucalyptus

Bronchitis

Inflammation of the mucous membrane in the bronchial tubes.

Description
Increases immune response to address possible infections and open the airways for symptomatic relief.

Suggested Duration
1-2 weeks

Cardamom, Black Pepper, Rosemary, Lime
Apply drop of each to chest and bottoms of feet 3-5x daily.

Respiratory Blend
Diffuse several drops; inhale 2 drops from cupped hands as needed.

Protective Blend Softgels +
Take 2 softgels 2x daily until symptoms subside.

Notes

Additional Support
• Arborvitae
• Oregano
• Melissa
• Eucalyptus

Calluses

Thickened or hardened part of the skin due to excess friction.

Description
Softens thickened skin for easy removal.

Suggested Duration
1-2 weeks

Melaleuca, Peppermint, Roman Chamomile
Apply a drop each to callused area 3x daily for 3 days.

After 3 days place feet in a cold water soak with 10 drops of each and use a pumice stone to remove the calluses.

Notes

Additional Support
• Oregano
• Basil
• Rosemary
• Lavender

Cancer

Neoplastic mass composed of abnormal cell growth resulting in a complex disease.

Description
Increases the immune response and slows the growth of abnormal cell proliferation.

Suggested Duration
1-3 years

Cellular Complex
Apply 2-4 drops to back of neck, spine, and bottoms of feet 4x daily.

Frankincense, Sandalwood, Turmeric, Lemongrass
Take a drop of each in a capsule 4x daily.

Detoxification Blend
Apply 2 drops diluted to sides of neck 3x daily.

Probiotic Complex
Take 2 capsules in the morning on an empty stomach.

Notes

Additional Support
• Detoxification Blend Softgels
• Detox Herbal Complex
• Digestive Blend Softgels
• Vitality Supplement Trio

Protocols

185

Cancer (Leukemia)
Malfunction of white blood cells in the body's blood. Often affects the bone marrow and lymphatic system.

Description
Improves the immune response and reduces a hyperactive immune system.

Suggested Duration
1-3 years

Cellular Complex
Apply 2-4 drops to back of neck, spine, and bottoms of feet 4x daily.

Frankincense, Sandalwood, Turmeric, Lemongrass
Take a drop of each in a capsule 4x daily.

Detoxification Blend
Apply 2 drops diluted to sides of neck 3x daily.

Probiotic Complex
Take 2 capsules in the morning on an empty stomach.

Notes
Additional Support
• Detoxification Blend Softgels
• Detox Herbal Complex
• Digestive Blend Softgels
• Vitality Supplement Trio

Candida
Fungal infection often caused by the overuse of antibiotics. Occurs frequently as vaginal yeast infections skin infections and oral thrush.

Description
Combats fungus overgrowth in gut, restores healthy flora.

Suggested Duration
2-3 months

Melaleuca, Lavender, Thyme, Clove
Dilute with a carrier oil and apply a drop of each to vaginal area 6x daily. (Follow the same protocol if infection is on the face or body.)

Probiotic Complex
Take 2 capsules in the morning and evening on an empty stomach.

Digestive Blend
2 softgels 2x daily after food.

Notes
Additional Support
• Arborvitae
• Yarrow
• Green Mandarin

Canker Sores
Viral infection that often occurs in the mouth but can also affect the lips.

Description
Decreases the expression of the virus and maintains a preventative regimen.

Suggested Duration
2-4 weeks

Melaleuca, Oregano, Clove
Dilute a drop each with FCO and apply directly to canker sore. Hold in mouth for 3 minutes. Apply 6x daily.

Combine 3 drops each to 20 drops of carrier oil and swish for 2 minutes daily for ongoing prevention.

Probiotic Complex
Take 2 capsules in the morning and evening on an empty stomach.

Protective Blend Softgels +
Take 2 softgels 2x daily.

Notes
Additional Support
• Digestive Blend Softgels
• Thyme

Celiac's
Autoimmune disorder affecting the small intestine.

Description
Promotes nutrient absorption, calms digestive system.

Suggested Duration
Ongoing

Digestive Enzymes
Take 2-3 capsules with meals.

Probiotic Complex
Take 2 capsules morning and evening on an empty stomach.

Digestive Blend
Rub on outside of stomach at onset of pain.

Metabolic Blend Softgels
Take 1-2 softgels 2-3x daily.

Notes
Additional Support
• Cinnamon
• Grapefruit
• Frankincense

Cholesterol (high)

Excess lipid molecules found in the blood, often the contributing cause of heart disease and heart attacks.

Description
Reduces the amount of cholesterol in the blood to prevent the formation of clots that may lead to heart conditions.

Suggested Duration
6-12 months

Yarrow, Rosemary, Frankincense
Take 2 drops each in a capsule 2x daily.

Vitality Trio
Take 2 of each bottle 2x daily.

Cellular Complex
Apply 2-4 drops to bottoms of feet 2x daily.

Probiotic Complex
Take 2 capsules morning and evening on an empty stomach.

Notes

Additional Support
• Digestive Blend Softgels
• Turmeric
• Lavender

Cold Sores

Inflamed blister in or near the mouth caused by herpes simplex virus.

Description
Combats viral infection, and promotes skin healing and pain relief.

Suggested Duration
As needed

Melaleuca & Melissa
Apply a drop of each diluted several times a day to combat the virus.

Helichrysum
Apply a drop diluted at night to help tissue heal.

Probiotic Complex
Take 2 capsules in the morning on an empty stomach.

Notes

Additional Support
• Arborvitae
• Black Pepper
• Protective Blend
• Frankincense

Colds (common)

Respiratory infection resulting in excess mucus, cough, and sinus issues.

Description
Provides antiviral and respiratory support.

Suggested Duration
5-10 days

Protective Blend Softgels +
Take 2 softgels 3x daily.

Protective Blend, Black Pepper, Melaleuca
Rub 2 drops each on bottoms of feet 3x daily.

Respiratory Blend
Rub onto chest and diffuse as needed.

Vitality Supplement Trio
Take 2 of each bottle 2x daily.

Notes

Additional Support
• Rosemary
• Cardamom
• Lime
• Litsea
• Energy & Stamina Complex

Constipation

Difficulty emptying bowels, usually associated with hardened feces.

Description
Stimulates proper digestive function and elimination.

Suggested Duration
2-3 months, then as needed

Digestive Enzymes
Take 2-3 capsules with meals.

Probiotic Complex
Take 2 capsules morning and evening on an empty stomach.

Clary Sage & Petitgrain
Rub 2-3 drops over stomach in a clockwise motion 3x daily.

Notes

Additional Support
• Bergamot
• Digestive Blend
• Cassia

Cough (chronic)
Chronic and involuntary respiratory expulsion.

Description
Increases immune response to address possible infections; opens the airways for symptomatic relief.

Suggested Duration
1-2 weeks

Cardamom & Lime
Gargle a drop each with water for 30 seconds, then swallow 3x daily.

Respiratory Blend, Rosemary, Black Pepper
Apply 2 drops each to chest and bottoms of feet 2x daily. Also diffuse several drops throughout the day.

Protective Blend Softgels +
Take 2 softgels 2x daily until symptoms subside.

Notes
Additional Support
• Oregano
• Melissa
• Arborvitae
• Eucalyptus

Crohn's Disease
Inflammatory disease of intestines, colon, and ileum.

Description
Reduces inflammation and swelling in the bowels.

Suggested Duration
6 months

GI Cleansing Complex
Take 1 softgel 1-2x daily for 2 weeks.

Peppermint, Basil, Frankincense
Take 1-2 drops each in capsule daily for 2 weeks after GI Cleansing Complex.

Probiotic Complex
Take 1 capsule w/each meal.

Digestive Blend
Take 1 softgel to ease discomfort 3-5x daily.

Notes
Additional Support
• Vitality Supplement Trio
• Ginger
• Marjoram

Cysts (ganglion)
Non-cancerous lumps that most commonly develop along the tendons or joints of your wrists or hands.

Description
Reduces the size or eliminates the cyst by softening the cyst and allowing the fluid to be absorbed and dispersed into the surrounding tissue.

Suggested Duration
2-4 weeks

Lemongrass, Oregano, Thyme, Cypress
Massage a drop of each diluted into the cyst 2x daily.

Then apply a small cloth soaked in caster oil over the cyst. Wrap tightly with tape or saran wrap overnight.

Notes
Additional Support
• Cellular Complex
• Yarrow
• Green Mandarin
• Lavender

Deodorant (body)
Unpleasant smell from pheromones or bacterial or mildew development.

Description
Helps manage bacteria and odor-causing toxicity.

Suggested Duration
4 weeks, then as needed

Cilantro
Take 2 drops in a capsule daily.

Detoxification Softgels
Take 1 softgel 2x daily.

Cleansing Blend
Use diluted with carrier oil under arms after showering.

Notes
Additional Support
• Joyful Blend
• Melaleuca
• Arborvitae
• Petitgrain

Depression
Experience of a more depressed mood and loss of interest in previously interesting activities.

Description
Increases mood by stimulation through senses.

Suggested Duration
3 months, then as needed

Bergamot, Melissa, Frankincense
Apply a drop of each to back of neck, spine and bottoms of feet 3x daily.

Joyful Blend
Diffuse several drops daily and inhale from cupped hands as needed.

Probiotic Complex
Take 2 capsules in the morning on an empty stomach.

Vitality Supplement Trio
Take 2 of each bottle 2x daily.

Notes

Additional Support
• Uplifting Blend
• Enlightening Blend
• Tangerine
• Hawaiian Sandalwood

Detox (full body)
Elimination of toxic substances accumulated in organs and tissues.

Description
Helps the body eliminate toxicity and free up filtering organs.

Suggested Duration
4 weeks

GI Cleansing Complex
Take 1 softgel w/each meal for 10 days (start with 1 a day, and work up to 3).

Detoxification Softgels
Take 1 softgel w/each meal.

Detox Herbal Complex
Take 1 capsule 2x daily.

Probiotic Complex
Take 1 capsule w/each meal during last 10 days.

Vitality Supplement Trio
Take 2 of each bottle 2x daily.

Notes

Additional Support
• Lemon (in water)
• Cilantro
• Grapefruit

Diabetes (type 1)
Autoimmune condition in which little or no insulin is produced by the pancreas.

Description
Stimulates cellular maintenance, helps balance blood sugar.

Suggested Duration
3-6 months, then as needed

Vitality Supplement Trio
Take 2 of each bottle 2x daily.

Rosemary, Cypress, Cassia
Take 1 drop each in capsule daily. Also rub diluted onto pancreas reflex points.

Geranium & Rosemary
Add 3 drops of each to a hot bath.

Notes

Additional Support
• Cellular Complex Blend
• Coriander
• Juniper Berry
• Bergamot

Diabetes (type 2)
Condition in which the body becomes resistant to insulin.

Description
Helps balance blood sugar, supports pancreas.

Suggested Duration
3-6 months, then as needed

Coriander, Cinnamon, Juniper Berry
Take 1-2 drops each in capsule daily.

Cellular Vitality Complex
Take 2 of each bottle 2x daily.

Detoxification Blend
Rub 2 drops onto pancreas reflex point or over pancreas daily.

Notes

Additional Support
• Cassia
• Metabolic Blend

Digestive Issues

Symptoms of gas, stomach ache, bloating, indigestion, and cramping.

Description
Relieves inflammation, gas, and discomfort in digestive system.

Suggested Duration
4 weeks, then as needed

Digestive Blend
Drink 1-2 drops with water, or rub over stomach to ease discomfort.

Digestive Enzymes
Take 1 capsule w/each meal.

Probiotic Complex
Take 2 capsules in the morning on an empty stomach.

Frankincense & Cardamom
Rub a drop of each onto stomach reflex points in the morning.

Notes

Additional Support
• Ginger
• Fennel
• Peppermint
• Yarrow

Ear Ache

Inflammation or infection of the middle ear usually caused by bacteria or virus.

Description
Provides assistance in dispersing the infection and draining the surrounding tissue.

Suggested Duration
2 weeks

Lavender, Basil, Melaleuca, Frankincense, Helichrysum
Apply a dab of each diluted around ear (do not place oils inside of ear).

Protective Blend Softgels +
Take 2 softgels 3x daily with food.

Probiotic Complex
Take 2 capsules in the morning on an empty stomach.

Notes

Additional Support
• Ginger
• Oregano

Eczema/Dermatitis

A condition of the skin causing patches of scales and dryness, often caused by bacterial infection.

Description
Reduces the infection, increases moisture, and promotes new skin cell growth.

Suggested Duration
3 months, then as needed

Arborvitae, Melaleuca, Frankincense
Combine 1-2 drops each with FCO and apply to the affected area 5x daily.

Apply a warm towel compress over the area after oils are applied in the evening.

Protective Blend Softgels +
Take 2 softgels 3x daily with food

Probiotic Complex
Take 2 capsules in the morning on an empty stomach.

Notes

Additional Support
• Myrrh
• Hawaiian Sandalwood

Endometriosis

A condition where uterine lining grows outside the uterus.

Description
Provides relief from pain and discomfort by increasing blood flow and circulation to the area.

Suggested Duration
1 year, then as needed

Clary Sage, Eucalyptus, Frankincense, Ylang Ylang
Apply a drop of each to lower abdomen 3x daily.

Cover with a hot compress towel after application in the evening.

Cellular Complex
Apply to abdomen 2x daily.

Probiotic Complex
Take 2 capsules in the morning on an empty stomach.

Notes

Additional Support
• Yarrow
• Hawaiian Sandalwood
• Myrrh
• Patchouli

Energy (low)

Fatigue caused by lack of sleep, toxicity, nervous issues, or regenerative issues.

Description

Increases energy by stimulation of the sympathetic nervous system, eliminating toxins, and inducing cellular pruning and regeneration.

Suggested Duration

6 months, then as needed

Peppermint, Bergamot, Lemongrass
Apply a drop of each to back of neck, spine and bottom of feet 3x daily.

Energy & Stamina Complex
Take 2 capsules 2x daily.

Probiotic Complex
Take 2 capsules in the morning on an empty stomach.

Omega Complex
Take 2 capsules 2x daily.

Notes

Additional Support
- Vitality Supplement Trio
- Frankincense
- Peppermint
- Tangerine
- Joyful Blend

Fibromyalgia

Condition where one experiences widespread muscle pain and tenderness.

Description

Decreases inflammation, promotes healthy cellular function.

Suggested Duration

1-3 years

Frankincense, Yarrow, Copaiba, Turmeric
Apply a drop of each to back of neck and bottoms of feet 2x daily.

Cellular Complex
Apply 2-4 drops to spine 2x daily. Also take 2 softgels 2x daily.

Soothing Blend
Massage lotion into inflamed areas 3x daily or as needed.

Probiotic Complex
Take 2 capsules in the morning on an empty stomach.

Melissa
Use 1 drop under tongue daily.

Notes

Additional Support
- Vitality Supplement Trio
- Energy & Stamina Complex
- Digestive Blend Softgels
- Detoxification Blend

Flu/Influenza

Viral infection of the respiratory passages.

Description

Combats viruses, boosts immune system, supports respiratory system.

Suggested Duration

5-10 days

Protective Blend, Melaleuca, Black Pepper
Rub 2 drops each on bottoms of feet 3x daily.

Protective Blend Softgels +
Take 2 softgels 3x daily.

Digestive Blend
Drink 1-3 drops in water, or rub over stomach to ease nausea & vomiting.

Respiratory Blend
Diffuse 8-10 drops. Sit/sleep near the diffuser. Also rub 2 drops over chest as needed.

Notes

Additional Support
- Melissa
- Cardamom
- GI Cleansing Complex

Focus & Concentration

Need for improved ability to remain on-task and mentally centered.

Description

Actives the parasympathetic nervous system and induces a more calm and focused mental state.

Suggested Duration

6 months

Vetiver, Frankincense, Wild Orange, Peppermint
Apply a drop of each to back of neck, spine and bottom of feet 3x daily.

Focus Blend
Apply to forehead and temples 2x daily and as needed.

Probiotic Complex
Take 2 capsules in the morning on an empty stomach.

Notes

Additional Support
- Sandalwood
- Ylang Ylang
- Roman Chamomile
- Siberian Fir

Protocols

Gout

Excess buildup of uric acid in the blood, often caused by poor dietary habits.

Description
Relieves pain, and disperse and dilutes the excess uric acid.

Suggested Duration
1 week

Frankincense, Turmeric, Lavender
Apply a drop of each to painful areas 3x daily.

Soothing Blend
Massage lotion into affected areas after above oils 3x daily.

Polyphenol Complex
Take 2 capsules 2x daily on an empty stomach.

Cellular Complex
Apply 2 drops to painful areas before bed each night.

Notes
Additional Support
- Yarrow
- Coriander
- Fennel
- Wintergreen

Headache

Continuous pain in the head or sinuses.

Description
Increases circulation and relieves pain.

Suggested Duration
As needed

Tension Blend
Apply roller regularly to forehead, neck and temples. Add a drop of Helichrysum if needed.

Polyphenol Complex
Take 2 capsules 2x daily on an empty stomach.

Cellular Complex
Rub 1-2 drops into bottoms of feet and spine 3x daily.

Notes
Additional Support
- Peppermint
- Frankincense
- Lavender
- Copaiba

Heartburn

Indigestion felt as a burning sensation in the chest.

Description
Balances stomach acid, eases pain of indigestion.

Suggested Duration
As needed

Digestive Blend
Drink 1-2 drops in water.

Digestive Enzymes
Take 1-3 capsules with each meal.

Cardamom
Rub 1-2 drops over stomach.

Notes
Additional Support
- Ginger
- Fennel
- Coriander

Hemorrhoids

Swollen veins that often lead to the formation of a small blood clot inside, or outside the anus.

Description
Reduces the inflammatory response to the veins, shrinks the size of the clot, and reduces pain.

Suggested Duration
8 weeks to 12 months

Melaleuca, Geranium, Juniper Berry, Frankincense
Apply a drop of each to the location of the hemorrhoids 3x daily. Dilute for sensitive skin.

Cellular Complex
Apply 2-4 drops with carrier oil to inside of legs from ankles to inner thighs 2x daily.

Notes
Additional Support
- Cypress
- Myrrh
- Sandalwood
- Patchouli

Hepatitis C

Viral infection that attacks the liver over several years.

Description
Combats bacterial overgrowth that becomes trapped in pores.

Suggested Duration
2-3 months

Helichrysum, Frankincense, Oregano
Apply a drop of each diluted to the sides of the lower back 6x daily. (If infection is on the face or body, follow the same protocol.)

Probiotic Complex
Take 2 capsules in the morning and evening on an empty stomach.

Digestive Blend
Take 2 softgels 2x daily after food.

Notes

Additional Support
• Neroli
• Thyme
• Greenland Moss
• Carrot Seed

Herniated Disc

Bulging of the central portion of a disc beyond the damaged outer rings.

Description
Increases circulation, reduces scar tissue, promotes healing.

Suggested Duration
6-12 months

Frankincense, Turmeric, Lavender
Apply 1 drop of each to painful areas 3x daily.

Soothing Blend
Apply lotion to affected area after above oils 3x daily.

Polyphenol Complex
Take 2 capsules 2x daily on an empty stomach.

Cellular Complex
Apply 2-4 drops to affected area before bed each night.

Notes

Additional Support
• Yarrow
• Copaiba
• Coriander
• Wintergreen

Herpes Simplex

Viral infection that often occurs in the mouth but can also affect the lips.

Description
Decreases the expression of the virus and maintains a preventative regimen.

Suggested Duration
1 week to 3 months

Cardamom, Melissa, Melaleuca
Apply a drop of each diluted directly to blister sore 6x daily.

Probiotic Complex
Take 2 capsules in the morning and evening on an empty stomach.

Omega Complex
2 softgels 2x daily.

Helichrysum
Apply a dab at night to help tissues heal.

Notes

Additional Support
• Clary Sage
• Geranium
• Lemon Myrtle

Immune Boost

Need for improved immune response to combat bacteria, viruses, and pathogens.

Description
Provides bacteria and virus-fighting agents, boosts immune system.

Suggested Duration
4 weeks

Protective Blend, Black Pepper, Melaleuca
Rub 2-4 drops each on bottoms of feet daily.

Probiotic Complex
Take 2 capsules in the morning on an empty stomach.

Vitality Supplement Trio
Take 2 of each bottle 2x daily.

Notes

Additional Support
• Frankincense
• Melissa
• Thyme

Infertility

Inability to conceive children.

Description
Supports the reproductive system and proper hormone production.

Suggested Duration
2-6 months

Full Body Detox
Follow instructions for Detox (full body).

Vitality Supplement Trio
Take 2 of each bottle 2x daily.

Clary Sage
Apply to reproductive reflex points 2x daily.

Yarrow
Take 2 drops under tongue 2x daily.

Notes

Additional Support
- Oil Touch Technique (receive weekly)
- Detoxification Blend

Irritable Bowels

A collection of symptoms relating to the GI tract often attributed to possible infection or damage to the intestinal mucosa.

Description
Relieves symptoms of gas, bloating, constipation, diarrhea, and belching.

Suggested Duration
3-6 months

Digestive Blend
Take 1 softgel with meals.

Cardamom & Turmeric
Drink a drop each in water to soothe discomfort as needed.

Probiotic Complex
Take 2 capsules in the morning and evening on an empty stomach.

Omega Complex
2 softgels 2x daily.

Lavender, Melaleuca, Frankincense, Digestive Blend
Apply a drop of each diluted over stomach 2x daily.

Notes

Additional Support
- Fennel
- Coriander
- Basil
- Lemongrass
- Caraway

Libido (low)

Decreased sex drive or sexual desire.

Description
Inspires an uninhibited sex drive.

Suggested Duration
2 weeks, then as needed

Inspiring Blend
Use a few drops diluted in massage, and diffuse several drops to inspire intimacy.

Ylang Ylang
Rub 1-2 drops on pulse points.

Clary Sage
Take 1-2 drops in capsule daily.

Notes

Additional Support
- Vitality Supplement Trio
- Energy & Stamina Complex
- Women's Perfume Blend

Lupus

Autoimmune disease marked by inflammation of the skin and organs.

Description
Induces the parasympathetic nervous system, eliminates antigens and latent infections, and reduces the immune response.

Suggested Duration
1-3 years

Frankincense, Yarrow, Copaiba, Turmeric
Apply a drop of each to back of neck and bottoms of feet 2x daily.

Cellular Complex
Apply 2-4 drops to spine 2x daily. Also take 2 softgels 2x daily.

Soothing Blend
Massage lotion into inflamed areas 3x daily or as needed.

Probiotic Complex
Take 2 capsules in the morning on an empty stomach.

Notes

Additional Support
- Vitality Supplement Trio
- Yarrow
- Detox Herbal Complex
- Digestive Blend Softgels
- Restful Complex

Lyme Disease

Inflammatory disease caused by bacteria transmitted by ticks.

Description
Induces the parasympathetic nervous system, eliminates antigens and latent infections, and reduces the immune response.

Suggested Duration
1-3 years

Cellular Complex
Apply 2-4 drops to spine, back of neck, and bottoms of feet 3x daily.

Cinnamon, Sandalwood, Turmeric, Clary Sage
Take a drop of each in a capsule 2x daily.

Detoxification Blend
Apply 2 drops to sides of neck 2x daily.

Probiotic Complex
Take 2 capsules in the morning on an empty stomach.

Copaiba Softgels
Take 1 softgel 3x daily.

Notes

Additional Support
- Vitality Supplement Trio
- Yarrow
- Detoxification Complex
- Restful Complex

Memory Issues

Difficulty recalling thoughts, names, events, and experiences.

Description
Increase the integrity of the gut lining and promote brain health.

Suggested Duration
1-3 years

Frankincense, Vetiver, Lavender, Rose
Apply a drop of each to back of neck 3x daily.

Probiotic Complex
Take 2 capsules in the morning on an empty stomach.

Cellular Complex
Apply 2-4 drops to spine and bottoms of feet 3x daily.

Copaiba Softgels
Take 1 softgel daily.

Notes

Additional Support
- Yarrow
- Rosemary
- Turmeric
- Sandalwood
- Clary Sage

Menopause

The ceasing of menstruation, typically between 45 and 50 years of age.

Description
Aids in hormone and mood balance, calms hot flashes.

Suggested Duration
4 months, then as needed

Women's Monthly Blend
Rub onto pulse points twice daily (avoid sun exposure for 12 hours after application).

Phytoestrogen Complex
Take 1 capsule 3x daily.

Peppermint
Apply a drop to back of neck to ease hot flashes.

Notes

Additional Support
- Vitality Supplement Trio
- Ylang Ylang
- Geranium

Menstruation (PMS)

The discharge of blood and other materials from the lining of the uterus.

Description
Balances mood and hormones during menstruation.

Suggested Duration
2 weeks as needed

Women's Monthly Blend
Rub onto pulse points and over ovaries (avoid sun exposure for 12 hours after application).

Balance
Rub behind ears to balance mood.

Phytoestrogen
Take 1 capsule 3x daily.

Notes

Additional Support
- Clary Sage
- Restful Blend
- Tension Blend

Protocols

195

Migraine

Recurrent throbbing headache accompanied by nausea and disturbed vision.

Description
Increases circulation and relieves pain.

Suggested Duration
1 day to 3 months

Tension Blend & Helichrysum
Apply roller and a drop of Helichrysum to forehead, neck, and temples at the early onset of discomfort.

Cellular Complex
Rub 2 drops onto bottoms of feet and spine 2x daily.

Frankincense, Turmeric, Lavender
Take a drop of each in a capsule 2x daily or as needed.

Polyphenol Complex
Take 2 capsules 2x daily on an empty stomach.

Notes

Additional Support
- Copaiba
- Marjoram
- Roman Chamomile
- Wintergreen

Mononucleosis

Viral disease with swelling of the lymph glands and prolonged lassitude.

Description
Provides antiviral support.

Suggested Duration
8-16 weeks

Thyme, Oregano, Protective Blend
Take 1-2 drops each in a capsule 3x daily.

Frankincense, Black Pepper
Rub 2 drops each to bottoms of feet.

Energy & Stamina Complex
Take 1-2 capsules twice daily.

Notes

Additional Support
- Vitality Supplement Trio
- Melissa
- Cassia

Mood Balance

Need for stabilized emotional state, often related to stress or hormone levels.

Description
Activates the parasympathetic nervous system and induces a more calm and focused mental state.

Suggested Duration
6 months

Frankincense, Lavender, Siberian Fir, Sandalwood
Apply a drop of each to back of neck, spine and bottom of feet 3x daily.

Focus Blend
Apply roller blend to temples and sides of neck 3x daily.

Probiotic Complex
Take 2 capsules in the morning on an empty stomach.

Restful Complex
Take 2 softgels before bed.

Notes

Additional Support
- Grounding Blend
- Ylang Ylang
- Roman Chamomile

Multiple Sclerosis

Nerve degeneration including the breakdown of the myelin sheath.

Description
Reduces symptoms of muscle weakness, muscle spasm and chronic pain.

Suggested Duration
1-3 years

Frankincense, Sandalwood, Turmeric, Clary Sage
Take a drop of each in a capsule 3x daily.

Detoxification Blend
Apply 2 drops to sides of neck 2x daily.

Probiotic Complex
Take 2 capsules in the morning on an empty stomach.

Cellular Complex
Apply 2-4 drops to spine, back of neck, and bottoms of feet 3x daily.

Notes

Additional Support
- Vitality Supplement Trio
- Yarrow
- Lavender
- Restful Complex
- Detox Herbal Complex

Muscle Aches

Inflammation and pain in one or more muscle region.

Description
Reduces inflammation, spasms, and pain in muscles.

Suggested Duration
2 weeks, then as needed

Massage Blend
Massage 2-4 drops into aching muscles 3x daily.

Polyphenol Complex
Take 1 capsule 3x daily.

Frankincense, Lemon
Take 1-2 drops each in capsule 2x daily.

Magnolia
Apply to affected muscles as needed throughout the day.

Notes

Additional Support
• Soothing Blend
• Cypress
• Douglas Fir
• Black Pepper

Neuropathy

Condition of weakness, numbness and tingling due to nerve damage.

Description
Increases blood flow, reduces pain and assists in repair of damaged nerves.

Suggested Duration
1-3 years

Cellular Complex & Vetiver
Apply 2-4 drops each to spine and bottoms of feet 4x daily.

Soothing Blend
Massage lotion into affected area after above oils 4x daily.

Frankincense, Copaiba, Turmeric, Black Pepper
Take a drop of each in a capsule 2x daily.

Probiotic Complex
Take 2 capsules in the morning on an empty stomach.

Notes

Additional Support
• Detox Herbal Complex
• Polyphenol Complex
• Rosemary
• Lavender

Nerve Damage

Dysfunction or breakdown of isolated nerves or the nervous system.

Description
Increases blood flow, reduces pain and assists in repair of damaged nerves.

Suggested Duration
3-6 months

Cellular Complex
Apply 2-4 drops to spine, bottom of feet, and affected areas 4x daily.

Vetiver & Frankincense
Apply 2 drops of each to bottoms of feet 2x daily.

Yarrow
Use 3-6 drops under the tongue 3x daily.

Notes

Additional Support
• Copaiba
• Wintergreen

Obsessive Compulsive Disorder

Excessive or obsessive thoughts that lead to compulsive behaviors

Description
Increases a general calming state due to the interaction of oils with neurotransmitters.

Suggested Duration
12 months

Roman Chamomile, Rose, Vetiver
Apply a drop of each to back of neck, spine and bottoms of feet 3x daily.

Probiotic Complex
Take 2 capsules in the morning on an empty stomach.

Melissa
Use a drop under the tongue daily.

Protective Blend
Drink 1 drop in water 2x daily.

Notes

Additional Support
• Frankincense
• Siberian Fir
• Sandalwood
• Lavender

Pets (anxiety)
Excessive uneasiness due to a variety of causes.

Description
Increases a general calming state due to the interaction of oils with neurotransmitters.

Suggested Duration
3 weeks, then as needed

Roman Chamomile, Lavender, OR Vetiver
Apply a drop diluted to coat of animal 2x daily.

Grounding Blend
Diffuse several drops during the day.

Restful Blend
Diffuse several drops at night.

Notes

Additional Support
- Frankincense
- Siberian Fir
- Sandalwood

Pets (fleas & bugs)
Fleas, ticks, and other pests.

Description
Prevents, removes, and repels fleas and various insects.

Suggested Duration
3 months, then as needed

Rosemary, Peppermint, Eucalyptus, Melaleuca
Add 10 drops of each to 20 oz spray bottle of water. Spray the solution on the coat of pet 3x daily.

Outdoor Blend
Combine 15 drops with carrier oil and apply to coat of pet 2x daily.

Notes

Plantar Fasciitis
Inflammation of the fascia attached to the from the heel to the metatarsal bones of the foot.

Description
Reduces inflammation and decreases pain.

Suggested Duration
Ongoing

Cellular Complex & Turmeric
Apply 2 each to affected area 3x daily.

Soothing Blend
Apply lotion to affected area 3x daily.

Polyphenol Complex
Take 2 capsules 2x daily on an empty stomach.

Notes

Additional Support
- Frankincense
- Rosemary
- Yarrow
- Wintergreen

Polio
Post-disease symptoms that include muscle weakness, fatigue and joint pain.

Description
Reduces pain, improves energy, and assists in cellular regeneration.

Suggested Duration
1-5 years

Cellular Complex Softgels
Take 2 softgels 2x daily.

Frankincense, Turmeric, Lavender
Apply a drop of each to spine, back of neck, and bottom of feet 3x daily.

Polyphenol Complex
Take 2 capsules 2x daily on an empty stomach.

Energy & Stamina Complex
Take 2 capsules 2x daily.

Notes

Additional Support
- Rosemary
- Yarrow
- Lemon Myrtle
- Sandalwood
- Wintergreen

Pregnancy (postnatal)
Care for mother after giving birth.

Description
Promotes pain relief, tissue healing, and emotional support after giving birth.

Suggested Duration
4-8 weeks

Helichrysum, Frankincense, Lavender
Apply 2 drops each diluted to areas with tearing 3x daily.

Ylang Ylang
Diffuse for mood balancing.

Phytoestrogen
Take 1 capsule 3x daily.

Helichrysum, Myrrh, Lavender
Massage 2 drops each diluted into stretch mark areas.

Notes

Additional Support
• Geranium
• Vitality Supplement Trio

Pregnancy (prenatal)
Care for mother during pregnancy.

Description
Relieves pregnancy sickness, provides vital nutrients, and provides emotional support.

Suggested Duration
9 months

Digestive Blend
Drink 2 drops or rub 2 drops over stomach to ease nausea.

Digestive Enzymes
Take 1-3 w/each meal.

Vitality Supplement Trio
Take 2 of each bottle 2x daily.

Bone Nutrient Complex
Take 1 capsule 3x daily.

Joyful Blend
Diffuse or wear daily.

Notes

Additional Support
• Ginger
• Grounding Blend
• Metabolic Blend
• Rose

Psoriasis
Skin disease marked by red, itchy, scaly patches.

Description
Relieves itchy, swollen skin, and promotes proper immune system function.

Suggested Duration
4-8 weeks

Helichrysum, Frankincense, Melaleuca, Lavender
Combine 10 drops each with carrier oil in roller bottle. Apply 3x daily.

Probiotic Complex
Take 2 capsules in the morning on an empty stomach.

Digestive Enzymes
Take 1-3 w/each meal.

Cellular Complex Blend
Take 1-2 softgels 3x daily.

Notes

Additional Support
• Copaiba
• Anti-Aging Blend
• Cedarwood

Rash
Patches of scales, dryness, pustules or redness of the skin.

Description
Reduces infection, calms inflammatory response, and promotes new skin cell growth.

Suggested Duration
2-4 weeks, then as needed

Arborvitae, Melaleuca, Frankincense
Combine a drop of each with carrier oil and apply 3-5x daily.

Apply a warm towel compress over the area after oils are applied in the evening.

Probiotic Complex
Take 2 capsules in the morning on an empty stomach.

Protective Blend Softgels +
Take 2 softgels 2x daily.

Notes

Additional Support
• Myrrh
• Sandalwood

Rheumatoid Arthritis

Often hereditary condition causing nodules on the fingers, pain, and stiffness.

Description
Combats bacterial overgrowth that becomes trapped in pores.

Suggested Duration
Ongoing

Copaiba, Turmeric, Frankincense
Apply a drop of each to affected areas 3x daily.

Soothing Blend
Massage lotion into affected areas after above oils 3x daily.

Polyphenol Complex
Take 2 capsules in the evening with food.

Cellular Complex Softgels
Take 2 softgels 3x daily.

Copaiba Softgels
Take 1 softgel daily.

Notes

Additional Support
• Marjoram
• Lemongrass

Scarring (uterine)

Condition where uterine lining grows outside the uterus.

Description
Relieves pain and discomfort by increasing blood flow and circulation to the area.

Suggested Duration
1 year, then as needed

Clary Sage, Frankincense, Ylang Ylang
Apply a drop of each to lower abdomen 2x daily. Cover with a hot compress towel with evening application.

Cellular Complex
Apply 2-4 drops to abdomen 2x daily.

Probiotic Complex
Take 2 capsules in the morning on an empty stomach.

Notes

Additional Support
• Yarrow
• Sandalwood
• Myrrh
• Patchouli

Sciatica

Condition often caused by injury, overuse, or general degradation to the sciatic nerve.

Description
Increases circulation, reduces scar tissue, promotes healing.

Suggested Duration
6-12 months

Cellular Complex
Apply 2-4 drops to bottoms of feet 2x daily.

Frankincense, Turmeric, Lavender
Massage a drop each into painful areas 2x daily.

Soothing Blend
Massage lotion into painful areas throughout the day as needed.

Polyphenol Complex
Take 2 capsules 2x daily on an empty stomach.

Notes

Additional Support
• Yarrow
• Copaiba
• Massage Blend

Seizures (myoclonic)

Disease where nerve cell activity is disturbed in the brain.

Description
Reduces the duration and frequency of seizures.

Suggested Duration
6-12 months, then as needed

Cellular Complex
Apply 2-4 drops to spine and bottoms of feet 4x daily.

Frankincense, Vetiver, Copaiba
Take a drop of each in a capsule or hold to the roof of mouth for 30 seconds 2x daily.

Probiotic Complex
Take 2 capsules in the morning on an empty stomach.

Immediately apply 4 drops of Frankincense to back of neck and bottoms of feet during seizure.

Notes

Additional Support
• Vitality Supplement Trio
• Yarrow
• Turmeric

Shingles

Viral infection that often occurs on the face or intercostal region.

Description
Decreases the expression of the viral infection, alleviates pain, and maintains a preventative regiment.

Suggested Duration
1 week to 3 months

Cardamom, Melissa, Lemon Myrtle, Melaleuca
Apply a drop of each with carrier oil to blisters 6x daily.

Probiotic Complex
Take 2 capsules morning and evening on an empty stomach.

Protective Blend
Take 2 capsules 2x daily after food.

Omega Complex
Take 2 softgels 2x daily.

Notes

Additional Support
• Seasonal Blend Softgels
• Siberian Fir
• Vitality Supplement Trio

Sinusitis

Bacterial infection resulting in pressure in the face, mucus discharge, and fatigue.

Description
Clears the bacterial infections and assists in the remediation of the symptoms.

Suggested Duration
1-4 weeks

Cardamom, Rosemary, Arborvitae, Melissa
Apply a drop of each with carrier oil over the maxillary sinus region 6x daily.

Probiotic Complex
Take 2 capsules morning and evening on an empty stomach.

Protective Blend
Take 2 capsules 2x daily after food.

Omega Complex
Take 2 softgels 2x daily.

Notes

Additional Support
• Myrrh
• Oregano
• Helichrysum

Sleep (insomnia)

Inability to fall or stay asleep.

Description
Induces a calming state that allows one to fall and stay asleep.

Suggested Duration
3 months, then as needed

Restful Blend Complex
Take 2 softgels 30 minutes before bed.

Restful Blend
Apply 2 drops to temples and bottoms of feet. Diffuse several drops near bedside.

Vetiver & Wild Orange
Take a drop of each under the tongue before bed.

Probiotic Complex
Take 2 capsules in the morning on an empty stomach.

Notes

Additional Support
• Frankincense
• Sandalwood
• Wild Orange

Sleep Apnea

Disorder with pauses in or periods of shallow breathing during sleep.

Description
Promotes open airways and more meaningful sleep.

Suggested Duration
Ongoing

Respiratory Blend
Diffuse 5-10 drops next to bedside at night. Also apply to sinus reflex points.

Protective Blend
Gargle 2 drops with water for 30 seconds, then swallow.

Restful Complex
Take 2 softgels 30 minutes before bed.

Notes

Additional Support
• Peppermint
• Rosemary
• Wintergreen

Smoking (stop)

Addiction to smoking cigarettes, vape pens, or other forms of nicotine.

Description
Helps curb cravings and smoking addiction, aids in detox.

Suggested Duration
6-12 weeks

Grapefruit
Drink 1-3 drops in water throughout the day.

Protective Blend
Swish 2 drops with water when cravings arise, especially after eating.

Black Pepper
Apply 1 drop to big toes 2x daily. Also inhale or diffuse throughout the day.

Detoxification Blend
Apply 2-4 drops to bottoms of feet 30 minutes before showering.

Notes
Additional Support
• Clove
• Detox Herbal Complex

Snoring

Disturbed vibrating or grunting sound in a person's breathing during sleep.

Description
Promotes open airways during sleep.

Suggested Duration
Ongoing

Respiratory Blend
Diffuse 5-10 drops near bedside at night. Also apply to chest, throat, and lung reflex points.

Protective Blend
Gargle 2 drops with water for 30 seconds, then swallow.

Lemon
Drink 1-3 drops in water before bed.

Notes
Additional Support
• Eucalyptus
• Rosemary
• Peppermint

Sore Throat

Pain in the throat due to inflammation from a virus or bacteria.

Description
Relieves pain and soreness in throat, provides antiviral and antibacterial support.

Suggested Duration
5-10 days

Lemon 10, Protective Blend 8, Helichrysum 2
Combine in small glass spray bottle with carrier oil. Apply as needed.

Lavender, Arborvitae
Massage 1-2 drops with carrier oil to outside of throat.

Notes
Additional Support
• Melissa
• Black Pepper
• Petitgrain

Stress

Emotional upset, physical malfunction, and mental stress.

Description
Increases a general calming state due to the interaction of oils with neurotransmitters.

Suggested Duration
4-8 weeks, then as needed

Grounding Blend
Apply 1-2 drops to back of ears, temples, and wrists often as needed.

Grapefruit, Tangerine, or Wild Orange
Diffuse several drops daily.

Probiotic Complex
Take 2 capsules in the morning on an empty stomach.

Restful Blend
Apply 2-4 drops to temples and bottoms of feet at bedtime. Diffuse several drops.

Notes
Additional Support
• Rose
• Roman Chamomile
• Siberian Fir
• Sandalwood

Sunburn

Reddening, inflammation, and sometimes blistering from sun overexposure.

Description
Relieves discomfort from sunburn, promotes healing.

Suggested Duration
3-7 days

Lavender, Yarrow, Helichrysum
Apply 2-4 drops with carrier oil or aloe to sunburnt skin 3-5x daily.

Peppermint
Add 5 drops to small glass spray bottle with water. Spritz to cool skin.

Notes

Additional Support
• Cedarwood
• Copaiba
• Roman Chamomile

Thrush

Infection of the mouth and throat from yeast-like fungus causing white patches.

Description
Provides anti-fungal support, eases oral discomfort.

Suggested Duration
1-3 weeks

Lemon, Melaleuca, Children's Omega-3
Combine 2 drops of each essential oil with 1 Tbs of omegas. Apply with clean finger to child's gums and tongue 2-3x daily.

Melaleuca & Lavender
Massage a drop into bottoms of child's feet 1x daily.

Notes

Additional Support
• Geranium
• Helichrysum

Thyroid (Hyper/ Grave's)

Autoimmune disorder resulting in excess of thyroid hormone.

Description
Assists with regulating the metabolism, detoxifying the body, and restoring balance.

Suggested Duration
1-3 years

Vetiver, Siberian Fir, Turmeric, Myrrh
Apply a drop of each to back of neck, spine, and throat 3x daily.

Probiotic Complex
Take 2 capsules in the morning on an empty stomach.

Grounding Blend
Apply 2-4 drops to bottoms of feet morning and night.

Detoxification Blend
Take 2 softgels 2x daily.

Notes

Additional Support
• Sandalwood
• Basil
• Detox Herbal Complex

Thyroid (Hypo/ Hashimoto's)

Autoimmune disorder resulting in insufficient thyroid hormone.

Description
Assists with regulating the metabolism, detoxifying the body, and restoring balance.

Suggested Duration
1-3 years

Myrrh, Turmeric, Clove, Lemongrass, Copaiba
Apply a drop of each to back of neck, spine, and throat 3x daily.

Probiotic Complex
Take 2 capsules in the morning on an empty stomach.

Energy & Stamina Complex
Take 2 capsules 2x daily.

Detoxification Blend
Take 2 softgels 2x daily.

Cellular Complex Softgels
Take 2 softgels 2x daily.

Notes

Additional Support
• Lemon Myrtle
• Rosemary
• Basil
• Vitality Supplement Trio

Protocols

Tinnitus

The feeling of noise or ringing in the ears.

Description
Soothes auditory canal and neurological auditory triggers.

Suggested Duration
3 months, then as needed

Frankincense, Lemongrass, Turmeric, Helichrysum
Apply a dab each to back of neck, spine, and around outside of ears 3x daily.

Energy & Stamina Complex
Take 2 capsules 2x daily.

Cellular Complex Softgels
Take 2 softgels 2x daily.

Notes
Additional Support
• Helichrysum
• Siberian Fir
• Sandalwood

Toenail Fungus

Infection often caused by the overuse of antibiotics.

Description
Combats fungus growth and provides preventative regimen.

Suggested Duration
1-3 months

Melaleuca, Arborvitae, Thyme
Combine oils in equal parts and apply a drop to affected area 3x daily (avoid surrounding skin.)

Probiotic Complex
Take 2 capsules in the morning on an empty stomach.

Protective Blend Softgels +
Take 2 softgels 2x daily.

Cellular Complex Softgels
Take 2 softgels 2x daily.

Notes
Additional Support
• Neroli
• Oregano
• Clove

Tourette's

Nervous system disorder that leads to repetitive vocalizations, limb or facial movement.

Description
Lessens the severity and occurrence of tics.

Suggested Duration
1-5 years

Rose, Clary Sage, Vetiver
Apply a drop each to back of neck, spine, and bottoms of feet 3x daily.

Focus Blend
Apply to temples and sides of neck 3x daily.

Probiotic Complex
Take 2 capsules in the morning on an empty stomach.

Cellular Complex Softgels
Take 2 softgels 2x daily.

Notes
Additional Support
• Frankincense
• Siberian Fir
• Roman Chamomile
• Vitality Supplement Trio

Urinary Tract Infection
Infection of the ureters from the kidneys to the bladder.

Description
Aids in combating bacterial infection and restoring regular immune defenses.

Suggested Duration
1-4 weeks

Oregano, Clove, Lemongrass, Frankincense
Take a drop each in a capsule 3-5x daily (discontinue Oregano and Lemongrass if more than 10 days).

Cellular Complex & Cypress
Rub 2 drops each over lower abdomen 2x daily. Dilute for sensitive skin.

Probiotic Complex
Take 2 capsules in the morning on an empty stomach.

Notes
Additional Support
• Arborvitae
• Thyme
• Protective Blend
• Melissa

Weight Loss (skin conditions) *Stretch marks and sagging skin after weight loss.*

Description
Improves appearance of scar tissue and helps restore skin elasticity.

Suggested Duration
8-12 weeks

Myrrh, Helichrysum, Frankincense, Yarrow
Massage 2 drops each with carrier oil into stretch marks 2x daily.

Metabolic Blend & Myrrh
Rub 3-5 drops each with carrier oil onto sagging skin. Cover oils with warm towel compress for 30 minutes before bed.

Notes

Additional Support
• Essential oil skincare line

Weight Loss *Excess weight usually due to the body's inability to access ketosis.*

Description
Assists with burning glucose and glycogen supplies at a faster rate in order to access the ketotic fat burning state.

Suggested Duration
3-6 months

Metabolic Blend
Apply 10-15 drops with carrier oil to abdomen and fatty areas at night.

Also drink 3-5 drops in water throughout the day.

Cellular Complex
Apply 2-4 drops of oil to lower abdomen 2x daily. Take 2 softgels 2x daily.

Detoxification Blend Softgels
Take 2 softgels 2x daily.

Notes

Additional Support
• Bergamot
• Coriander
• Fennel
• Lemon Myrtle

Wrinkles *Age effects or trauma to the overall integrity of the skin.*

Description
Restores skin integrity and appearance of fine lines and wrinkles.

Suggested Duration
Ongoing

Green Mandarin, Frankincense, Rose
Massage a drop of each into affected areas morning and night.

Anti-Aging Blend
Apply over wrinkles 2x daily.

Omega Complex
Take 2 softgels 2x daily.

Cellular Complex Softgels
Take 2 softgels 2x daily.

Notes

Additional Support
• Sandalwood
• Arborvitae
• Myrrh
• Blue Tansy
• Essential oil skincare line

Yeast Infection *Fungal infection often caused by the overuse of antibiotics.*

Description
Combats fungal infection and restores balance in the gut and affected areas.

Suggested Duration
2-3 months

Melaleuca, Lavender, Thyme, Clove
Apply 1 drop of each diluted to vaginal area 6x daily. (If infection is on the face or body follow the same protocol.)

Probiotic Complex
Take 2 capsules morning and evening on an empty stomach.

Protective Blend Softgels +
Take 2 softgels 2x daily after food.

Notes

Additional Support
• Arborvitae
• Green Mandarin
• Yarrow

Protocols

Section 7

Lifestyle Protocols

Lifestyle Protocols

Take your wellness experience to the next level with Lifestyle Protocols.

You've used the Ailments section and the Protocols by Ailments to troubleshoot health challenges. Now use Lifestyle Protocols to uplevel the parts of your life you want to enhance.

Choose a Lifestyle Protocol that matches where you want to go next with your wellness. Do the protocol for the suggested time, then evaluate your progress.

If you're satisfied, move onto the next Lifestyle Protocol that stands out to you. If you feel you have more work to do, stick with the one you're on!

You can't go wrong with choosing a Lifestyle Protocol. Each one will take you in a positive direction.

After all, anything that points you toward a natural solutions lifestyle is the right direction!

BTW - if things are good right now, use the *Good Life* protocol!

Abundance Generator

Sometimes life calls you to focus on more abundance. Whether it's abundance in money, health, or life-satisfaction, this protocol will help you draw good things to you.

Protocol Benefits
- Opens your first chakra (money & stability)
- Grounds your energy to the present moment
- Opens your mind to the story of new possibilities
- Creates an emotional set point for gratitude in your day

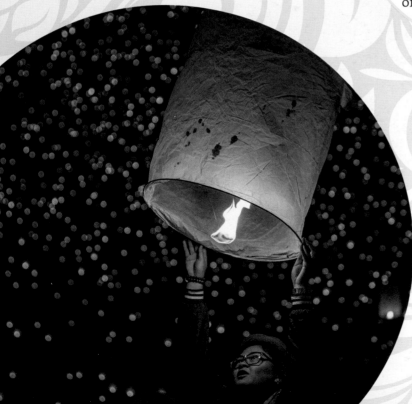

Time frame
Do this protocol for *4 weeks*. Then reevaluate or switch to another Lifestyle Protocol.

First Chakra

Grounding Blend
Massage 2 drops into the heels of your feet each morning and night.

Vetiver & Rosemary
Add a drop of each to floor of your shower in the morning.

Dreamstorm

Get a special notebook to dreamstorm in once a day. It's best to do it first thing in the morning before the world takes over your attention.

Spend 10-15 minutes writing what you're grateful for and what you're excited to see unfold in your life.

Then review what you've written just before going to bed.

Abundant Atmosphere

Wild Orange
Diffuse 6-8 drops every day.

Joyful Blend
Breathe a couple drops from your palms while focusing on your abundant future periodically each day.

Lifestyles

209

Addiction Recovery

Regain the satisfaction of being in control of your desires, cravings, and where you derive satisfaction in life with this protocol.

Protocol Benefits
- Helps curb cravings
- Uses activity as a healthy distraction
- Fortifies self-concept

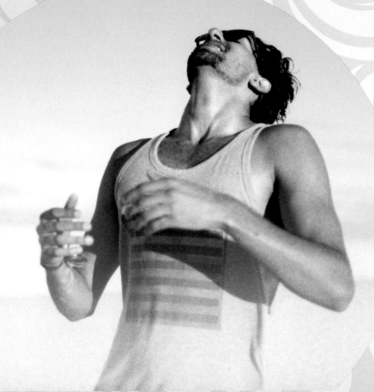

Craving Control

Black Pepper
Rub a drop on bottoms of feet (especially big toes), morning and night.

Grapefruit
Drink 4-8 drops in a glass or stainless steel water bottle throughout the day.

Cleansing Blend
Diffuse 4-6 drops daily.

Time frame
Use this protocol for *8 weeks.* Then reevaluate to determine if you'll continue or move onto another Lifestyle Protocol.

Active Distraction

Daily Physical Activity
Use walking, running, weight lifting, yoga, or other daily physical activity to keep endorphins and spirits high.

Energy & Stamina Complex
Take 2 capsules 30 minutes before physical activity.

Respiratory Blend
Rub 2 drops onto chest before and during physical activity.

Confident Reflection

Centering Blend
Rub a drop over your heart during times of weakness.

Visualizing
Visualize yourself whole and complete while using the Centering Blend each day.

Age *Defier*

Aging is nothing more than the process of returning to childhood in many cultures. For those who choose youth over the temptation to slow down, this protocol keeps vitality from fading too quickly.

Protocol Benefits
- Decrease pain & inflammation
- Support cellular & organ health
- Improve digestion & elimination
- Reverse the appearance of aging

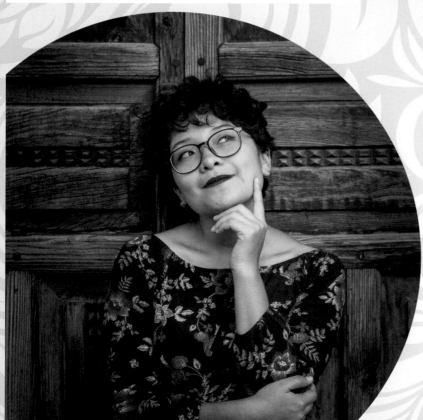

Pain Reducer

Polyphenol Complex
Take 2 capsules whenever pain arises, or take 1 capsule 3x daily.

Soothing Blend
Massage a few drops into sore areas as often as needed.

Frankincense
Take a drop under the tongue. Also diffuse several drops.

Time frame
Use this protocol for *12 weeks,* then as desired for continued anti-aging benefits.

Energy & Cellular Health

Vitality Supplement Trio
Take 2 of each bottle 2x daily.

Energy & Stamina Complex
Take 2 capsules 30 minutes before yoga or working out.

Invigorating Blend
Inhale 2-4 drops from cupped hands as needed. Also diffuse several drops.

Youthful Skin & Complexion

Anti-Aging Blend
Roll on this blend daily to reduce age spots and wrinkles.

Essential Oil Skincare
Use oil-infused skincare products daily to provide anti-aging nutrients.

Brain & Memory Booster

Cellular Complex
Take 2 softgels 2x daily.

Peppermint & Rosemary
Diffuse several drops of each daily. Also massage a couple drops onto back of neck.

The *Athlete*

Life is about the hustle. For athletes of any kind, the hustle is sustainable when you care for your body and all the systems that make the machine work.

Protocol Benefits
- Eases stress on joints and connective tissue
- Soothes sore muscles & speeds recovery
- Provides full-body energy
- Boosts mood and motivation to increase likelihood of sticking with your routine

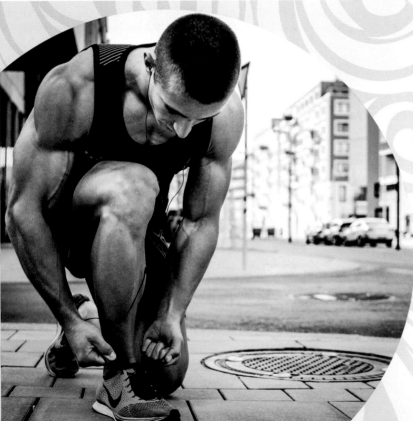

Muscle & Joint Support

Polyphenol Complex
Take 2 capsules before working out.

Soothing Blend
Massage a few drops into muscles as a pre-workout. Also massage into sore areas post-workout.

Lemongrass
Rub 2 drops diluted into ligaments & joints that have been worked hard.

Respiratory System Support

Respiratory Blend
Rub 2 drops onto chest before and during exercise.

Eucalyptus
Add 2 drops onto your shower floor during your post-workout shower.

Time frame
Use this protocol for *12 weeks* during training, then as desired to continually support your active lifestyle.

Full Body Energy Supply

Vitality Supplement Trio
Take 2 of each bottle 2x daily.

Energy & Stamina Complex
Take 2 capsules 30 minutes before yoga or working out.

Lemon & Grapefruit
Drink 4-6 drops in a glass or stainless steel water bottle.

Mood & Motivation Elevator

Encouraging Blend
Inhale 2 drops from your palms to prepare mentally for your routine.

Peppermint
Put a small dab on your tongue.

Lifestyles

Auto-Immune *Recovery*

This protocol facilitates DNA repair, addresses unhealthy inflammatory issues, and gently supports regular immune function.

Protocol Benefits
- Focuses on long-term damaged DNA repair
- Helps balance and calm unhealthy inflammation
- Supports healthy immune function without stimulating hyper immune activity.

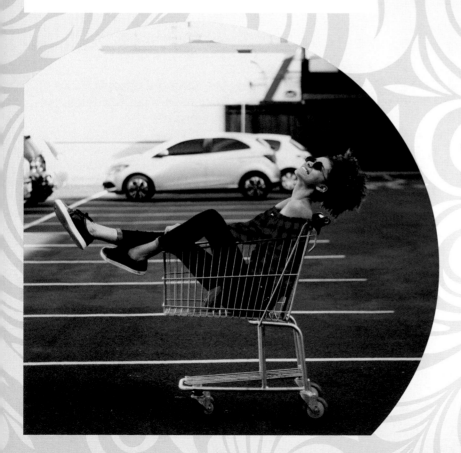

Damaged DNA Repair

Cellular Complex Softgels
Take 2 softgels 2-3x daily.

Cellular Complex
Rub 2-4 drops into spine and or the bottoms of your feet every night before bed.

Time frame
Do this protocol for *12 weeks*. Then reevaluate or switch to another Lifestyle Protocol.

Inflammation Regulation

Vitality Supplement Trio
Take 2 of each bottle twice daily.

Polyphenol Complex
Take 1 capsule 3x daily.

Frankincense, Turmeric & Copaiba
Use a drop of each under your tongue 2-3x daily. Also rub on the bottoms of feet as needed.

Grounding Blend
Rub 2 drops on the bottoms of feet daily.

Immune System Fortification

Probiotic Complex
Take 1 capsule 3x daily with meals.

Protective Blend
Diffuse 4-6 drops daily, and rub 2 drops onto bottoms of feet in the morning.

Babies: *Healthy & On Track*

A healthy and happy baby brings happiness to the whole home. Use this protocol to address the basic elements of infant health.

Protocol Benefits
• Boosts baby's immune system
• Calms tummy troubles & solves digestive issues
• Keeps skin soothed and soft
• Helps baby feel calm and peaceful

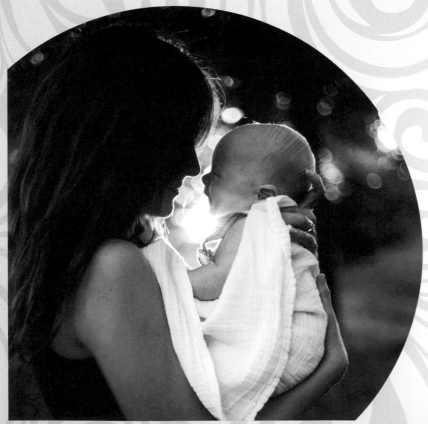

Bolstered Immune System

Protective Blend
Diffuse 4-6 drops in the home daily to keep baby's immune system high. Rub a dab onto feet once a day for immune boost.

Lemon
Use as a gentle sanitizer on your hands and on commonly used objects.

Time frame
Use this protocol on an ***ongoing basis*** to maintain baby's health. Troubleshoot specific ailments in the other sections of this book as needed.

Healthy Tummy

Digestive Blend
Massage a drop diluted with 1 Tbs coconut oil onto baby's tummy to calm digestive trouble (diarrhea, constipation, and tummy ache).

Bergamot
Rub a drop onto baby's feet 1-2x a day to stimulate healthy digestive function.

Happy Skin & Bums

Lavender & Roman Chamomile
Combine a drop of each with 1 Tbsp coconut oil, and rub onto baby's bum 2-3x daily.

Also combine a drop of each into lotion to soothe baby's skin.

Peaceful Mood

Lavender & Wild Orange
Let baby breathe a drop of each from your hands to soothe crying.

Reassuring Blend
Diffuse 4-6 drops in baby's room to calm baby's temper.

Babies: *Healthy Connections*

Sometimes baby can be inconsolable, detached, or overly attached. Healthy emotional connections set baby up for better overall health and a calmer home experience.

Protocol Benefits
- Promotes healthy maternal bond
- Promotes healthy paternal bond
- Calms anxiety and increases peaceful environment at home

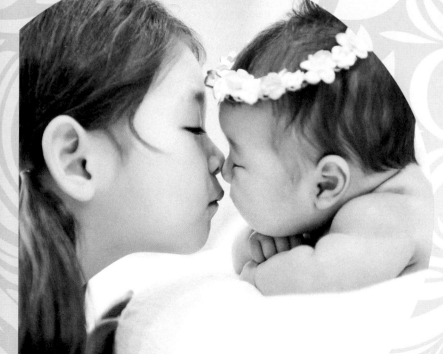

Soothing
Maternal Bond

Myrrh & Geranium
Diffuse 2 drops of each during cuddle time with mom. Also rub a drop of each diluted over baby's back.

This is especially powerful during nursing or while singing to baby.

Time frame
Do this protocol for *2 weeks*. Then reevaluate or switch to another Lifestyle Protocol.

Soothing
Paternal Bond

Patchouli & Frankincense
Diffuse 2 drops of each during cuddle time with dad. Also rub a drop of each diluted over baby's back.

This can be especially important if dad works out of the home.

Peaceful
& Soothing Home

Reassuring Blend or Comforting Blend
Diffuse 4-6 drops of either blend to promote a peaceful atmosphere.

Combine with the power of music (classical music or new age piano) for powerful impact.

Babies: *Immunity-boosting*

This protocol is focused on babies who need extra support in developing a strong immune system.

Protocol Benefits
- Combats harmful pathogens in the air
- Sanitizes common surfaces naturally
- Improves immune system at the gut level
- Supercharges immune system through direct application

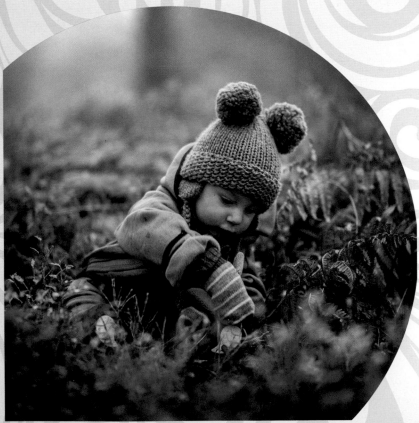

Clean & Safe Environment

Cleansing Blend
Diffuse 4-6 drops to cleanse impurities from the air.

Lemon & Protective Blend
Combine several drops of each with water and a Tbs rubbing alcohol in a glass spray bottle to make a natural sanitizing surface cleaner.

Time frame
Do this protocol for *8 weeks.* Then reevaluate or switch to a different protocol.

Healthy Gut for Healthy Immunity

Bergamot
Rub a drop neat onto baby's feet 1-2x daily.

Children's Probiotic
Dissolve 1/2 sachet into baby's bottle once a day to improve immune system at the gut level (do not heat).

Immunity Supercharge

Protective Blend & Melaleuca
Dilute a drop of each in 1 Tbs FCO. Rub onto baby's spine and bottoms of feet 2-3x daily.

Frankincense
Rub a drop into baby's spine nightly for full-body cellular support.

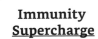

Lifestyles

Beautifying

Beauty is a concept that starts from an internal perception. Use this protocol to nourish beauty on the outside and a healthy self-concept on the inside.

Protocol Benefits
- Uses oil-infused skincare to maintain healthy skin
- Repairs sun damage and signs of aging
- Provides extra nourishment to skin
- Encourages a healthy internal self-concept

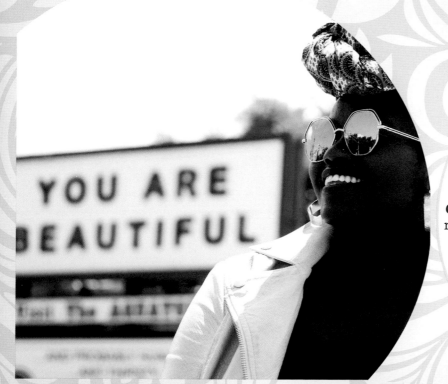

Beautiful Self-Concept

Captivating Blend
Apply to wrists and over heart during meditation, journaling, or while speaking positive affirmations in the mirror when you first wake up and right before bed.

Neroli & Rose
Wear as a perfume, remembering a few things you like about yourself each time you notice the fragrance.

Time frame
Do this protocol for *12 weeks*. Then reevaluate, considering whether to continue your line of skincare products or to try another line of oil-infused skincare.

Skin Enhancement

Anti-Aging Blend
Massage into age spots, fine lines, and wrinkles daily as needed.

Omegas + Essential Oils
Double your daily dose of the omega + essential oil complex to provide extra nourishment to your skin.

Natural Skincare

Oil-Infused Skincare
Use essential oil-infused skincare products daily to naturally protect skin from premature aging, to maintain suppleness, and to improve skin color.

Cleanser: Use during morning shower and to remove makeup before bed.

Toner: Apply to restore skin nutrients after cleansing.

Moisturizer: Apply directly after toner.

Serum: Apply to improve fine lines and wrinkles as needed.

Brainiacs: *Mental Health*

This protocol supports healthy brains of all ages. It focuses on stimulating healthy neurological activity, brain chemistry, and a general sense of alertness.

Protocol Benefits
• Provides nutrients for brain and gut health
• Activates healthy neurological activity
• Stimulates mental activity aromatically
• Enhances memory

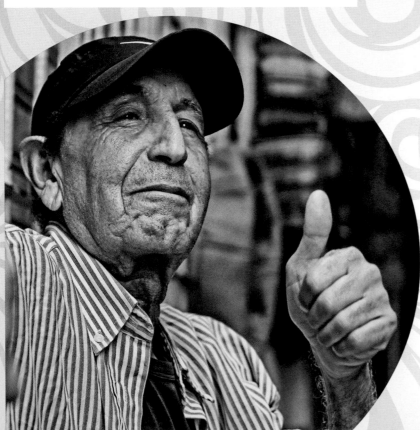

Brain 1 & Brain 2 Fuel

Vitality Supplement Trio
Take 2 of each bottle 2x daily.

Cellular Complex Softgels
Take 2 softgels 2-3x daily.

Probiotic Complex
Take 1 capsule 3x daily to enhance the gut (the 2nd brain) and support neurotransmitter production.

Aromatic Stimulant

Basil, Lavender, & Lime
Diffuse 2 drops of each to stimulate the mind and senses in the afternoons.

Time frame
Use this protocol for *12 weeks.* Then reevaluate to continue use or switch to a different Lifestyle Protocol.

Neurological Activator

Vetiver
Rub a drop onto bottoms of feet and behind ears daily.

Cellular Complex
Massage 2 drops into spine or bottoms of feet daily.

Memory Enhancement

Rosemary & Peppermint
Diffuse several drops of each daily. Also massage a couple drops onto back of neck.

Peppermint
Use a drop of Peppermint on the tongue to awaken the mind as needed.

Frankincense
Hold a drop on your thumb to the roof of your mouth once daily.

Cancer Combat

The body has the power to heal itself. While essential oils do not cure cancer, they facilitate a healthy alkaline environment, encourage proper cellular apoptosis, and support morale while combating cancer. These add up to a powerful cancer regimen.

Protocol Benefits
- Facilitates damaged DNA repair
- Promotes alkalinity & anti-carcinoma support
- Provides crucial and alkalizing nutrition
- Boosts morale & encouragement

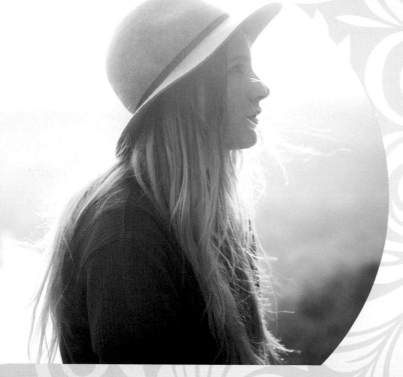

Damaged DNA Repair

Cellular Complex Softgels
Take 2 softgels 2-3x daily.

Cellular Complex
Massage 2 drops into spine and bottoms of feet twice daily.

Time frame
Do this protocol for *16 weeks*. You may increase the frequency of any of the components. Reevaluate and continue as needed.

Alkalinity & Anti-carcinoma Assist

Frankincense
Rub 2-4 drops Frankincense over or close to affected areas 4-8 times daily.

Sandalwood, Frankincense, & Siberian Fir: Diffuse 2 drops of each throughout the day.

Cinnamon & Lemon
Drink 1 drop Cinnamon & 4 drops Lemon in water throughout the day.

Cellular Nutrition & Fuel

Vitality Supplement Trio
Take 2 capsules of each bottle twice daily.

Plant-Based Diet
Move to a completely plant-based diet. Avoid processed foods. Consume as much raw produce as possible.

Morale Booster

Joyful Blend
Diffuse several drops or inhale from cupped hands as often as needed.

Confidence Overhaul

Self-confidence comes not from external validation, but from within. Use this protocol to process self-defeating emotions and patterns, to center your self-perception, and to reinforce a strong self-concept.

Protocol Benefits
• Grounds and centers your energy
• Opens your heart to vulnerability and possibility
• Redefines your perception of yourself and your future

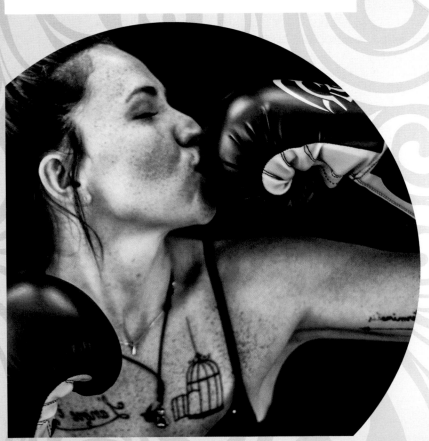

Grounding & Centering

Grounding Blend
Apply 2 drops to the bottoms of your feed each morning. Begin the day with prayer or gratitude, even if it's brief.

Centering Blend
Diffuse 4-6 drops in the home or office to keep your attention focused within.

Time frame
Use this protocol for **21 days**. Then reevaluate and decide to continue or switch to a different Lifestyle Protocol.

Heart Opener

Captivating Blend
Apply over your heart 2-3x daily. Place your hand over your heart, and speak out loud a few things you appreciate about yourself.

Renewing or Comforting Blend
Inhale a couple drops of either blend when you need to surrender old self-defeating patterns.

Self-Concept Reinforcement

Redefining Your Future Self
Spend 15 minutes each day visualizing or journaling about your ideal future self. Learn to define yourself not by what you see now, but by whom you know you're growing into.

Your Favorite Oil or Blend
Reinforce your concept of the new self by enjoying your favorite oil each time you do this exercise.

Emotional Detox

There are seasons to renew, and there are seasons to detox. Use this protocol to protect your energetic boundaries, purge pain and negativity from your body and energy, and to claim a more joyful state.

Protocol Benefits
- Cleanses the energy in your environment
- Trains your mind and soul to expect a new emotional set point
- Purges negativity from your physical body

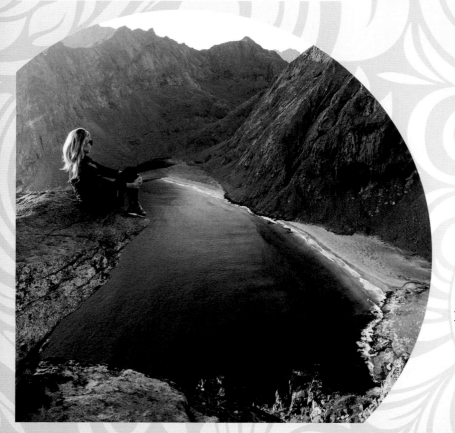

Purified Environment

Cleansing Blend
Diffuse 4-6 drops daily, especially during meditation and journaling.

Melaleuca
Apply a drop to wrists after interactions with less-than-healthy relationships. This oil assists with "energetic vampirism."

Time frame
Use this protocol for **21 days**. Then reevaluate and decide to continue or switch to a different Lifestyle Protocol.

Joy Infusion

Joyful Blend
Add a couple drops to the floor of your shower each morning.

Encouraging Blend
Diffuse 4-6 drops or inhale a couple drops from your palms to elevate your mood.

Lemon, Lime, Grapefruit, Tangerine
Add 2 drops each to a glass or stainless steel water bottle. Contemplate a joyful emotional set point as you enjoy.

Negativity Purge

Soothing Blend
Use a few drops during daily exercise, focusing on allowing your body to release old pain and negative emotions.

Exercise that gets your heart rate up is ideal for this kind of release.

The *Good Life*

This is the master of all the Lifestyle Protocols. It addresses the fundamentals of continued health and wellness. Use it on its own or in addition to any other protocol.

Protocol Benefits
- Provides crucial nutrients to cells, organs, & body systems
- Promotes a sustainable healthy emotional state
- Allows the body to rejuvenate through meaningful sleep
- Increases energy naturally

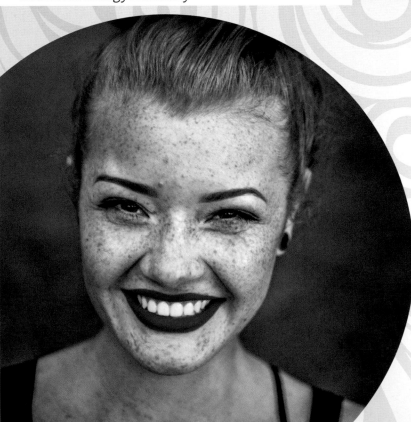

Physical
Wellness First

Vitality Supplement Trio
Take 2 of each bottle 2x daily.

Digestive Enzymes
Take 1-3 capsules with each meal.

Probiotic Complex
Take 1 capsule with each meal.

Cellular Complex Softgels
Take 1 softgel with each meal.

Meaningful
Relaxation & Sleep

Restful Blend
Diffuse several drops, and rub a drop onto your temples before bed each night.

Restful Complex
Take 2 softgels 30 minutes before bed.

Time frame
Treat this as an ***ongoing*** protocol. Use it in conjunction with any other protocol.

Emotional
Well-Being

Grounding Blend
Rub a drop onto the bottoms of feet each morning.

Invigorating or Joyful Blend
Give yourself 60-second emotional resets throughout the day as you pause to breathe a couple drops from your palms.

Energy
Enhancement

Lemon
Drink a few drops in water throughout the day.

Peppermint & Rosemary
Put a dab on your tongue for a quick pick-me-up.

Gut Repair

Every body function is connected to the gut. A large part of the immune system is housed there, crucial neurotransmitters are produced, and nutrient assimilation happens. Repairing the gut repairs the mind and body.

Protocol Benefits
- Tames discomfort like gas, bloating, and indigestion
- Decreases inflammation
- Promotes internal tissue healing
- Encourages long-term mending and health

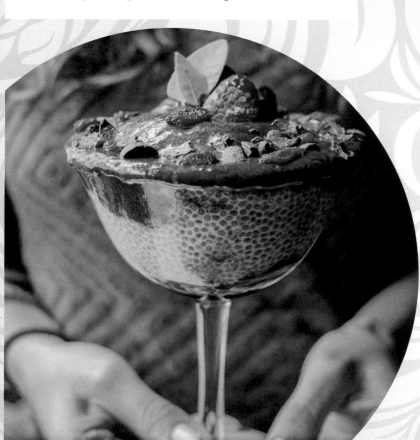

Tummy Tamer

Digestive Blend
Drink a few drops in water or in a capsule, or rub two drops on the outside of the stomach for any stomach discomfort.

Digestive Enzymes
Take 1-3 capsules with each meal to experience easier digestive function.

Time frame
Use the Tummy Tamer on an ***ongoing basis.*** Use the Inflammation Challenger and the Long-term repair during separate ***10-day sprees.***

Inflammation Challenger

Frankincense & Lemongrass
Take 2 drops each in a capsule 1-3 times a day. Only use Lemongrass internally for 10 days at a time (taking 2 week break before continuing).

Helichrysum
Drink 2 drops in water or a capsule, or rub outside stomach to ease inflammation and promote internal tissue healing.

Long-term Repair

GI Cleansing Complex
Purge the gut of Candida, fungus overgrowth, and unhealthy bacteria by taking 1 softgel with each meal for 10 days. Start with only 1 a day, and work your way to 3.

Bone Broth
Make homemade bone broth or buy from the health food store. Sip warm in a mug morning and night to nourish the gut. It's wise to cut inflammatory foods during this process as well (dairy, sugar, etc.)

Lifestyles

Home Holistic *Nurse*

Being the healer in your home means having the confidence to remedy the small things that can take away from enjoying life. Be prepared with this protocol to feel more empowered with your family's wellness.

Protocol Benefits
• Help the family feel peaceful and happy
• Remedy life's little emergencies
• Keep everyone's immune systems high

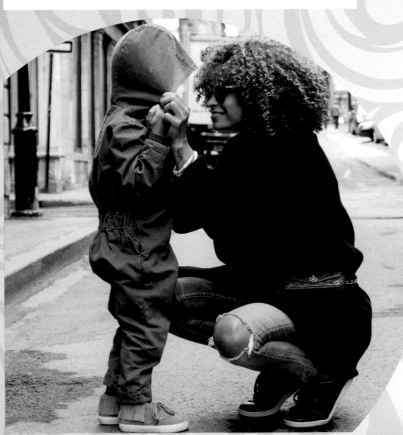

Happy Moods
All Around

Wild Orange
Diffuse several drops or let your child inhale from his/her own hands.

Reassuring Blend
Apply a dab to the temples to calm quarrels and upset.

Time frame
This protocol is meant to be used on an *ongoing basis*. It can be used in conjunction with other protocols geared toward more specific wellness goals.

Life's
Little Emergencies

Melaleuca
Use as an antiseptic and disinfectant for cuts and scrapes.

Lavender
Use to soothe rashes, bumps, bruises, and tears.

Digestive Blend
Use to ease tummy aches and pain.

Helichrysum
Use to help cuts and scrapes heal.

Preventative
Wisdom

Protective Blend
Massage 2 drops diluted into sore joints and connective tissue.

Lemon
Add a few drops to a pitcher of water at dinner time to gently cleanse impurities.

Kids: *Focused Energy*

Kids need energy to grow, play, and enjoy. Sometimes that energy simply needs to be focused in the right place at the right time. Use this protocol to help your child enjoy being a kid while also learning to focus in the right times.

Protocol Benefits
- Provides crucial nutrients to the brain and gut
- Grounds child's energy and improves focus & concentration
- Encourages energy that isn't hyperactive

Kid's Brain Fuel

Children's Omega-3
Use a double dose of Omegas to provide the brain with plenty of healthy fatty acids.

Children's Probiotic
Use 1-2 sachets daily to provide the gut (the 2nd brain) with plenty of healthy flora.

Time frame
Use this protocol for *4 weeks.* Then reevaluate and determine whether to continue or switch to another Lifestyle Protocol.

Powerful Focus

Focus Blend
Roll onto the back of your child's neck when attention spans are short and focus is needed.

Grounding Blend
Rub a drop onto your child's feet each morning.

Balanced Energy

Wild Orange & Lavender
Diffuse 3 drops of each to stimulate a healthy level of energy that doesn't feel hyperactive.

Also combine 10 drops of each with FCO in a roller bottle for your child to use during playtime.

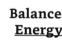

Kids: *Healthy & On-Track*

Healthy is an easier state to maintain when you've got the right components to support continued health! Use this protocol as a regular lifestyle standard to keep kids healthy and happy.

Protocol Benefits
- Provides crucial nutrients easy to miss in many modern diets
- Boost encouragement and focus
- Increase immunity

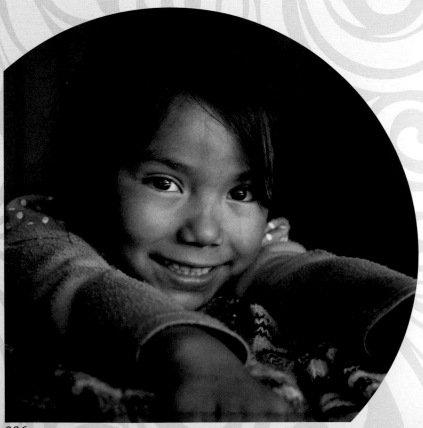

Amazing
Kid's Nutrition

Children's Chewable
Take 1 daily for fundamental nutrients and a healthy body.

Children's Omega-3
Take 1-2 Tbs daily by spoon, or mix into juice or a smoothie.

Children's Probiotic
Consume 1 sachet daily to support healthy digestive & immune function.

Time frame
Treat this as an *ongoing* protocol. It can be used in conjunction with other protocols targeted at more specific wellness goals.

Healthy
Mind & Mood

Invigorating Blend
Let your child breathe a couple drops from cupped hands to encourage a positive outlook and happy countenance.

Focus Blend
Roll onto the back of your child's neck to improve focus, especially during study and chore time.

Healthy
Immunity

Protective Blend
Rub a drop onto the bottoms of feet each morning to keep your child's immune system high.

Also diffuse several drops after school, and use Protective Blend surface cleaner to keep common areas germ-free naturally.

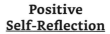

Love Life Boost

Whether seeking new love or fortifying an existing relationship, this protocol is designed to help you view yourself as beautiful and desirable, and to turn up the heat and attraction too.

Protocol Benefits
- Reinforces a positive self-concept
- Plumps lips to be more irresistible
- Leverages natural aphrodisiacs to boost attraction

Positive Self-Reflection

Captivating Blend
Roll over heart daily. Enjoy the aroma as you speak out loud a few things you appreciate about yourself that you believe others will value too.

Rose
Roll over your wrists and heart while journaling about or visualizing your ideal relationship.

Time frame
Use this protocol for *2 weeks.* Then reevaluate or switch to a different Lifestyle Protocol.

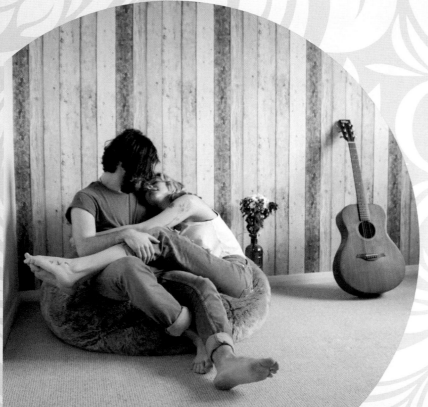

Tempting Aphrodisiacs

Fat Lips
Combine 2 drops each of Cinnamon, Geranium, and Cardamom with FCO in a small roller or empty 5ml bottle. This will plump your lips and make kissing a new adventure.

Inspiring Blend
This blend is full of natural aphrodisiacs. Use it as a perfume, diffuse in the bedroom, or use with FCO in an intimate massage.

Ylang Ylang
This natural aphrodisiac serves as a beautiful perfume or cologne for men and women. Wear daily for increased sex appeal.

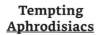

Lifestyles

227

Mindfulness

To find your true self, go within. Turn anxiety & stress into peaceful introspection. This protocol takes your attention away from the outside world and to your inner world for self-discovery and more authentic personal expression.

Protocol Benefits
- Centers your mind and heart for meditation
- Turns your focus inward
- Clarifies the energy in your environment

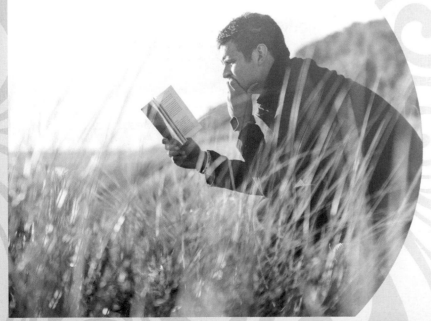

Centered Meditation

Vetiver & Ginger
Massage a drop of each onto the bottoms of feet, especially the big toes before meditation.

Steadying Blend
Use a drop on wrists and temples during meditation, personal development reading, and journaling.

Time frame
Do this protocol for *4 weeks*. Then reevaluate or switch to another Lifestyle Protocol.

Focused Introspection

Grapefruit & Siberian Fir
Rub a drop of each over your heart as you breathe deeply, taking your attention within. Use these moments to remind yourself what is real and what is perceived about yourself.

Sandalwood
Diffuse 4-6 drops during prayer, meditation, yoga, or chants.

Clarified Energy

Purify & Lemongrass
Diffuse 3-4 drops each daily to keep the energy in your space clean and open to new opportunity and discovery.

Musclemen: *trimming, toning, bulking*

Building muscle happens from breaking down muscle tissue and refortifying it with the right macros, and this protocol supports components that make this process happen smoothly.

Protocol Benefits
- Manage inflammation while building muscle
- Cut body fat efficiently
- Support muscle development and recovery

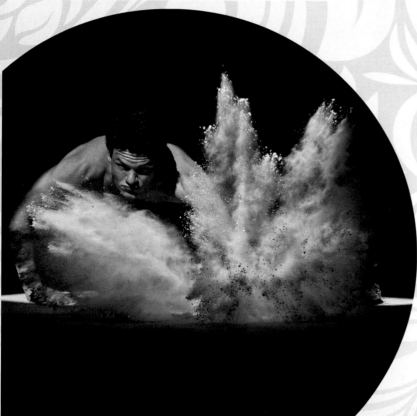

Inflammation Manager

Polyphenol Complex
Take 2 capsules before working out.

Soothing Blend
Massage a few drops into sore areas as often as needed.

Lemongrass
Take a drop under the tongue. Also diffuse several drops.

Time frame
Use this protocol for *4 weeks,* then reevaluate or switch to another Lifestyle Protocol.

Body Fat Eliminator

Trim Shake
Use as directed in a shake or smoothie twice daily. Use in tandem with your preferred protein powder.

Grapefruit
Drink 4 drops in a glass or stainless steel water bottle daily to activate fat-burning enzymes produced by the liver.

Metabolic Blend
Drink a few drops in water or chew Metabolic Blend Gum to address cravings.

Muscle Longevity

Siberian Fir & Marjoram
Massage a couple drops of each with FCO into fatigued muscles to restore and recover quickly.

Pain & Inflammation-away

Turn pain into peace by addressing inflammation at every level. This protocol is ideal for people with both temporary and chronic conditions.

Protocol Benefits
- Ease inflammation from the inside-out
- Soothe muscles, joints, & connective tissue
- Support healthy inflammatory response at a cellular and nervous system level

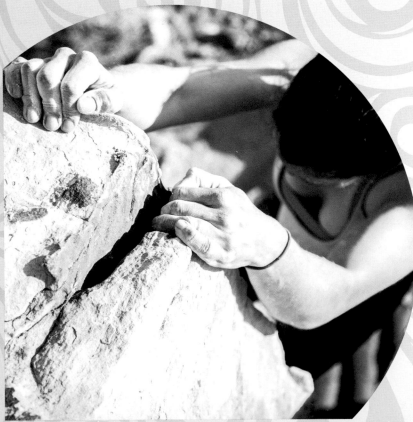

Internal Inflammation Reduction

Polyphenol Complex
Take 2 capsules whenever pain arises, or take 1 capsule 3x daily.

Frankincense & Copaiba
Use a drop of each under the tongue 2-3x daily.

Cellular Complex Softgels
Take 1 softgel with each meal.

Time frame
Do this protocol for *8 weeks*. Then reevaluate or switch to another Lifestyle Protocol.

Muscle, Joint, & Connective Tissue Help

Soothing Blend
Massage a few drops into painful areas as often as needed.

Massage Blend
Massage a few drops with FCO to pull tension out of muscles.

Lemongrass
Rub a couple drops with FCO to soothe painful joints and ligaments.

Body Restoration

Vitality Supplement Trio
Take 2 of each bottle twice daily to powerfully address inflammation on a cellular level.

Vetiver
Rub a drop into the bottoms of feet or spine for nervous system support.

Teens: *Clear Skin*

Acne and blemishes arise from bacterial issues, hormone imbalance, or toxicity overload. This protocol addresses all three simultaneously.

Protocol Benefits
- Addresses bacterial issues on the surface
- Uses oil-infused skincare to safely address cosmetic issues
- Pulls toxicity overwhelm from endocrine system
- Helps balance hormone levels

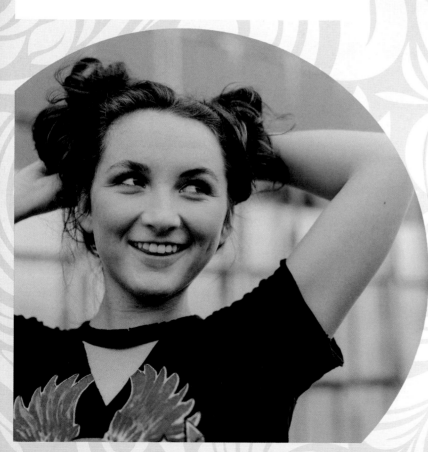

Topical Repair

Skin Clearing Blend
Apply a dab to affected areas.

Melaleuca
Alternate the Skin Clearing Blend with Melaleuca to see which oil your skin responds best to.

Helichrysum
Gently apply a dab to damaged skin.

Toxicity Reduction

Detoxification Softgels
Take 1-2 softgels with each meal.

Detoxification Blend
Rub a drop onto bottoms of feet 20 minutes before showering to pull toxins out of the body.

Time frame
Use this protocol for *8 weeks.* Then reevaluate and continue use as needed.

Oil-Infused Skincare Products

Use an essential oil-infused skincare face wash and moisturizer to help skin recover from acne and blemishes.

Hormone Balance

Ylang Ylang & Jasmine
Apply a dab of each to pulse points in the evening or in stressful moments.

Full Body Detox
Consider doing the 30-day Full Body Detox in this book to reset hormone balance in the body.

Teens: *Studious*

Students thrive when focus becomes easy. This protocol helps students laser in on what's important so they can keep priorities and also enjoy life outside of study.

Protocol Benefits
• Encourages focus & concentration
• Fuels the brain and body for optimal performance
• Fosters an environment conducive to productive studying

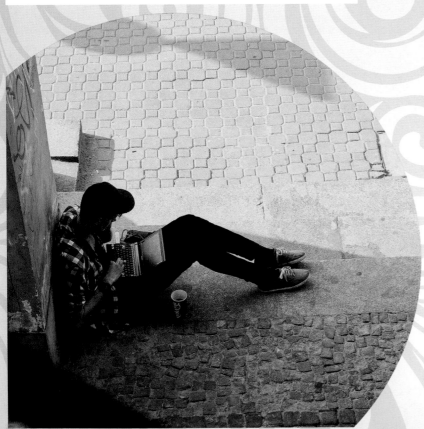

Focus Promoter

Focus Blend
Roll onto the back of neck and temples to improve state concentration.

Grounding Blend
Rub a couple drops onto the bottoms of feet after showering each morning.

Time frame
Do this protocol for *4 weeks*. Then reevaluate or continue on an ongoing basis.

Brain & Body Fuel

Vitality Supplement Trio
Take 2 of each bottle 2x daily.

Energy & Stamina Complex
Take 1-2 capsules 30 minutes before study time.

Probiotic Complex
Take 1 capsule with each meal.

Studious Environment

Rosemary, Peppermint, & Lime
Diffuse 3 drops of each to promote memory retention and focus during study.

Trauma Recovery

Trauma of any kind - abuse, injury, or abrupt life transitions - can leave a sense of being broken or incomplete. Use this protocol to begin the process of realizing your wholeness, your perfection, and your possibility.

Protocol Benefits
- Provides body and mind with essential nutrients for physical and emotional recovery
- Boosts endorphins and positive mood neurotransmitters
- Facilitates the creation of a new story for the future

Whole Body Support

Vitality Supplement Trio
Take 2 of each bottle twice daily to provide crucial bio-available nutrients to cells, organs, and body systems.

Polyphenol Complex
Take 1 capsule 3x daily to support a healthy inflammatory response.

Cellular Complex Blend
Massage 2 drops into the spine each night.

Time frame
Do this protocol for *8 weeks*. Then reevaluate or switch to another Lifestyle Protocol.

Return To True Self

Encouraging Blend
Diffuse several drops and inhale from cupped hands to return to a healthy sense of self.

Melissa
Use a drop under the tongue each day to improve serotonin production.

Writing A New Story

Enlightening Blend
Rub a couple drops over your heart and apply to pulse points.

Use this blend while journaling. Identify any self-defeating stories you might be telling yourself, and transform them into a story that empowers you to move into a future of new and improved possibility.

Consider working with a coach or counselor to guide your thoughts and processes.

Weight Loss

Remember that healthy weight is subjective, not universal. Determine a weight goal you'll feel highly encouraged by, and use this protocol to help you achieve it.

Protocol Benefits
- Curb cravings naturally
- Keep your spirits & motivation high
- Release toxicity overload to eliminate the need for toxin-protecting fat stores

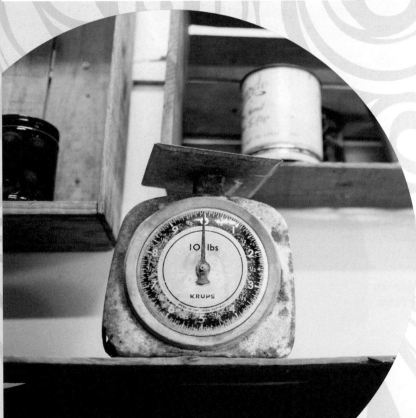

Craving Control

Metabolic Blend Softgels
Take 2-3 softgels 2-3x daily. Also chew Metabolic Blend gum.

Metabolic Blend
Massage several drops with FCO over fatty areas 30 minutes before showering.

Grapefruit
Drink a few drops in water throughout the day.

Time frame
Do this protocol for *8 weeks.* Then reevaluate or switch to a different Lifestyle Protocol.

Internal Motivation

Lime & Rosemary
Diffuse 3 drops of each, or inhale a drop from your palms as needed.

Energy & Stamina Complex
Take 2 capsules 30 minutes before exercise to boost energy and determination.

Vitality Supplement Trio
Take 2 of each bottle 2x daily.

Endocrine, Organ, & Tissue Detox

Detoxification Complex
Take 1 capsule with each meal.

Detoxification Blend Softgels
Take 1 softgel with each meal.

Metabolic Blend
Massage several drops with FCO over fatty areas 30 minutes before showering. Wrap with BPA-free plastic wrap for improved results.

Whole Heart Healing

Whether life has presented a few bumps or it's simply time to return to wholeheartedness, hearts can always use healing.

Protocol Benefits
• Release crippling grief and sadness
• Transition anger and resentment into constructive emotions
• Return the heart to a state of hopefulness and renewal

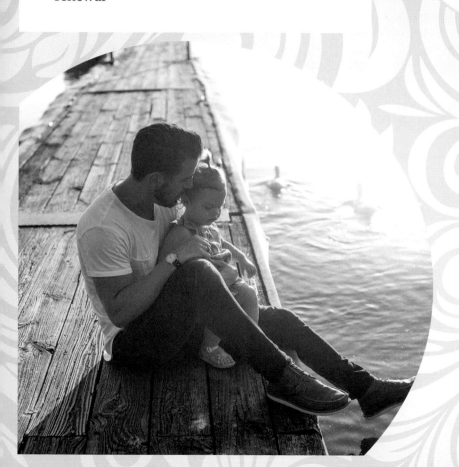

Grief Release

Comforting Blend
Rub a couple drops over the heart and also the pads of your feet. Breathe deeply, envisioning surrendering grief and pain to a higher power.

Time frame
Do this protocol for *8 weeks*. Then reevaluate or switch to another Lifestyle Protocol.

Anger & Resentment Transition

Wintergreen, Thyme, & Lemongrass
Place a dab of each on the corner of a paper where you can write out the negative emotions you'd like to transition.

Write silent letters that you can tear up or burn. Write to release, and then write to reposition your feelings into something constructive.

Heart & Soul Restoration

Renewing Blend
Rub a couple drops over the heart, and inhale from cupped hands during prayer and meditation.

Hopeful Blend
Wear as a perfume or cologne during the day, turning your thoughts to appreciation when you notice the aroma.

Whole Life Detox

You know it's time to purge what isn't serving when life gives you feedback in the form of conflict, health challenges, or difficulty seeing things differently. Use this protocol to jump start detoxing your life from many angles.

Protocol Benefits
- Remove toxicity from relationships
- Pull toxicity from your physical body
- Turn heart toxicity into connection with your heart
- Find a cooperative attitude through attitude detox

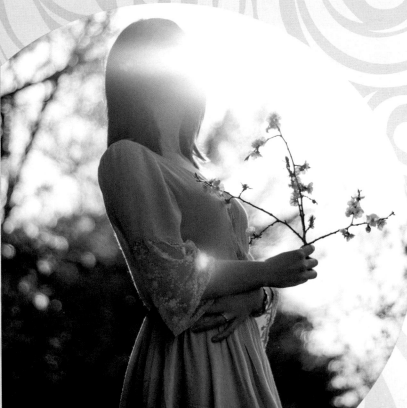

Relationship Detox

Frankincense & Roman Chamomile
Breathe a drop of each from cupped hands as you contemplate relationships to determine their truth and purpose.

Douglas Fir
Diffuse several drops to facilitate surrendering unhealthy patterns.

Time frame
Use this protocol for *2 weeks.* Then reevaluate or switch to another Lifestyle Protocol.

General Physical Detox

Vitality Supplement Trio
Take 2 of each bottle twice daily.

Detoxification Complex
Take 1 capsule with each meal.

Detoxification Blend Softgels
Take 1 softgel with each meal.

Heart & Spirit Detox

Jasmine
Apply to pulse points and over heart to encourage a true sense of self.

Geranium & Arborvitae
Diffuse 2 drops each to reconnect to your heart center.

Attitude Detox

Bergamot & Cypress
Diffuse 3 drops each and apply to the bottoms of feet to encourage flexibility in perception while staying true to ethics and values.

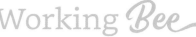

Working *Bee*

There is a season for diligent work, and this protocol supports being eagerly engaged in a worthy cause. Use it to be your best self so you can make your greatest contributions.

Protocol Benefits
- Keeps energy and focus grounded
- Supports the body with crucial nutrients for optimal performance and sustained energy
- Assists with mental clarity and creativity

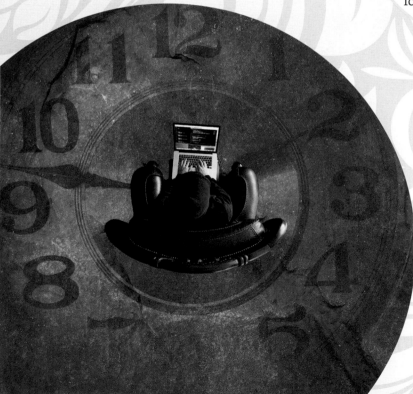

Time frame
Do this protocol for *4 weeks* or during intense periods of work and tight deadlines.

Energy Grounding

Grounding Blend
Rub 2 drops on bottoms of feet each morning to promote focus.

Patchouli, Bergamot, & Clary Sage
Diffuse 2 drops each during long work hauls to balance the soul.

Body Care & Maintenance

Vitality Supplement Trio
Take 2 of each bottle twice daily.

Energy & Stamina Complex
Take 2 capsules 30 minutes before yoga or working out.

Polyphenol Complex
Take 2 capsules before working out, or 1 capsule 3x daily on non-workout days.

Clarity & Creativity Spree

Peppermint & Frankincense
Hold a dab of each to the roof of your mouth for 30 seconds.

Invigorating Blend
Diffuse several drops or inhale from cupped hands every few hours.

The *Yogi*

The Yogi yields a silent-but-powerful energy. He is dedicated to his practice and to his peace of mind. Above all else, he is committed to presence in every moment.

Protocol Benefits
- Increase presence of mind
- Maintain balanced energy
- Support muscles, joints, & connective tissue
- Boost physical and mental energy

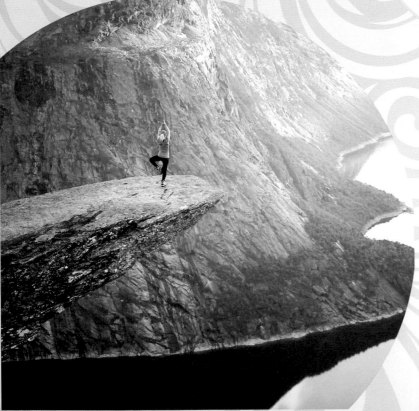

Intention, <u>Prep, &</u> <u>Centerdness</u>

Steadying Blend
Apply a drop to bottoms of feet while setting intentions for your practice and in salutation poses.

Centering Blend
Rub a drop over the heart to bring your focus back to your center and the present moment.

Enlightening Blend
Diffuse several drops and apply to pulse points to bring enlightenment to your most challenging poses and your most peaceful moments.

Time frame
Use this protocol on an *ongoing basis* as long as it serves your practice. Experiment using different oils during practice after a few weeks.

Zen for Joints <u>& Ligaments</u>

Lemongrass
Massage 2 drops diluted into sore joints and connective tissue.

Soothing Blend
Massage oil or rub to soothe muscles after a workout or yoga practice.

Physical <u>Stamina</u>

Vitality Supplement Trio
Take 2 of each bottle twice daily.

Energy & Stamina Complex
Take 2 capsules 30 minutes before yoga or working out.

Polyphenol Complex
Take 2 capsules before working out, or 1 capsule 3x daily on non-workout days.

Section 8

Emotions & *Energy*

How to Use *Emotions & Energy*

This section addresses emotional and energetic health with an *emotional guidance scale* as a measuring stick.

The emotional guidance scale was developed by authors Esther and Jerry Hicks. The bottom of the scale indicates the lowest forms of emotion and energy, whereas the top of the scale represents the highest forms.

The premise of the scale is that making large leaps from a low point to a high point is usually impractical. Instead, take an honest emotional inventory. Find where you are, and see what it will take to progress upward just a little bit.

This is the fastest way to improve your emotions.

Each stage of the guidance scale includes oils to help you **process** the level where you are, as well as oils to help you **progress** to the next level. The last oil listed in each step is also the first oil of the following step.

You'll also find powerful intentions you can speak or write as you use the suggested oils. These are designed to help meet you where you are in the moment, and to gently guide you to the next level.

Remember that you can't do it wrong. Discover what works for you, and enjoy climbing one step at a time.

For a comprehensive emotional guide, purchase Emotions & Essential Oils *by Enlighten.*

Emotions

Emotional Guidance Scale

Identify where you are on the scale. Use the suggested oils to process where you are and gently progress up the scale.

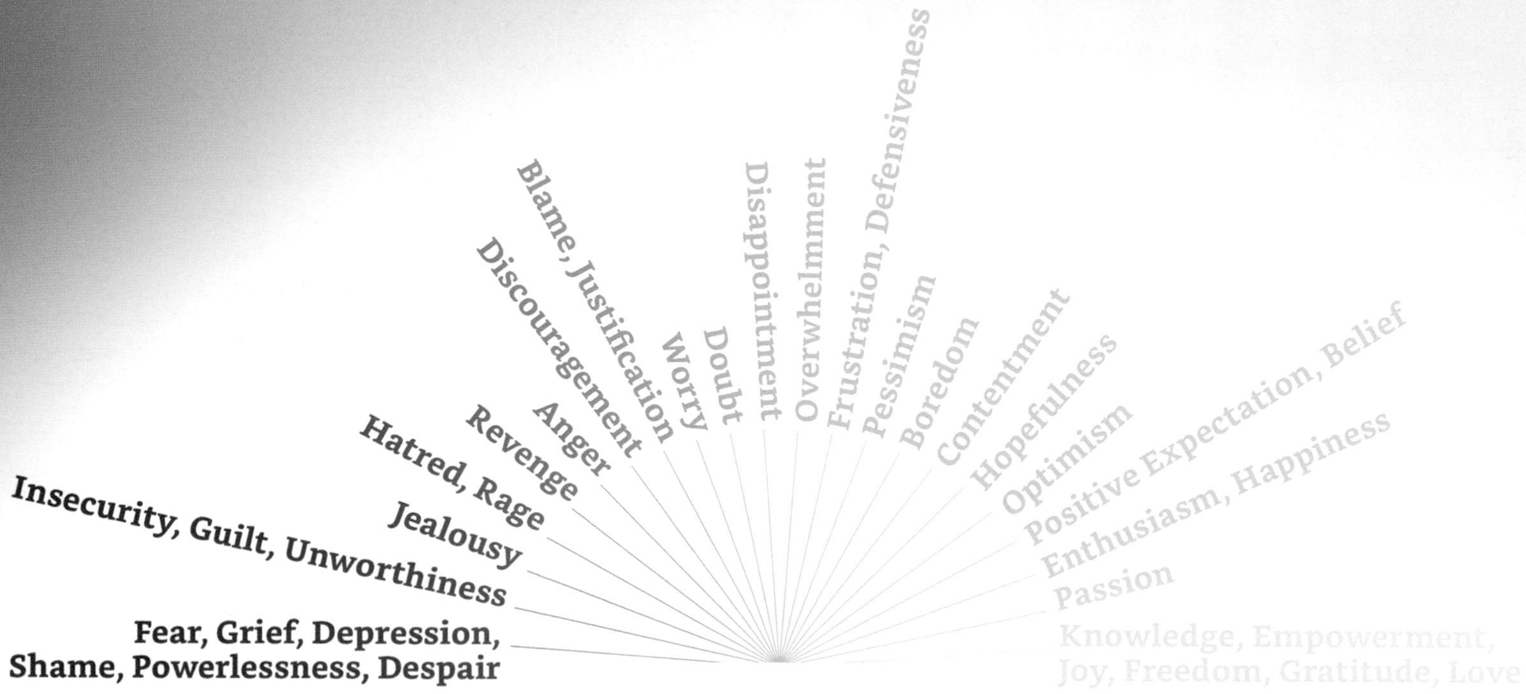

Fear, Grief, Depression, Shame, Powerlessness, Despair

Insecurity, Guilt, Unworthiness

Jealousy

Hatred, Rage

Revenge

Anger

Discouragement

Blame, Justification

Worry

Doubt

Disappointment

Overwhelmment

Frustration, Defensiveness

Pessimism

Boredom

Contentment

Hopefulness

Optimism

Positive Expectation, Belief

Enthusiasm, Happiness

Passion

Knowledge, Empowerment, Joy, Freedom, Gratitude, Love

Fear, Grief, Depression, Despair, Powerlessness, Shame

" I can be okay right here, right now, for at least the next few moments. Then I can take the next few moments after that. I am safe. I can hold on.

Oils to *Process*

Grounding Blend
Rub 2 drops onto the bottoms of feet morning and evening to bring a sense of safety. However things may be, you are at least safe in the present moment.

Helichrysum
Apply to your wrists and solar plexus (above your naval) to initiate healing from shame and despair.

Metabolic Blend
Add 4 drops to your glass or stainless steel water bottle throughout the day to help ease any desire to self-sabotage.

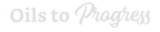

Oils to *Progress*

Melissa
Hold a drop to the roof of your mouth for 30 seconds to stimulate serotonin and dopamine production and receptivity, resulting in a lightened countenance.

Bergamot
Diffuse several drops throughout the day to begin returning to a sense of who you truly are.

Frankincense
Use a drop under your tongue 2-3 times daily to combat depression by facilitating proper neurotransmitter activity.

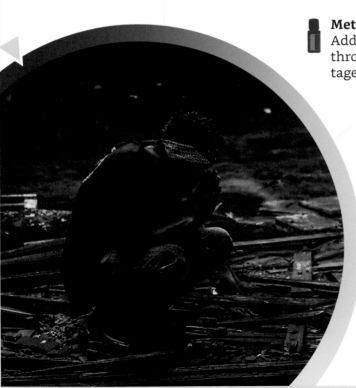

Emotions

Insecurity, Guilt, Unworthiness

Oils to *Process*

Frankincense & Myrrh
Insecurity and guilt can frequently be adopted from mother or father. Use Frankincense (father) or Myrrh (mother) on your wrists as you write out your feelings in a letter you can burn.

Jasmine
Apply over your heart, gently breathing in permission to be who you are.

Spearmint
Diffuse a few drops to lift the feeling of being unseen.

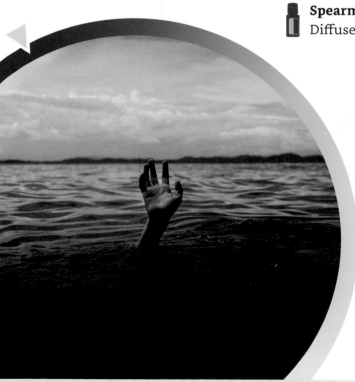

Oils to *Progress*

Reassuring Blend
Apply a couple drops to pulse points during prayer, song, or meditation. Focus on turning thoughts about what's wrong into simply noticing the peace in the present moment.

Peppermint
Rub a drop over your heart to breathe life back into your heart.

Lemon
Inhale a few drops from your palms, offering your higher self permission to guide you to a truer self-concept.

Emotions

Jealousy

Oils to *Process*

Lemon
Inhale a few drops from cupped hands to diffuse sharp feelings of jealousy or envy, including envy of the emotional state of others.

Birch
Add a few drops to a bath or shower. Allow yourself to release feelings of being unsupported.

Black Pepper
Diffuse a few drops to help clear emotional dishonesty and the temptation to mask insecurities with materialism.

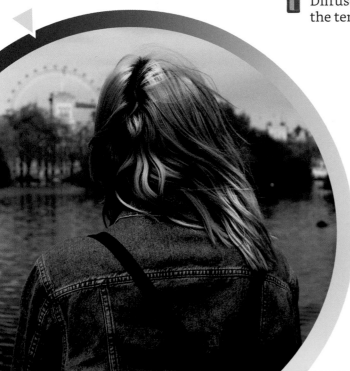

Oils to *Progress*

Cinnamon
Put a dab on your tongue. Focus on exhaling jealousy and rejection of self.

Cedarwood
Massage a couple drops into the back of your neck and temples. Ask that you be met with a sense of community and support of those who really matter to you.

Cassia
Diffuse a few drops to transform feelings of embarrassment, humiliation, or being judged into a sense of self-assurance.

Emotions

Hatred/Rage

Oils to *Process*

Cassia
Diffuse a few drops, allowing the warmth to calm hatred and rage. Begin to see that your true desire is to feel safe and heard from within.

Thyme
Add a couple drops to your shower. Focus on washing away bitterness, resentment, and emotional bondage.

Melaleuca
Inhale a drop from your palms with the intention of releasing relationships that breach healthy boundaries.

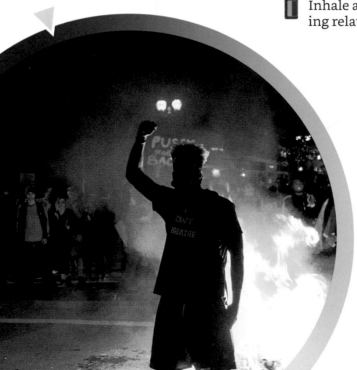

Oils to *Progress*

Juniper Berry
Diffuse several drops to dilute irrational fears that become expressed as hate toward others.

Soothing Blend
Massage a few drops with FCO or lotion into sore and tense muscles where you may be storing unresolved pain.

Wintergreen
Inhale a drop from cupped hands with the intention of learning to surrender the need to control.

Emotions

245

Revenge

Oils to *Process*

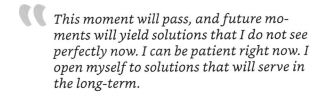

Wintergreen
Inhale a drop from your palms, visualizing negative emotions leaving your body and being absorbed by the earth or the sun.

Clary Sage
Put a dab over your third eye (between and right above your eyebrows), and ask the question, "Is there potentially another way to look at this scenario?"

Oregano
Add a toothpick swirl to a cup of hot tea. Acknowledge the desire for revenge, and then give it permission to fade.

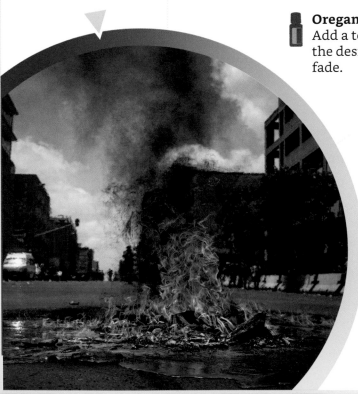

Oils to *Progress*

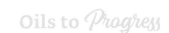

Grounding Blend
Apply a drop behind and over your ears. Allow out-of-control feelings to begin to settle.

Comforting Blend
Apply a drop to your pulse points and heart. Notice the slight improvement that comes from turning your attention from the outside world inward. Notice the inner pain that is asking to be acknowledged.

Cardamom
Drink a drop in water. Allow the sensation to remind you of what it feels like to be objective, to feel more responsible in your self-control.

Emotions

Anger

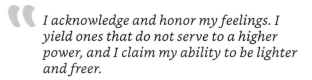
Oils to *Process*

Cardamom
Diffuse a couple of drops. Let the aroma become the sensation of releasing angry feelings in a non-harmful way.

Reassuring Blend
Apply a drop to your pulse points and heart. Turn your thoughts from whatever makes you angry, and focus just for a few moments only on your breath.

Grounding Blend
Apply a drop to your temples and the bottoms of your feet. Remember that feelings are temporal, and that even your anger is okay to acknowledge.

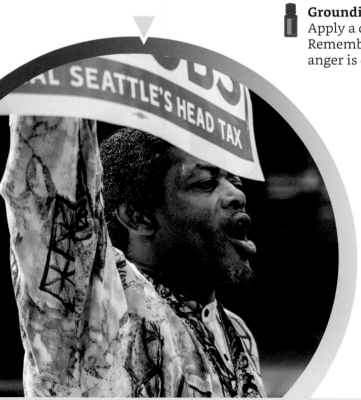

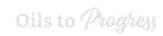

Oils to *Progress*

Douglas Fir
Inhale a few drops from your palms. Offer an intention to forgive any patterns of anger that have been passed from generations before you, and to be the end of that pattern.

Detoxification Blend
Apply a couple drops to the bottoms of your feet 20 minutes before showering. Let your shower help wash away both physical and emotional toxicity.

Cleansing Blend
Diffuse several drops to cleanse the energy of your space, and to begin cleansing emotion that has been harming more than it has been helping.

Emotions

Discouragement

Oils to *Process*

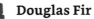

Douglas Fir
Inhale a few drops from cupped hands, remembering that patterns of the past do not determine the future.

Wild Orange
Diffuse several drops. Sense that there may be more opportunities and possibilities - even ones you aren't yet aware of.

Helichrysum
Apply a drop over your heart. Honor your hurt. Allow your feelings to be for the moment.

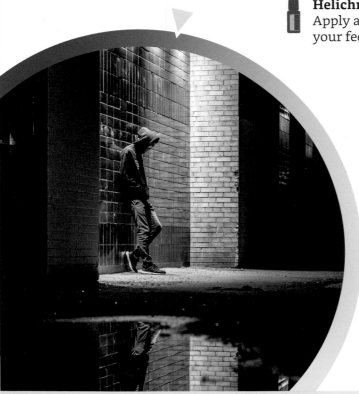

Oils to *Progress*

Uplifting Blend
Diffuse several drops, simply letting the beautiful aroma be enough in the now-moment.

Captivating Blend
Apply to your wrists and over your heart. Let yourself flow a little more effortlessly between breaths.

Eucalyptus
Inhale a drop from your palms. Allow feelings of being defeated or wanting to disappear from life to turn into trust that you can find a way to heal your life.

Emotions

Blame, Justification

Oils to *Process*

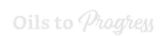

Eucalyptus
Inhale a couple drops from your palms, and rub a bit over your chest. Open your airways as you open your heart and surrender just a little bit of blame.

Ginger
Use a drop on the floor of your shower or in a bath. Gently release the desire to make others responsible for your experiences.

Focus Blend
Apply to the back of your neck. Write a page of ideas of things you (not others) can do for your situation.

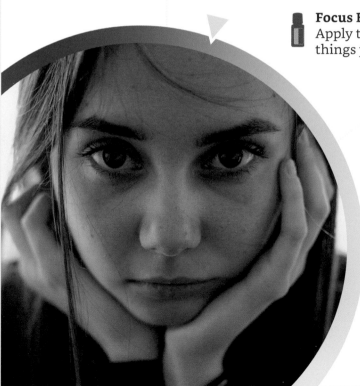

Oils to *Progress*

Clove
Diffuse a couple drops, focusing on releasing feelings of being controlled and being co-dependent. Ask what it feels like to be in charge of your own feelings.

Cilantro
Use a toothpick swirl in cooking or add a bit to your diffuser blend. Let the taste symbolize feeling easier in your relationships.

Cypress
Inhale a couple drops from your palms, asking what it looks like to be more in flow.

Worry

Oils to *Process*

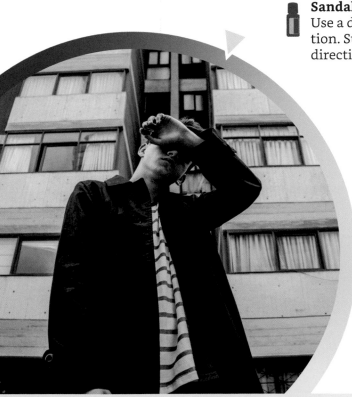

Cypress
Diffuse several drops, noticing the motion and flow of your breath. Remember that things work themselves out, and that life continues on.

Melaleuca
Inhale a drop from your palms. Release any unhealthy expectations you have of others.

Sandalwood
Use a drop on your temples during prayer and meditation. Surrender to higher guidance, and focus on the direction you want to go.

Oils to *Progress*

Rosemary
Diffuse a few drops as you learn to trust in a higher consciousness that has more answers and greater wisdom than your mind has alone.

Cilantro
Rub a drop to the bottoms of your feet before showering to detox the need to be in control.

Cellular Complex Blend
Massage a few drops into your spine or bottoms of your feet to transform your body and emotions into operating with health and vitality.

Emotions

Doubt

Oils to *Process*

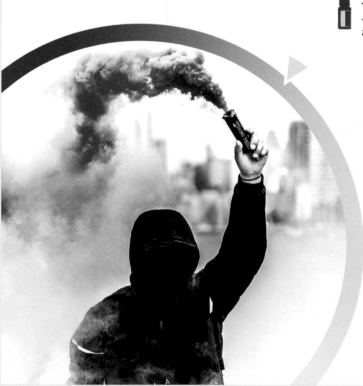

Cellular Complex Blend
Massage a few drops into your spine and your feet to support whole-body cellular health and emotional transformation.

Lemongrass
Diffuse a few drops to cleanse doubt from your energy, and commit to cleaning it up from your vocabulary.

Anti-Aging Blend
Apply around your eyes and forehead to invite spiritual insight about how the greater good is unfolding.

Oils to *Progress*

Rose
Apply to your pulse points and over your heart to begin replacing self-doubt with divine love. Forces bigger than you have your best interest at heart.

Rosemary
Diffuse several drops to open your mind to ways you can transition from doubt into greater possibility.

Fennel
Dab a bit onto your tongue, and appreciate how this oil represents personal responsibility. All you can do is keep your agreements and do your best in any given day.

Disappointment

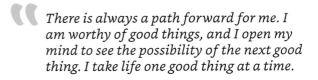

There is always a path forward for me. I am worthy of good things, and I open my mind to see the possibility of the next good thing. I take life one good thing at a time.

Oils to *Process*

Fennel
Put a dab on your tongue, and consider the gift of being responsible for your life.

Cedarwood
Massage a few drops into your neck and shoulders, as well as anywhere you may have skin conditions. Remember that this aroma symbolizes community and the people who have your back.

Lemongrass
Diffuse several drops to cleanse disappointment from the air.

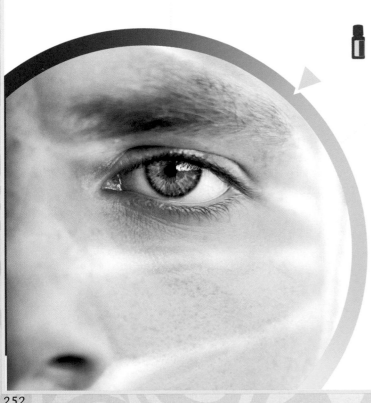

Oils to *Progress*

Arborvitae
Rub a drop onto your wrists and temples, looking for the connection between what you thought was disappointing and where you hope the road will take you.

Skin Clearing Blend
Apply to skin conditions where chronic disappointment may be manifesting physically.

Ylang Ylang
Wear as a perfume or cologne to remind yourself of your ability to be both intellectual and intuitive as you discover the way forward.

Overwhelmment

Oils to *Process*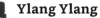

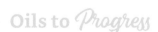

Ylang Ylang
Diffuse a few drops to soften your mood and emotional state.

Digestive Blend
Drink a couple drops in water to help your physical digestion as well as your ability to digest emotions.

Protective Blend
Rub a couple drops on the bottoms of your feet to provide a protective energetic boundary as you prioritize and determine those things you will do best.

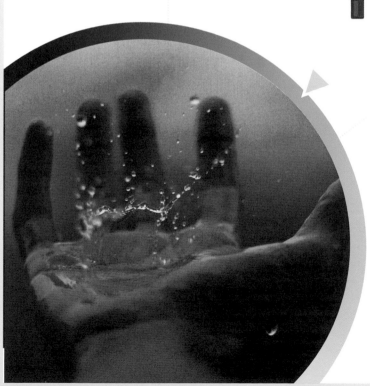

Oils to *Progress*

Tension Blend
Massage onto muscles and areas where overwhelm has turned into pain and tension.

Basil
Diffuse a few drops with your favorite citrus oils to bring about a sense of renewal and refreshment.

Women's Monthly Blend
Apply to your wrists to help balance hormones and to experience the safety that lies in being vulnerable and say no to things that no longer serve (For men too. Be careful of photosensitivity for 48 hours.)

Emotions

253

Frustration, Irritation, Impatience, Defensiveness

> *It's safe to be calm, and it's safe to be heard. I allow myself to see the humanity in others and in myself. I allow myself to be soft in my interactions with others.*

Oils to *Process*

Women's Monthly Blend
Apply to pulse points (be careful of photosensitivity) to remember that force is the slowest way to bring about lasting change.

Vetiver
Apply a drop to the bottoms of your heels and behind your ears to calm the temptation to use irritation as a replacement for constructive communication.

Oregano
Add a toothpick swirl to a hot herbal tea to soothe desires to control others.

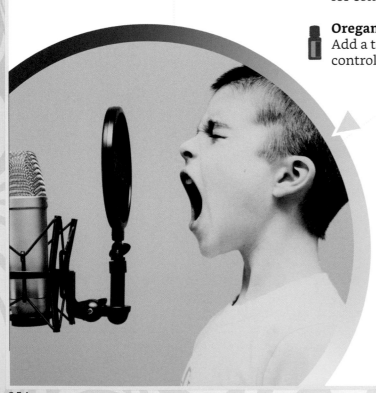

Oils to *Progress*

Respiratory Blend
Breathe a few drops from your palms, and rub some onto your chest. Inhale and exhale deeply as you release frustration through your breath.

Restful Blend
Rub a couple drops onto your temples and over your pillow to help you sleep peacefully and wake in a state of forgiveness.

Roman Chamomile
Diffuse a few drops to see the higher purpose in the things you're experiencing now.

Pessimism

> *I release the past and surrender to what's unseen. I allow my mind to be calm, and to know that everything always works out.*

Oils to *Process*

Roman Chamomile
Rub a drop over your forehead to encourage constructive insights that are authentic to the greater good.

Black Pepper
Use a drop in cooking or on the bottoms of your feet to release any sense of being controlled.

Vetiver
Apply a drop to your heels and behind your ears to root your attention to the present, rather than allowing it to run wild with unpleasant possibilities.

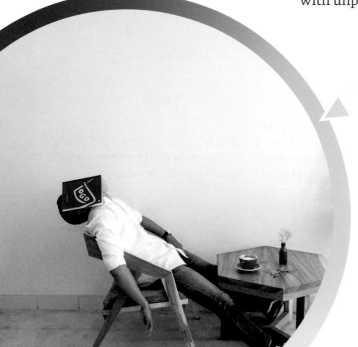

Oils to *Progress*

Wild Orange
Diffuse several drops throughout the day to regain the sense that there is enough abundance and prosperity.

Uplifting Blend
Breathe a couple drops from your palms as you shift pessimistic thoughts to thoughts that feel just a little lighter.

Peppermint
Hold a drop to the roof of your mouth to awaken your mind to other possibilities and outcomes.

Boredom

" *I allow my thoughts to be peaceful and centered. I am easily seeing encouraging things on the horizon, and I lean into it.*

Oils to *Process*

Peppermint
Inhale a drop from cupped hands to find a bit of heartiness in this moment.

Cedarwood
Rub a couple drops onto pulse points, especially during journaling. This helps increase a sense of community and desire to connect with others.

Jasmine
Apply to pulse points to increase a sense of safety and desire to open up in close & intimate relationships.

Oils to *Progress*

Detoxification Blend
Rub a couple drops on the bottoms of your feet 20 minutes before showering to pull out toxins that cause you to feel sluggish.

Invigorating Blend
Inhale a few drops from your hands throughout the day to bring your energy a little bit higher.

Inspiring Blend
Add a few drops to your body lotion to add inspiration to your day.

Contentment

> *I am deeply present. I surrender to what is here and now, and I allow myself to be nurtured at every level.*

Oils to *Process*

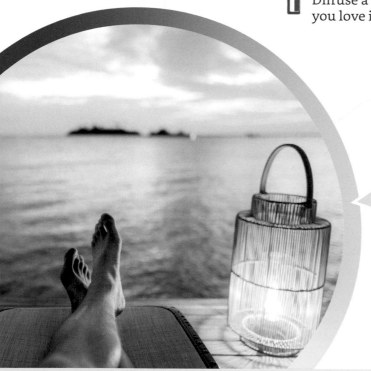

Inspiring Blend
Diffuse a few drops to transition any agitation or lack of control into knowing that the present moment is all that matters.

Geranium
Rub a drop over your heart to indulge in a few things you appreciate about yourself in the here and now.

Roman Chamomile
Diffuse a couple drops or use in the bath to soak up what you love in the present moment.

Oils to *Progress*

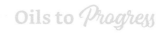

Lemon
Use 4 drops in your drinking water throughout the day to add a little more light to your day-to-day experiences.

Sandalwood
Use a drop on the temples and wrists during gratitude prayers and meditation to see the divine unfolding through every hopeful feeling.

Anti-Aging Blend
Apply around eyes and forehead to better sense the hope embedded in every variant of the future.

Emotions

257

Hopefulness

Oils to *Process*

Anti-Aging Blend
Apply this around your eyes and forehead to transition any remaining disparity into hopefulness.

Clary Sage
Use this oil in a bath to relax into seeing more of where you can allow hope to guide your life.

Restful Blend
Rub a couple drops onto your temples and over your pillow before bed to ease any troubled thoughts, drifting off with the intention to wake more hopeful.

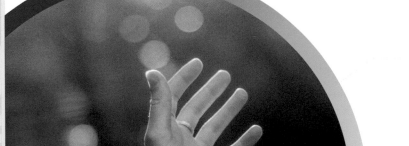

Oils to *Progress*

Grapefruit
Drink a few drops in your glass or stainless steel water bottle throughout the day to facilitate a healthy relationship with your body and your mind.

Helichrysum
Apply a dab over the third eye (between and slightly above your eyebrows) to better see how hope can turn into continuous optimism.

Hopeful Blend
Apply to pulse points and over the heart to feel the warmth of a more hopeful countenance.

Optimism

Oils to *Process*

Hopeful Blend
Apply to pulse points to gently invigorate the senses to recall feelings of seeing improvement and progress.

Cardamom
Inhale a drop from your palms to soothe remaining parts of the ego that want to stay focused on limitation rather than possibility.

Siberian Fir
Apply a few drops over your heart to lift any recurring family patterns of pessimism.

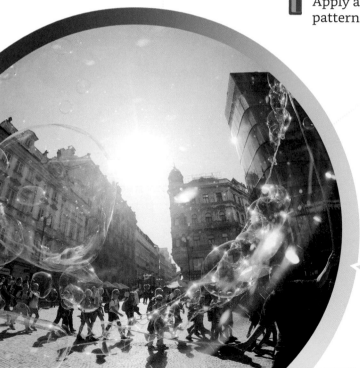

Oils to *Progress*

Melissa
Rub a drop onto the bottoms of your feet, focusing on the big toe, to shed light on the silver lining in every scenario.

Bergamot
Diffuse several drops to encourage a strong sense of self, knowing optimistic possibilities arise from within.

Tangerine
Put a few drops in your drinking water throughout the day to bring an air of fun to problem solving.

Emotions

Positive Expectation, Belief

Oils to *Process*

Tangerine
Diffuse several drops to keep a sense of playfulness. Remember that it can be fun and easy to expect positive things to unfold.

Peppermint
Rub a drop over the heart to improve buoyancy and a sense of optimism.

Uplifting Blend
Inhale a couple drops from cupped hands to find and lift those parts of you that doubt the future.

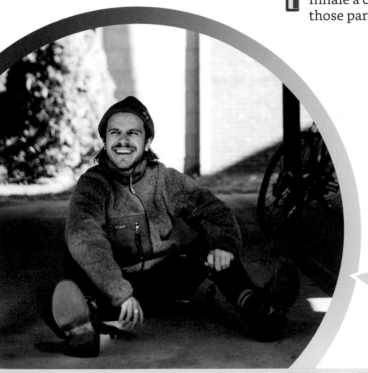

Oils to *Progress*

Invigorating Blend
Diffuse several drops to invigorate the senses and see good things coming in your physical and spiritual surroundings.

Bergamot
Rub a drop over your solar plexus (just over your naval) to ignite belief in yourself. Belief in self opens belief to unlimited possibilities outside the self. (Avoid direct sunlight for 48 hours.)

Wild Orange
Inhale a couple drops from your hands to remember that abundance and well-being exist in unlimited supply.

Emotions

Enthusiasm, Eagerness, Happiness

" *There is a space for happiness in every moment. I am worthy of happy feelings, and I show up in beautiful, eager pursuit of genuine happiness daily.*

Oils to *Process*

Wild Orange
Diffuse several drops to tap into the unlimited happiness that exists in the spaces you create your life in.

Lavender
Rub a couple drops over your throat to open your communication center and your willingness to speak enthusiasm.

Basil
Inhale a drop from your palms to ease self-limiting patterns of staying the same instead of being renewed.

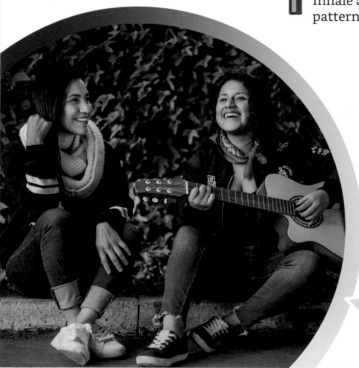

Oils to *Progress*

Melissa
Hold a drop on the roof of your mouth to stimulate serotonin and dopamine production, boosting your feelings of elation.

Respiratory Blend
Rub a few drops over your heart to breathe new life into your daily experiences.

Encouraging Blend
Diffuse several drops to raise the vibration of your space, and to fuel the high energy of enthusiasm.

Passion

> *It is safe to be me, to be completely in love with who I am. What I love matters. I am free to pursue my true desires.*

Oils to *Process*

Encouraging Blend
Diffuse several drops to acknowledge places where limited thinking gets in the way of passionately pursuing life.

Rosemary
Use a few drops in the shower or in a diffuser to inspire receptivity of new passionate possibilities.

Women's Perfume Blend
Apply to pulse points to tap into instinctive guidance. Sometimes you don't know all the answers; you only know what feels right.

Oils to *Progress*

Inspiring Blend
Wear on pulse points as a perfume or cologne.

Jasmine
Apply over heart, taking several moments to breathe deeply and enjoy the building excitement that comes with living your passions.

Uplifting Blend
Use a few drops in water, or rub onto the bottoms of your feet 20 minutes before showering. A clean vessel (body) is conducive to a more passionate lifestyle.

Love, Joy, Knowledge, Empowerment, Freedom, Gratitude

Oils to *Process*

Uplifting Blend
Diffuse several drops to expand your knowing that all is well, joyful, purposeful, and divinely guided.

Arborvitae
Use a dab on the temples during gratitude prayers and gratitude journaling.

Ylang Ylang
Apply a drop to wrists and pulse points on the neck while doing something you love like singing in the car or shower.

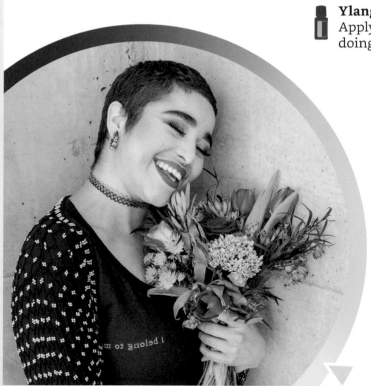

Oils to *Progress*

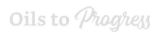

Joyful Blend
Inhale a drop from cupped hands during moments of reflection and appreciation.

Lime
Drink a few drops in a glass of ice water to sink further into your zest for life.

Rose
Apply over the heart to connect more deeply to unconditional self-love and love of others.

Emotions

Section 9

Science & Research

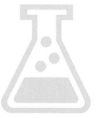

How to Use *Science & Research*

While anecdotal evidence of essential oil benefits can be a powerful demonstration of what oils can do, science provides answers as to *why* they do what they do.

As of the publishing of this book, over 3,000 peer-reviewed studies have been documented by universities, hospitals, and research groups to discover and demonstrate the efficacy of essential oils and their constituents. These studies can be found in rapidly growing numbers through resources like www.pubmed.com and www.aromaticscience.com.

The treasure of essential oils is their chemistry. Each oil contains a unique and robust chemistry set, and each chemical constituent provides various therapeutic benefits.

This section provides a breakdown of essential oils by common property and which naturally occurring chemical constituents provide the associated therapeutic benefits of each property. The science shared in this section has been drawn from the research and resources cited in the references section in this book.

Begin exploring this section by first becoming familiar with the common therapeutic properties oils have.

For a comprehensive and accessible scientific expansion on the chemistry of essential oils, purchase "Essential Oils Unlocked" by PJ Hanks.

Therapeutic Properties *Glossary*

The following are the most common therapeutic properties of essential oils. The pages that follow expand on common chemical constituents that provide each of these therapeutic properties, and in which essential oils they can be found.

Analgesic	Reduces pain sensation	**Aphrodisiac**	Increases sexual desires
Anti-allergenic	Reduces allergic response	**Astringent**	Firms tissues, reduces secretions
Antiarthritic	Useful in treating arthritis	**Cardiotonic**	Vitalizes cardiovascular system
Antibacterial	Kills or prevents bacterial growth	**Carminative**	Reduces gas or bloating
Anticarcinogenic	Inhibits development of cancer cells	**Decongestant**	Reduces congestion and opens airways
Anticonvulsant	Reduces convulsions	**Digestive Stimulant**	Aids in proper digestive processes
Antidepressant	Alleviates depression symptoms	**Disinfectant**	Fights the spread of germs
Antiemetic	Eases nausea and vomiting	**Expectorant**	Removes excess mucus
Antifungal	Prevents fungal growth	**Immunostimulant**	Stimulates immune system activity
Anti-infectious	Prevents uptake of infection	**Nervine**	Beneficial effect on nerves
Anti-inflammatory	Alleviates inflammation	**Regenerative**	Promotes body tissue regeneration
Antioxidant	Destroys or inhibits growth of parasites	**Restorative**	Promotes restoration of body systems
Anti-parasitic	Alleviates pain and stiffness	**Rubefacient**	Increases circulation & skin redness
Anti-rheumatic	Reduces damage from free radicals	**Sedative**	Relaxes psychological and physical activity
Antispasmodic	Prevents or relieves spasms & convulsions	**Soporific**	Induces sleep
Antitumoral	Inhibits growth of tumors	**Stomachic**	Stimulates digestion & appetite
Antitussive	Relieves coughs	**Tonic**	Encourages feelings of vitality
Antiviral	Inhibits replication of viral RNA	**Vasodilator**	Relaxes blood vessels, lowers blood pressure

Other therapeutic properties that have not been reviewed in this section due to redundancy or because less research has been done include anaphrodisiac, anti-carcinoma, anticatarrhal, anticoagulant, antimicrobial, antimutagenic, antiputrescent, antiseptic, antitoxic, calmative, cleanser, cytophylactic, deodorant, detoxifier, diuretic, emmenagogue, energizing, galactagogue, grounding, insecticidal, invigorating, laxative, mucolytic, neuroprotective, purifier, refreshing, relaxing, revitalizer, steroidal, stimulant, uplifting, vasoconstrictor, vermicide, vermifuge, and warming.

Science

Chemistry of *Essential Oils*

Essential oils are comprised of chemical compound groups. Each compound group is comprised of individual chemical constituents. Compound groups are defined by both the number of carbon atoms they have and the type of functional group assigned to them.

Constituents tend to have similar and complimentary therapeutic properties with other constituents found in their same group.

Monoterpene Hydrocarbons   Therapeutic properties include detoxifying, anti-inflammatory, antiseptic, sedative, insecticidal, anti-tumoral, restorative, and mood-enhancing.

Sesquiterpene Hydrocarbons   Therapeutic properties include anti-inflammatory, anti-microbial, analgesic, digestive stimulant, vasodilator, endocrine support, and calmative.

Chamazulene   Chamazulene is not a naturally occurring constituent in plants, but rather occurs during distillation as the constituent Matricene decomposes. Therapeutic properties include antioxidant and regenerative.

Monoterpene Alcohols   Therapeutic properties include antiseptic, anti-fungal, anti-microbial, analgesic, antioxidant, antispasmodic, and integumentary restorative.

Sesquiterpene Alcohols   Therapeutic properties include anti-microbial, anti-inflammatory, endocrine support, nervine, astringent, vasodilator, antispasmodic, sedative, and soporific.

Aldehydes   Therapeutic properties include calmative, anti-microbial, anti-inflammatory, analgesic, nervine, and hypotensive.

Esters   Therapeutic properties include calmative, analgesic, antispasmodic, anti-fungal, and nervine.

Ketones   Therapeutic properties include mucolytic, regenerative, analgesic, sedative, and anti-inflammatory.

Oxides   Therapeutic properties include anti-microbial, expectorant, mucolytic, and analgesic.

B-Caryophyllene

Constituent Details
- Sesquiterpene Alkene
- This constituent is a member of the cannabinoid family

Common Oils
- Copaiba (45-65%)
- Black Pepper (8-46%)
- Ylang Ylang (5-25%)
- Melissa (1-22%)
- Clove (0.6-20%)
- Thyme (0.1-15%)
- Frankincense (0.1-10%)

Methyl Salicylate

Constituent Details
- Ester

Common Oils
- Birch (98%)
- Wintergreen (98%)

Analgesic

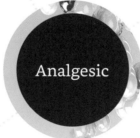

Reduces pain sensation

a-Pinene

Constituent Details
- Monoterpene Alkene

Common Oils
- Frankincense (25-65%)
- Cypress (20-65%)
- Juniper Berry (24-55%)
- Coriander (5-20%)
- Helichrysum 5-20%
- Rosemary (5-20%)
- Siberian Fir (5-20%)
- Black Pepper (1-20%)
- Fennel (1-15%)

d-3-Carene

Constituent Details
- Monoterpene Alkene

Common Oils
- Cypress 7-30%
- Siberian Fir 5-20%
- Black Pepper 0.01-21%

de Cássia da Silveira E, *Int J Mol Sci*, 2017 | Zalachoras, *Planta Medica*, 2010 | Jimenez, *Die Pharmazie*, 1989

Constituent Details
• Monoterpene Alkene Aldehyde

Common Oils
• Lemongrass (25-36%)
• Melissa (9-26%)
• Lemon (0.4-2%)
• Wild Orange (<1.3%)
• Geranium (0-1.1%)

Neral

Citral

Constituent Details
• Monoterpene Aldehyde

Common Oils
• Litsea (70-85%)
• Lemongrass (65-85%)
• Petitgrain (36%)
• Lime (6-9%)
• Lemon (2-5%)

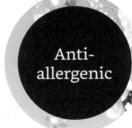

Anti-allergenic

Reduces allergic response

Geranial

Constituent Details
• Monoterpene Alkene Aldehyde

Common Oils
• Lemongrass (36-55%)
• Melissa (12-38%)
• Lemon (0.5-4.3%)
• Lime (2.2-3.9%)
• Wild Orange (<1.8%)

Mckay, *Phytotherapy Research*, 2006
Emílio-Silva, *Inflammation*, 2017

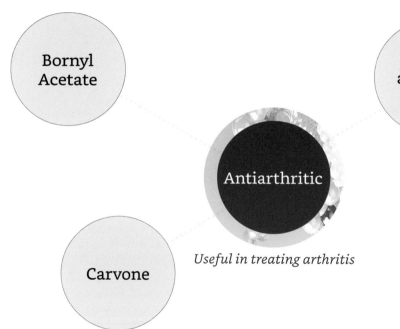

Constituent Details
· Monoterpene Ester

Common Oils
· Siberian Fir (20-40%)

Bornyl Acetate

a-Pinene

Constituent Details
· Monoterpene Alkene

Common Oils
· Frankincense (25-65%)
· Cypress (20-65%)
· Juniper Berry (24-55%)
· Coriander (5-20%)
· Helichrysum 5-20%
· Rosemary (5-20%)
· Siberian Fir (5-20%)
· Black Pepper (1-20%)
· Fennel (1-15%)

Antiarthritic

Useful in treating arthritis

Carvone

Constituent Details
· Monoterpene Ketone

Common Oils
· Spearmint (20-80%)
· Dill (40-65%)

Naseri, *Iran Journal of Pharmaceutical Research*, 2012
Kim, *The American Journal of Chinese Medicine*, 2015

Science

Constituent Details
• Monoterpene Phenol

Common Oils
• Oregano (60-80%)
• Thyme (0.2-16%)

Carvacrol

Constituent Details
• Monoterpene Alkene

Common Oils
• Melaleuca (10-55%)
• Cumin (3-35%)
• Lime (5-20%)
• Marjoram (0.5-20%)
• Lemon (3-16%)
• Bergamot (3-12%)
• Coriander (0.1-10%)

g-Terpinene

Benzyl Acetate

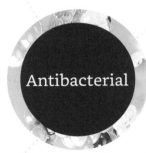

Antibacterial

Kills or prevents bacterial growth

Limonene

Constituent Details
• Ester

Common Oils
• Jasmine (5-25%)

Constituent Details
• Monoterpene Alkene

Common Oils
• Grapefruit (90-97%)
• Tangerine (80-99%)
• Wild Orange (80-97%)
• Lemon (55-75%)
• Lime (40-70%)
• Dill (30-55%)
• Bergamot (20-55%)
• Spearmint (5-30%)
• Black Pepper (9-25%)
• Frankincense (5-20%)

p-Cymene

Constituent Details
• Monoterpene Alkene

Common Oils
• Thyme (3-35%)
• Cumin (3-20%)

Magi, *Frontiers in Microbiology*, 2015 | Cristani, *Journal of Agricultural and Food Chemistry*, 2007 | Rath, *Indian Journal of Pharmaceutical Sciences*, 2008

Science

Lanceol

Constituent Details
• Sesquiterpene Alcohol

Common Oils
• Hawaiian Sandalwood (2-16%)
• Indian Sandalwood (1.5-1.7%)
• Helichrysum (.2%)
• Clary Sage (.1%)

Constituent Details
• Monoterpene Alkene

Common Oils
• Wild Orange (83-95%)
• Grapefruit (84-95%)
• Tangerine (87-91%)
• Dill (35-68%)
• Bergamot (27-52%)
• Helichrysum (10.7%)

Limonene

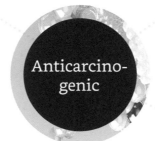

Anticarcino-genic

Inhibits development of cancer cells

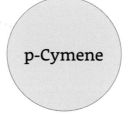

p-Cymene

Constituent Details
• Monoterpene Alkene

Common Oils
• Thyme (18-37%)
• Cumin (5-17%)
• Frankincense (0.7-11%)
• Oregano (3-10%)
• Coriander (0-8.4%)
• Rosemary (2.4-6%)
• Marjoram (2.2-5.3%)

Chen, *Oncology Letters,* 2013 | Elson, *Carcinogenesis,* 1988 | Marchese, *Materials,* 2017

Science

Constituent Details
• Phenol

Common Oils
• Thyme (48-62%)
• Oregano (0.3-4%)
• Blue Tansy (0.8-1.8%)

Limonene

Constituent Details
• Monoterpene Alkene

Common Oils
• Grapefruit (90-97%)
• Wild Orange (80-97%)
• Black Pepper (16-24%)
• Spearmint (9-21%)
• Frankincense (5-20%)
• Neroli (6-17%)
• Helichrysum (10.7%)

Thymol

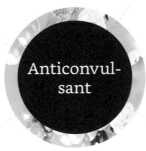

Anticonvul-sant

Reduces convulsions

a-Thujene

E-Anethole

Constituent Details
• Monoterpene Ketone

Common Oils
• Frankincense (1-19.3%)
• Juniper Berry (1.8%)

Constituent Details
• Ether

Common Oils
• Fennel (58-92%)
• Star Anise (71-91%)

Karimzadeh, *BMC Complementary and Alternative Medicine*, 2012
Aliabadi, *International Journal of Medical Laboratory*, 2016
Viana, *Biological & Pharmaceutical Bulletin*, 2000

Constituent Details
• Ester

Common Oils
• Jasmine (5-25%)

Benzyl Acetate

Constituent Details
• Monoterpene Ether

1,8-Cineole

Common Oils
• Eucalyptus (55-85%)
• Rosemary (30-60%)
• Cardamom (25-50%)
• Basil (6-6.7%)
• Peppermint (1-10%)
• Spearmint (0.1-10%)
• Frankincense (0-2.9%)

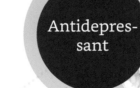

Antidepressant

Alleviates depression symptoms

Constituent Details
• Monoterpene Alcohol

Common Oils
• Lemongrass (25-50%)
• Melissa (1-32%)

Neral

a-Phellandrene

Constituent Details
• Monoterpene Alkede

Common Oils
• Dill (6.5%)
• Frankincense (0-5.9%)

Piccinelli, *Nutritional Neuroscience*, 2014
Kim, *Evidence-Based Complementary and Alternative Medicine*, 2014

Constituent Details
• Monoterpene Alcohol

Common Oils
• Rose (10-30%)
• Geranium (5-25%)
• Lemongrass (1-15%)

Geraniol

Gurjunene

Constituent Details
• Sesquiterpene Alkene

Common Oils
• Spikenard (3-13%)

Neryl Acetate

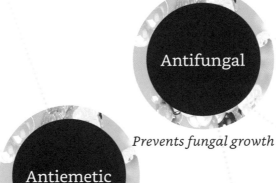

Antifungal

Prevents fungal growth

Constituent Details
• Monoterpene Ester

Common Oils
• Helichrysum (25-50%)

Menthol

Antiemetic

Constituent Details
• Monoterpene Alcohol

Common Oils
• Peppermint (19-54%)

Eases nausea and vomiting

Ocimene

Sabinene

Menthone

Constituent Details
• Monoterpene Ketone

Common Oils
• Peppermint (8-31%)
• Geranium (0.1-2.4%)
• Spearmint (0.1-1.7%)

Constituent Details
• Monoterpene Alkene

Common Oils
• Lavender (0.3-10%)

Constituent Details
• Monoterpene Alkene

Common Oils
• Blue Tansy (10-30%)
• Douglas Fir (5-25%)
• Marjoram (0.4-33%)
• Juniper Berry(0.0-30%)
• Black Pepper (0.1-23%)

Oz, *Frontiers in Pharmacology,* 2017
Sadraei, *Research in Pharmaceutical Sciences,* 2013

Djihane, *Saudi Pharmaceutical Journal,* 2017
Valente, *Food and Chemical Toxicology,* 2013
Flach, *Planta Medica,* 2002

Constituent Details
• Monoterpene Alkene

Common Oils
• Cypress (7-30%)
• Siberian Fir (5-20%)
• Black Pepper (0.01-21%)

d-3-Carene

Limonene

Constituent Details
• Monoterpene Alkene

Common Oils
• Tangerine (80-99%)
• Grapefruit (90-97%)
• Wild Orange (80-97%)
• Lemon (55-75%)
• Lime (40-70%)
• Dill (30-55%)
• Bergamot (20-55%)
• Spearmint (5-30%)
• Black Pepper (9-25%)
• Frankincense (5-20%)

Anti-infectious

Prevents uptake of infection

Geranial

Constituent Details
• Monoterpene Aldehyde

Common Oils
• Lemongrass (25-50%)
• Melissa (10-47%)

Kon KV, *Expert Rev Anti Infect Ther*, 2012
Astani, *Iranian Journal of Microbiology*, 2014

Science

Constituent Details
• Monoterpene Ketone

Common Oils
• Blue Tansy (5-20%)
• Rosemary (5-15%)
• Coriander (2-8%)

Camphor

Methyl Salicylate

Constituent Details
• Ester

Common Oils
• Birch (98%)
• Wintergreen (98%)

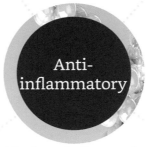

Anti-inflammatory

Alleviates Inflammation

Constituent Details
• Monoterpene Alkene

Common Oils
• Siberian Fir (10-30%)
• Ginger (1-10%)

Camphene

B-Caryophyl-lene

Constituent Details
• Sesquiterpene Alkene

Common Oils
• Copaiba (45-65%)
• Black Pepper (8-46%)
• Ylang Ylang (5-25%)
• Melissa (1-22%)
• Clove (0.6-20%)
• Thyme (0.1-15%)
• Frankincense (0.1-10%)

Oliveira-Tintino, *Phytomedicine*, 2018
Bayala, *PLoS ONE*, 2014

Constituent Details
• Sesquiterpene Alkene

Common Oils
• Copaiba (2-12%)
• Basil (1-7%)

Bergamotene

Constituent Details
• Sesquiterpene Alkene

Common Oils
• Copaiba (45-65%)
• Black Pepper (8-46%)
• Ylang Ylang (5-25%)
• Melissa (1-22%)
• Clove (0.6-20%)
• Thyme (0.1-15%)
• Frankincense (0.1-10%)

B-Caryophyl-lene

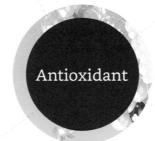

Antioxidant

Reduces damage from free radicals

Camphene

Constituent Details
• Monoterpene Alkene

Common Oils
• Siberian Fir (10-30%)
• Ginger (1-10%)

Cinnamalde-hyde

Constituent Details
• Aldehyde

Common Oils
• Cassia (75-97%)
• Cinnamon (45-80%)

Pandey, *Medicines*, 2017
Li, *Journal of Food Science and Technology*, 2017

Science

Constituent Details
- Phenylpropenoid Ether

Common Oils
- Clove (0.2%)
- Basil (0.1%)
- Melaleuca (.06%)

Methyleuge-nol

Limonene

Constituent Details
- Monoterpene Alkene

Common Oils
- Tangerine (80-99%)
- Grapefruit (90-97%)
- Wild Orange (80-97%)
- Lemon (55-75%)
- Lime (40-70%)
- Dill (30-55%)
- Bergamot (20-55%)
- Spearmint (5-30%)
- Black Pepper (9-25%)
- Frankincense (5-20%)

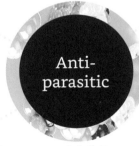

Anti-parasitic

Destroys or inhibits growth of parasites

p-Cymene

Constituent Details
- Monoterpene Hydrocarbon

Common Oils
- Thyme (18-37%)
- Oregano (4-9%)
- Coriander (0-8%)
- Rosemary (1-6%)
- Marjoram (2-5%)

Sena-Lopes, *Plos One*, 2018
Gomes, *American Journal of Plant Sciences*, 2014
Escobar, *Memórias Do Instituto Oswaldo Cruz*, 2010

Constituent Details
• Monoterpene Ester

Common Oils
• Siberian Fir (20-40%)

Constituent Details
• Monoterpene Aldehyde

Common Oils
• Lemongrass (25-50%)
• Melissa (10-47%)

Bornyl Acetate

Geranial

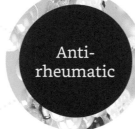

Anti-rheumatic

Alleviates pain & stiffness

Methyl Salicylate

Constituent Details
• Ester

Common Oils
• Birch (98%)
• Wintergreen (98%)

Shakeel-u-Rehman, *EC Microbiology*, 2018
Mitoshi, *International Journal of Molecular Medicine*, 2014

Science

Constituent Details
- Monoterpene Ketone

Common Oils
- Blue Tansy (5-20%)
- Rosemary (5-15%)
- Coriander (2-8%)

B-Caryophyl-lene

Constituent Details
- Sesquiterpene Alkene

Common Oils
- Copaiba (24-53%)
- Black Pepper (9-30%)
- Ylang Ylang (1-21%)
- Melissa (0.3-19%)
- Clove (0.6-12%)
- Lavender (1-5%)
- Cinnamon (1-5%)
- Helichrysum (5%)

Camphor

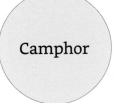

Antispasmodic

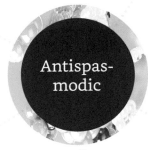

Prevents or relieves spasms, convulsions, & contractions

Linalyl Acetate

Constituent Details
- Monoterpene Ester

Common Oils
- Clary Sage (45-73%)
- Lavender (25-46%)
- Bergamot (17-40%)
- Marjoram (7-10%)
- Neroli (0.6-10%)
- Cardamom (6.5%)

Benzyl Benzoate

Constituent Details
- Ester

Common Oils
- Jasmine (8-20%)
- Ylang Ylang (4-14%)
- Cassia (1%)
- Cinnamon (1%)

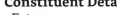

Leonhardt, *Fundam Clin Pharmacol*, 2010 | Andrade, *Journal of Medicinal Plants Research*, 2011 | Astudillo, *Phytotherapy Research*, 2004

Constituent Details
· Monoterpene Ketone

Common Oils
· Frankincense (1-19.3%)
· Juniper Berry (1.8%)

a-Terpinene

Constituent Details
· Monoterpene Alkene

Common Oils
· Melaleuca (5-13%)
· Marjoram (3-5.9%)
· Roman Chamomile (0-4.5%)
· Juniper Berry (0-2.6%)
· Douglas Fir (2%)

a-Thujene

Antitumoral

Inhibits growth of tumors

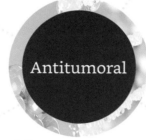

Carvacrol

Constituent Details
· Monoterpene Phenol

Common Oils
· Oregano (61-83%)
· Marjoram (76-81%)
· Thyme (41%)

a-Pinene

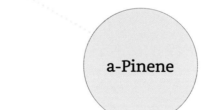

Constituent Details
· Monoterpene Alkene

Common Oils
· Frankincense (41-80%)
· Juniper Berry (24-55%)
· Cypress (20-52%)
· Rosemary (19-35%)
· Helichrysum (21.7%)

Yin, *Cytotechnology*, 2011 | Biswas, *Evidence-Based Complementary and Alternative Medicine*, 2011 | Fernandes, *Bioactive Essential Oils and Cancer*, 2015

Science

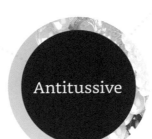

1,8-Cineole

Constituent Details
· Monoterpene Ether

Common Oils
· Eucalyptus (60-64%)
· Rosemary (39-57%)
· Cardamom (26-44%)
· Melaleuca (15%)
· Basil (6-6.7%)

Khusimol

Constituent Details
· Sesquiterpene Alcohol

Common Oils
· Vetiver (5-15%)

Antitussive

Relieves Coughs

Menthol

Constituent Details
· Monoterpene Alcohol

Common Oils
· Peppermint (20-60%)

Takaishi, *Molecular Pain*, 2012
Jirovetz, *Scientia Pharmaceutica*, 2003
Laude, *Pulmonary Pharmacology*, 1994

Science

Constituent Details
• Monoterpene Aldehyde

Common Oils
• Lemongrass (25-50%)
• Melissa (10-47%)
• Wild Orange (1.8%)

Geranial

Constituent Details
• Monoterpene Alcohol

Common Oils
• Rose (10-30%)
• Geranium (5-25%)
• Lemongrass (1-15%)
• Melissa (1-8.1%)
• Neroli (0.8-3%)
• Ylang Ylang (0-3%)
• Eucalyptus (0.2-2%)

Geraniol

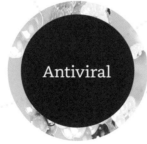

Antiviral

Prevents the replication of viral RNA

Lindestrene

Constituent Details
• Sesquiterpene Ether

Common Oils
• Myrrh (1-20%)

Citral

Constituent Details
• Monoterpene Alkene Aldehyde

Common Oils
• Lemongrass (77-90%)
• Melissa (<64%)
• Lime (4-6%)
• Orange (1.5%)

Pourghanbari, *VirusDisease*, 2016
Farhath, *Avicenna Journal of Phytomedicine*, 2013
Astani, *Phytotherapy Research*, 2009

Science

Benzyl Acetate

Constituent Details
· Ester

Common Oils
· Jasmine (5-25%)

Nerol

Constituent Details
· Monoterpene Alkene Aldehyde

Common Oils
· Helichrysum (14.6%)
· Rose (0.8-8%)
· Melissa (0.6-1.3%)
· Neroli (0.3-1.3%)
· Geranium (0-1.2%)

Aphrodisiac

Increases sexual desires

Carvacrol

Constituent Details
· Monoterpene Phenol
· Increases concentration of Follicle Stimulating Hormone and Testosterone

Common Oils
· Oregano (61-83%)
· Thyme (41%)

Phytol Acetate

Constituent Details
· Diterpenoid Alkene Alcohol

Common Oils
· Jasmine (7-12%)

Ali, *Asian Pacific Journal of Tropical Biomedicine*, 2015

Science

Astringent

Firms tissues & organs, reduces secretions

Fenchone

Constituent Details
· Monoterpene Ketone

Common Oils
· Fennel (1-20%)

a & B-Santalol

Constituent Details
· Sesquiterpene Alcohol

Common Oils
· Hawaiian Sandalwood (10-60%)
· Indian Sandalwood (10-60%)

d-3-Carene

Constituent Details
· Monoterpene Alkene

Common Oils
· Cypress (7-30%)
· Siberian (Fir 5-20%)
· Black Pepper (0.01-21%)

Phytol

Constituent Details
· Alcohol

Common Oils
· Jasmine (3-50%)

Sripathi, *National Product Research*, 2017
Raina AP, *Journal of Medicinal Plants Research*, 2013

Science

Constituent Details
• Sesquiterpene Alkene

Common Oils
• Copaiba (45-65%)
• Black Pepper (8-46%)
• Ylang Ylang (5-25%)
• Melissa (1-22%)
• Clove (0.6-20%)
• Thyme (0.1-15%)
• Frankincense (0.1-10%)

B-Caryophyl-lene

Linalyl Acetate

Constituent Details
• Monoterpene Ester

Common Oils
• Clary Sage (40-75%)
• Petitgrain (40-65%)
• Lavender (25-45%)
• Bergamot (10-45%)

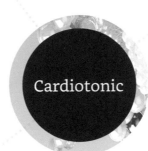

Cardiotonic

Vitalizes cardiovascular system, tones the heart

Constituent Details
• Phenol/Phenylpropanoid

Eugenol

Common Oils
• Clove (63-95%)
• Cinnamon (1-10%)

Lavdeep, *Pharmacologia*, 2013
Khair-Ul-Bariyah, *Pakistan Journal of Chemistry*, 2012
Unnikrishnan, *International Ayurvedic Medical Journal*, 2015

Constituent Details
• Monoterpene Ester

Common Oils
• Siberian Fir (20-40%)
• Douglas Fir (10%)

Bornyl
Acetate

Constituent Details
• Phenylpropene

Common Oils
• Fennel (50-90%)

Anethole

Menthol

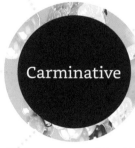

Carminative

Reduces gas or bloating

Curcumene

Constituent Details
• Monoterpene Alcohol

Common Oils
• Peppermint (20-60%)

Constituent Details
• Sesquiterpene Alkene

Common Oils
• Helichrysum (2-20%)
• Ginger (0.1-10%)

Zingiberene

Constituent Details
• Sesquiterpene Alkene

Common Oils
• Ginger (20-40%)

Peana, *Phytomedicine*, 2002
Mustafa, *Journal of Essential Oil Research*, 2005

Science

Constituent Details
• Monoterpene Ester

Common Oils
• Siberian Fir (20-40%)
• Douglas Fir (10%)

Bornyl
Acetate

Constituent Details
• Monoterpene Ether

Common Oils
• Eucalyptus (55-85%)
• Rosemary (30-60%)
• Cardamom (25-50%)
• Basil (6-6.7%)
• Peppermint (1-10%)
• Spearmint (0.1-10%)

1,8-Cineole

Camphene

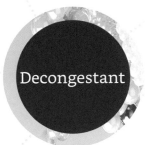

Decongestant

Reduces congestion and opens airways

Constituent Details
• Monoterpene Alkene

Common Oils
• Siberian Fir (10-30%)
• Ginger (1-10%)

B-Pinene

Constituent Details
• Monoterpene Alkene

Common Oils
• Douglas Fir (20-40%)
• Cumin (4-35%)
• Lime (10-25%)
• Lemon (6-18%)
• Black Pepper (2-20%)
• Bergamot (3-12%)
• Blue Tansy (2-10%)

Camphor

Constituent Details
• Monoterpene Ketone

Common Oils
• Blue Tansy (5-20%)
• Rosemary (5-15%)
• Coriander (2-8%)

Juergens, *Drug Research*, 2014
Santos, *Phytotherapy Research*, 2000
Peana, *Phytomedicine*, 2002

Science

B-Caryophyl-lene

Constituent Details
• Sesquiterpene Alkene

Common Oils
• Copaiba (45-65%)
• Black Pepper (8-46%)
• Ylang Ylang (5-25%)
• Melissa (1-22%)
• Clove (0.6-20%)
• Thyme (0.1-15%)
• Frankincense (0.1-10%)

Anethole

Constituent Details
• Phenylpropene

Common Oils
• Fennel (50-90%)

Digestive Stimulant

Aids in proper digestive processes

Linalyl Acetate

Constituent Details
• Monoterpene Ester

Common Oils
• Clary Sage (40-75%)
• Petitgrain (40-65%)
• Lavender (25-45%)
• Bergamot (10-45%)

Cinnamalde-hyde

Constituent Details
• Aldehyde

Common Oils
• Cassia (75-97%)
• Cinnamon (45-80%)

Asano, *Biochem Biophys Res Commun*, 2016
Dahham, *Molecules*, 2015

Constituent Details
• Sesquiterpene Alkene

Common Oils
• Patchouli (2-25%)

Aromadend-rene

a-Cedrene

Constituent Details
• Sesquiterpene Alkene

Common Oils
• Cedarwood (10-47%)

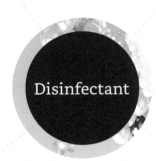

Disinfectant

Fights the spread of germs

Citronellyl Formate

d-3-Carene

Constituent Details
• Monoterpene Ester

Common Oils
• Geranium (1-15%)

Constituent Details
• Monoterpene Alkene

Common Oils
• Cypress (7-30%)
• Siberian Fir (5-20%)
• Black Pepper (0.01-21%)

Mulyaningsih, *Phytomedicine*, 2010
Mulyaningsih, *Pharm Biol*, 2011
Ouedrhiri, *Environ Sci Pollut Res Int*, 2017

Science

Constituent Details
• Sesquiterpene Ether

Common Oils
• Myrrh (15-35%)

Curzerene

Constituent Details
• Monoterpene Alcohol

Common Oils
• Peppermint (20-60%)

Menthol

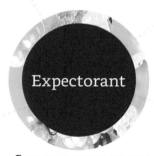

Expectorant

Removes excess mucus

a-Pinene

Constituent Details
• Monoterpene Alkene

Common Oils
• Frankincense (25-65%)
• Cypress (20-65%)
• Juniper Berry (24-55%)
• Coriander (5-20%)
• Helichrysum 5-20%
• Rosemary (5-20%)
• Siberian Fir (5-20%)
• Black Pepper (1-20%)
• Fennel (1-15%)

Terpinyl Acetate

Constituent Details
• Monoterpene Ester

Common Oils
• Cardamom (25-50%)

Rivas da Silva, *Molecules*, 2012
Yang, *Molecules*, 2011

Science

Bornyl Acetate

Constituent Details
- Monoterpene Ester

Common Oils
- Siberian Fir (20-40%)
- Douglas Fir (10%)

Eugenol

Constituent Details
- Phenol/Phenylpropanoid

Common Oils
- Clove (63-95%)
- Cinnamon (1-10%)

Immuno-stimulant

Stimulates immune system activity

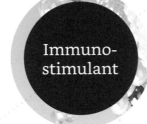

Myrcene

Common Oils
- Juniper Berry (0-25%)
- Tangerine (0.5-8%)
- Wild Orange (0.5-5%)

Constituent Details
- Monoterpene Alkene

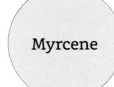

Chamazulene

Constituent Details
- Sesquiterpene Poly-alkene

Common Oils
- Blue Tansy (17-38%)
- Yarrow (19.7%)
- Roman Chamomile (0-4.4%)

Neral

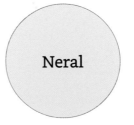

Constituent Details
- Monoterpene Alcohol

Common Oils
- Lemongrass (25-50%)
- Melissa (1-32%)

Dibazar, *Journal of Immunotoxicology*, 2015
Uyeda, *Asian Pacific Journal of Allergy and Immunology*, 2016

Constituent Details
· Monoterpene Alkene

Common Oils
· Tangerine (80-99%)
· Grapefruit (90-97%)
· Wild Orange (80-97%)
· Lemon (55-75%)
· Lime (40-70%)
· Dill (30-55%)
· Bergamot (20-55%)
· Spearmint (5-30%)
· Black Pepper (9-25%)
· Frankincense (5-20%)

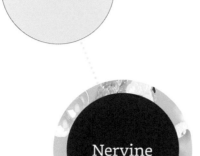

Limonene

Nervine

Beneficial effect on nerves

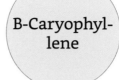

B-Caryophyl-lene

Constituent Details
· Sesquiterpene Alkene

Common Oils
· Copaiba (45-65%)
· Black Pepper (8-46%)
· Ylang Ylang (5-25%)
· Melissa (1-22%)
· Clove (0.6-20%)
· Thyme (0.1-15%)
· Frankincense (0.1-10%)

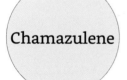

Chamazulene

Constituent Details
· Sesquiterpene Poly-alkene

Common Oils
· Blue Tansy (2-15%)

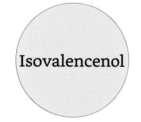

Isovalencenol

Constituent Details
· Sesquiterpene Alcohol
· This Constituent is responsible for much of Vetiver's beautiful perfume-like aroma

Common Oils
· Vetiver (5-20%)

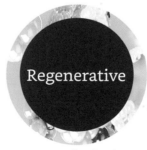

Regenerative

Promotes body tissue regeneration

Constituent Details
· Monoterpene Alkene

Camphene

Common Oils
· Siberian Fir (10-30%)
· Ginger (1-10%)

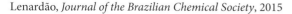
Lenardão, *Journal of the Brazilian Chemical Society*, 2015

Viveros-Paredes, *Pharmaceuticals*, 2017
Tiwari, *Toxicology in Vitro*, 2009

Science

Constituent Details
• Sesquiterpene Ether

Common Oils
• Myrrh (15-35%)

Curzerene

Linalool

Constituent Details
• Monoterpene Alcohol

Common Oils
• Coriander (60-75%)
• Basil (40-80%)
• Lavender (20-47%)
• Petitgrain (15-30%)
• Clary Sage (8-40%)
• Cilantro (10-35%)
• Bergamot (3-20%)

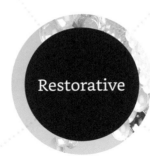

Restorative

Promotes restoration and recovery of body systems

Chamazulene

Citronellol

Constituent Details
• Sesquiterpene Poly-
alkene

Common Oils
• Blue Tansy (17-38%)
• Yarrow (19.7%)
• Roman Chamomile (0-
4.4%)

Constituent Details
• Monoterpene Alcohol

Common Oils
• Geranium (30-45%)
• Rose (20-40%)

Chien, *Evidence-Based Complementary and Alternative Medicine*, 2012
Al-Mobeeriek, *Clinical, Cosmetic and Investigational Dentistry*, 2011
Bowles, *International Journal of Aromatherapy*, 2002

Science

Constituent Details
• Monoterpene Alkene

Common Oils
• Juniper Berry (0-25%)
• Tangerine (0.5-8%)
• Wild Orange (0.5-5%)

Myrcene

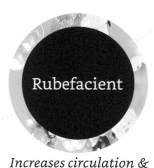

Rubefacient

Increases circulation & skin redness

Linalyl Acetate

Constituent Details
• Monoterpene Ester

Common Oils
• Clary Sage (40-75%)
• Petitgrain (40-65%)
• Lavender (25-45%)
• Bergamot (10-45%)

Constituent Details
• Sesquiterpene Alcohol

Common Oils
• Cedarwood (9-40%)

Cedrol

Constituent Details
• Monoterpene Alcohol

Common Oils
• Coriander (60-75%)
• Basil (40-80%)
• Lavender (20-47%)
• Petitgrain (15-30%)
• Clary Sage (8-40%)
• Cilantro (10-35%)
• Bergamot (3-20%)

Linalool

Fura-noeudesma 1,3-Diene

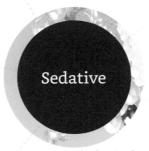

Sedative

Relaxes psychological & physiological activity

Constituent Details
• Sesquiterpene Ether

Common Oils
• Myrrh (15-45%)

Terpineol

Constituent Details
• Monoterpene Alcohol

Common Oils
• Eucalyptus (1-15%)
• Petitgrain (1-12%)

Isoamyl Tiglate

Constituent Details
• Ester
• This compound is responsible for much of Roman Chamomile's fragrant aroma.

Common Oils
• Roman Chamomile (5-40%)

Han, *Biochimie Open*, 2017
Kagawa, *Planta Medica*, 2003
Sharafzadeh, *Journal of Applied Pharmaceutical Science*, 2011

Science

Constituent Details
· Ester

Common Oils
· Jasmine (5-25%)

Benzyl Acetate

Cedrol

Constituent Details
· Sesquiterpene Alcohol

Common Oils
· Cedarwood (9-40%)

Soporific

Induces sleep

Isobutyl Angelate

Constituent Details
· Ester

Common Oils
· Roman Chamomile (5-40%)

Takeda, *Evidence-Based Complementary and Alternative Medicine*, 2017
Cho, *Evidence-Based Complementary and Alternative Medicine*, 2013
Sayowan, *Journal of Health Research*, 2013

Science

Constituent Details
• Phenylpropene

Common Oils
• Fennel (50-90%)

Anethole

Limonene

Constituent Details
• Monoterpene Alkene

Common Oils
• Tangerine (80-99%)
• Grapefruit (90-97%)
• Wild Orange (80-97%)
• Lemon (55-75%)
• Lime (40-70%)
• Dill (30-55%)
• Bergamot (20-55%)
• Spearmint (5-30%)
• Black Pepper (9-25%)
• Frankincense (5-20%)

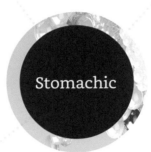

Stomachic

Stimulates digestion & appetite

Curcumene

Constituent Details
• Sesquiterpene Alkene

Common Oils
• Helichrysum (2-20%)
• Ginger (0.1-10%)

Yamahara, *Yakugaku Zasshi*, 1992
Asano, *Biochemical and Biophysical Research Communications*, 2016

Chamazulene

Constituent Details
• Sesquiterpene Polyalkene

Common Oils
• Blue Tansy (17-38%)
• Yarrow (19.7%)
• Roman Chamomile (0-4.4%)

Geranial

Constituent Details
• Monoterpene Aldehyde

Common Oils
• Lemongrass (25-50%)
• Melissa (10-47%)

Citronellol

Constituent Details
• Monoterpene Alcohol

Common Oils
• Geranium (30-45%)
• Rose (20-40%)

Tonic

Encourages feelings of vitality

Jatamansone

Constituent Details
• Sesquiterpene Ketone

Common Oils
• Spikenard (3-20%)

Farnesene

Constituent Details
• Sesquiterpene Alkene

Common Oils
• Ylang Ylang (5-15%)
• Ginger (0.1-10%)

Bastos, *Basic & Clinical Pharmacology & Toxicology,* 2009
Mckay, *Phytotherapy Research,* 2006
Nishteswar, *AYU,* 2014

Science

Bulnesene

Constituent Details
· Sesquiterpene Alkene

Common Oils
· Patchouli (1-20%)

Constituent Details
· Phenylpropene

Common Oils
· Fennel (50-90%)

Anethole

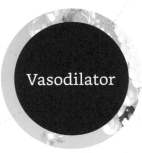

Vasodilator

Relaxes blood vessels, lowers blood pressure

Citronellol

Cinnamalde-hyde

Constituent Details
· Monoterpene Alcohol

Common Oils
· Geranium (30-45%)
· Rose (20-40%)

Constituent Details
· Aldehyde

Common Oils
· Cassia (75-97%)
· Cinnamon (45-80%)

Tognolini, Pharmacological Research, 2007
Soares, *Life Sciences*, 2007
Ribeiro-Filho, *European Journal of Pharmacology*, 2016

Section 10

References & Credits

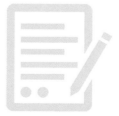

Photography Credits

Thank you to the up-and-coming artists on Unsplash for putting their work into the world. The following artists' beautiful photography is found throughout Advanced Oil Magic.

INTRO

Joshua Fuller
Eddie Hooiveld
Yasin Hoşgör
Liana Mikah
Katherine Hanlon
Holger Link
Ian Wagg
Joshua Coleman

AILMENTS

Mehrshad Rajabi
Christin Hume
Rizky Subagja
Jeshoots.com
Evelyn Mostrom
Iler Stoe
Julie Johnson
Nik MacMillan
Stacey Rozells
Annie Spratt
Omar Lopez
Andrew Pons
A Fox
Oliver Sjöström
Tanja Heffner
Andrii Podilnyk
Fabio Spinelli
Xavier Mouton Photographie
Edward Virvel
Kelly Sikkema

Artem Bali
Matteo Vistocco
Rawpixel

SINGLE OILS

Tamara Garcevic
Francesca Hotchin
Milan Popovic
Grace Ho
Matteo Vistocco
Taya Iv
Aziz Acharki
Roberto Nickson
Neil Rosenstech
Miroslava
Taylor Kiser
Simon Matzinger
Daiga Ellaby
Pablo Lancaster Jones
Rawpixel
Element5 Digital
Juliane Liebermann
Andrew Neel
Alex Geerts
Attentie Attentie
Edward Boulton
Artem Bali
Andrés Medina
Alexandra Golovac
Dan Gold
James Sutton
Mike Kenneally
Tracey Hocking

Bin Thiều
Georgia de Lotz
Kyle Loftus
Alex Blăjan
Christin Hume
Kelly Sikkema
Rose Elena
Rhand McCoy
Ryan Christodoulou
Alexandre Croussette
Becca Tapert
Icons8 team
Benjamin Voros
Zuza Reinhard
Aiony Haust
Daryn Stumbaugh
Anthony Tran
Yuvraj Singh
Cristian Palmer
Matheus Frade
Joanna Kosinska
Max Bender
Marvin Meyer
Anna Sullivan
Roberto Salinas
Laura Marques
Chris Jarvis
Julie Johnson
Dan Gold
Les Anderson
Edward Virvel
Clem Onojeghuo
Geert Pieters
Nathan Peterson
Mi Pham

Matthew LeJune
Severin Höin
Joseph Barrientos
Faye Cornish
Lyndon Li
Paulius Dragunas
Toa Heftiba
Thomas Heintz
Lera Freeland
Alexander Michl
Kirill Zakharov
Easton Oliver
Willian Justen de Vasconcellos
Kyle Loftus
Dominik Jirovský
Shari Sirotnak
Sebastien Gabriel
Huan Minh
Jason Briscoe
Giulia Bertelli
Charlotte Karlsen
Eric Nopanen
Joseph Pearson
Daniel Silva Gaxiola
Kinga Cichewicz

OIL BLENDS

Olivia Bauso
Marvin Meyer
Daiga Ellaby
Alora Griffiths
Kevin Grieve

Atikh Bana
Jason Leung
Victor Vorontsov
Jon Moore
Annie Spratt
Kelly Sikkema
Caroline Hernandez
Ben White
Michael Podger
Kiana Bosman
Blake Meyer
Robert Collins
Justin Young
Thao Le Hoang
Naomi Koelemans
Ricardo Resende
Sharon McCutcheon
Charles Deluvio
Hilary Hahn
Sarah Shaffer
Raul Petri
Heather Schwartz
Nick West
Rodion Kutsaev
Ksenya von Shlezinger
Loverna Journey

SUPPLEMENTS

Ben White
Jared Erondu
Jenn Evelyn-Ann
Rawpixel
Tim Tiedemann

Brooke Lark
Vincent Foret
Jay Wennington
Shangyou Shi
Clique Images
Tomas Anton Escobar
Ja Ma
Albert Melu
Joshua Yu
Taylor Kiser
Brooke Lark
Erwan Hesry
Annie Spratt
Ivan Jevtic
Kinga Cichewicz
Alexandr Podvalny

Vitaliy Paykov
Annie Spratt
Hutomo Abrianto
Sharon Garcia
Warren Wong
JC Gellidon
Ian Espinosa
Ian Dooley
Pawel Janiak
Tim Mossholder
Andy Omvik
Marek Mucha

Sebastián León Prado
Sai De Silva
Toa Heftiba
Mari Lezhava
Ben White
Lopez Robin
Brooke Cagle
Kevin Ku
Calum MacAulay
Caleb Jones

AILMENT PROTOCOLS

Qingbao Meng

EMOTIONS & ENERGY

Anders Jildén
Geetanjal Khanna
Feliphe Schiarolli
Simon Migaj
Savs
Dev
Jason Rosewell
Bruce Mars
Fotografia.ges

LIFESTYLE PROTOCOLS

Julia Caesar
Austin Neill
Brandon Bynum
Darius Bashar
Alexander Redl
Laura Marques
Julie Johnson
Myung-Won Seo
Janko Ferlič
Paola Aguilar
Hannah Grace
Aziz Acharki
Karl Fredrickson
Chad Madden
Matheus Ferrero
Manuel Meurisse
Jorge Barahona
Brook Anderson

Bibliography

Aromatic Science. AromaticScience, LLC. Web. July, 2017. <www.aromaticscience.com>

AromaTools. Modern Essentials: a Contemporary Guide to the Therapeutic Use of Essential Oils. AromaTools, 2018.

Enlighten Alternative Healing. Emotions and Essential Oils: A Modern Resource for Healing: Emotional Reference Guide. 4th ed., Enlighten Alternative Healing, 2017.

Harding, Jennie: The Essential Oils Handbook. Duncan Baird Publishers Ltd, 2008.

Lawless, Julia: The Encyclopedia of Essential Oils: The Complete Guide to the Use of Aromatic Oils In Aromatherapy, Herbalism, Health, and Well Being. Conari Press, 2013.

Schiller, Carol & Schiller, David: The Aromatherapy Encyclopedia: A Concise Guide to Over 395 Plant Oils. Basic Health Publications Inc, 2008.

Schnaubelt, Kurt. The Healing Intelligence of Essential Oils: the Science of Advanced Aromatherapy. Healing Arts Press, 2011.

Tisserand, Robert, et al. Essential Oil Safety: A Guide for Health Care Professionals. 2nd ed., Churchill Livingstone/Elsevier, 2014.

Total Wellness Publishing. The Essential Life: A Simple Guide to Living the Wellness Lifestyle. Total Wellness Publishing, 2017.

Worwood, Valerie Ann. The Complete Book of Essential Oils and Aromatherapy, Revised and Expanded: Over 800 Natural, Nontoxic, and Fragrant Recipes to Create Health, Beauty, And Safe Home and Work Environments. New World Library, 2016.

References

Al-Mobeeriek, Azizah. "Effects of Myrrh on Intra-Oral Mucosal Wounds Compared with Tetracycline- and Chlorhexidine-Based Mouthwashes." *Clinical, Cosmetic and Investigational Dentistry*, 2011, p. 53., doi:10.2147/cciden.s24064.

Ali, B., Al-Wabel, N. A., Shams, S., Ahamad, A., Khan, S. A., & Anwar, F. (2015, August). Essential oils used in aromatherapy: A systemic review. *Asian Pacific Journal of Tropical Biomedicine*, 5(8), 601-611. doi:https://doi.org/10.1016/j.apjtb.2015.05.007

Aliabadi, Ali, et al. "Effects of Thymol on Serum Biochemical and Antioxidant Indices in Kindled Rats." *International Journal of Medical Laboratory*, vol. 3, no. 1, Feb. 2016, pp. 43-49.

Almeida, Reinaldo Nóbrega De, et al. "Essential Oils and Their Constituents: Anticonvulsant Activity." *Molecules*, vol. 16, no. 3, 2011, pp. 2726-2742., doi:10.3390/molecules16032726.

Andrade, Luciana N. "Spasmolytic Activity of p-Menthane Esters." *Journal of Medicinal Plants Research*, vol. 5, no. 32, 2011, doi:10.5897/jmpr11.1074.

Asano T., Aida S., Suemasu S., et al. "Anethole Restores Delayed Gastric Emptying and Impaired Gastric Accommodation in Rodents." *Biochem Biophys Res Commun*. 2016;472(1):125-30

Asano, Teita, et al. "Anethole Restores Delayed Gastric Emptying and Impaired Gastric Accommodation in Rodents." *Biochemical and Biophysical Research Communications*, vol. 472, no. 1, 2016, pp. 125-130., doi:10.1016/j.bbrc.2016.02.078.

Astani, Akram, and Paul Schnitzler. "Antiviral Activity of Monoterpenes Beta-Pinene and Limonene against Herpes Simplex Virus in Vitro." *Iranian Journal of Microbiology*, vol. 6, no. 3, June 2014, pp. 149-155.

Astani, Akram, et al. "Comparative Study on the Antiviral Activity of Selected Monoterpenes Derived from Essential Oils." *Phytotherapy Research*, 2009, doi:10.1002/ptr.2955.

Astudillo, Adela, et al. "Antispasmodic Activity of Extracts and Compounds Of Acalypha Phleoides Cav." *Phytotherapy Research*, vol. 18, no. 2, 2004, pp. 102-106., doi:10.1002/ptr.1414.

Bastos, Joana F. A., et al. "Hypotensive and Vasorelaxant Effects of Citronellol, a Monoterpene Alcohol, in Rats." *Basic & Clinical Pharmacology & Toxicology*, vol. 106, no. 4, July 2009, pp. 331-337., doi:10.1111/j.1742-7843.2009.00492.x.

Bayala, Bagora, et al. "Chemical Composition, Antioxidant, Anti-Inflammatory and Anti-Proliferative Activities of Essential Oils of Plants from Burkina Faso." *PLoS ONE*, vol. 9, no. 3, 2014, doi:10.1371/journal.pone.0092122.

Biswas, Raktim, et al. "Thujone-Rich Fraction Of Thuja Occidentalis Demonstrates Major Anti-Cancer Potentials: Evidences From In Vitro Studies on A375 Cells." *Evidence-Based Complementary and Alternative Medicine*, vol. 2011, 2011, pp. 1-16., doi:10.1093/ecam/neq042.

Bowles, E Joy, et al. "Effects of Essential Oils and Touch on Resistance to Nursing Care Procedures and Other Dementia-Related Behaviours in a Residential Care Facility." *International Journal of Aromatherapy*, vol. 12, no. 1, July 2002, pp. 22-29., doi:10.1054/ijar.2001.0128.

Chen, Yingli, et al. "Composition and Potential Anticancer Activities of Essential Oils Obtained from Myrrh and Frankincense." *Oncology Letters*, vol. 6, no. 4, Aug. 2013, pp. 1140-1146., doi:10.3892/ol.2013.1520.

Chien, Li-Wei, et al. "The Effect of Lavender Aromatherapy on Autonomic Nervous System in Midlife Women with Insomnia." *Evidence-Based Complementary and Alternative Medicine*, vol. 2012, 2012, pp. 1-8., doi:10.1155/2012/740813.

Cho, Mi-Yeon, et al. "Effects of Aromatherapy on the Anxiety, Vital Signs, and Sleep Quality of Percutaneous Coronary Intervention Patients in Intensive Care Units." *Evidence-Based Complementary and Alternative Medicine*, vol. 2013, 2013, pp. 1-6., doi:10.1155/2013/381381.

Cristani, Mariateresa, et al. "Interaction of Four Monoterpenes Contained in Essential Oils with Model Membranes: Implications for Their Antibacterial Activity." *Journal of Agricultural and Food Chemistry*, vol. 55, no. 15, 2007, pp. 6300-6308., doi:10.1021/jf070094x.

Dahham, S.S., Tabana, Y.M., Iqbal, M.A., et al. "The Anticancer, Antioxidant and Antimicrobial Properties of the Sesquiterpene β-Caryophyllene from the Essential Oil of Aquilaria crassna." *Molecules*. 2015;20(7):11808-11829.

de Cássia da Silveira E, Sá R, Lima TC et al. Analgesic-Like Activity of Essential Oil Constituents: An Update. *Int J Mol Sci*. 2017 Dec 9;18(12). pii: E2392. doi: 10.3390/ijms18122392.

Djihane, Bouzid, et al. "Chemical Constituents of Helichrysum Italicum (Roth) G. Don Essential Oil and Their Antimicrobial Activity against Gram-Positive and Gram-Negative Bacteria, Filamentous Fungi and Candida Albicans." *Saudi Pharmaceutical Journal*, vol. 25, no. 5, 2017, pp. 780-787., doi:10.1016/j.jsps.2016.11.001.

Elson, Charles E., et al. "Anti-Carcinogenic Activity of d-Limonene during the Initiation and Promotion/Progression Stages of DMBA-Induced Rat Mammary Carcinogenesis." *Carcinogenesis*, vol. 9, no. 2, 1988, pp. 331-332., doi:10.1093/carcin/9.2.331.

Emílio-Silva, Maycon T., et al. "Antipyretic Effects of Citral and Possible Mechanisms of Action." *Inflammation*, vol. 40, no. 5, 2017, pp. 1735-1741., doi:10.1007/s10753-017-0615-4.

Escobar, Patricia, et al. "Chemical Composition and Antiprotozoal Activities of Colombian Lippia Spp Essential Oils and Their Major Components." *Memórias Do Instituto Oswaldo Cruz*, vol. 105, no. 2, 2010, pp. 184-190., doi:10.1590/s0074-02762010000200013.

Farhath, Seema, et al. "Immunomodulatory Activity of Geranial, Geranial Acetate, Gingerol, and Eugenol Essential Oils: Evidence for Humoral and Cell-Mediated Responses." *Avicenna Journal of Phytomedicine*, vol. 3, no. 3, 2013, pp. 224-230.

Fernandes, Janaina. "Antitumor Monoterpenes." *Bioactive Essential Oils and Cancer*, 2015, pp. 175-200., doi:10.1007/978-3-319-19144-7_8.

Flach, Adriana, et al. "Chemical Analysis and Antifungal Activity of the Essential Oil Of Calea Clematidea." *Planta Medica*, vol. 68, no. 9, 2002, pp. 836-838., doi:10.1055/s-2002-34414.

Gomes, Marcos S., et al. "Use of Essential Oils of the Genus Citrus as Biocidal Agents." *American Journal of Plant Sciences*, vol. 05, no. 03, Feb. 2014, pp. 299-305., doi:10.4236/ajps.2014.53041.

Han, Xuesheng, et al. "Chemical Composition Analysis and in Vitro Biological Activities of Ten Essential Oils in Human Skin Cells." *Biochimie Open*, vol. 5, 2017, pp. 1-7., doi:10.1016/j.biopen.2017.04.001.

Jimenez, J, et al. "Comparative Study of Different Essential Oils of Bupleurum Gibraltaricum Lamarck." *Die Pharmazie*, vol. 44, no. 4, 1 Apr. 1989, pp. 284-287.

Jirovetz, L., et al. "Medicinal Used Plants from India: Analysis of the Essential Oils of Sphaeranthus Indicus Flowers, Roots and Stems with Leaves." *Scientia Pharmaceutica*, vol. 71, 2003, pp. 251-259.

Juergens, U. "Anti-Inflammatory Properties of the Monoterpene 1.8-Cineole: Current Evidence for Co-Medication in Inflammatory Airway Diseases." *Drug Research*, vol. 64, no. 12, 2014, pp. 638-646., doi:10.1055/s-0034-1372609.

Kagawa, D, et al. "The Sedative Effects and Mechanism of Action of Cedrol Inhalation with Behavioral Pharmacological Evaluation." *Planta Medica*, vol. 69, no. 7, July 2003, pp. 637-641., doi:10.1055/s-2003-41114.

Karimzadeh, Fariba, et al. "Anticonvulsant and Neuroprotective Effects of Pimpinella Anisum in Rat Brain." *BMC Complementary and Alternative Medicine*, vol. 12, no. 1, 2012, doi:10.1186/1472-6882-12-76.

Khair-Ul-Bariyah, S., et al. "Ocimum Basilicum: A Review on Phytochemical and Pharmacological Studies." *Pakistan Journal of Chemistry*, vol. 2, no. 2, 2012, pp. 78-85., doi:10.15228/2012.v02.i02.p05.

Kim, Dae-Seung, et al. "Alpha-Pinene Exhibits Anti-Inflammatory Activity Through the Suppression of MAPKs and the NF-KB Pathway in Mouse Peritoneal Macrophages." *The American Journal of Chinese Medicine*, vol. 43, no. 04, 2015, pp. 731-742., doi:10.1142/s0192415x15500457.

Kim, Ka Young, et al. "The Effect of 1,8-Cineole Inhalation on Preoperative Anxiety: A Randomized Clinical Trial." *Evidence-Based Complementary and Alternative Medicine*, vol. 2014, 2014, pp. 1-7., doi:10.1155/2014/820126.

Kon KV, Rai MK. Plant essential oils and their constituents in coping with multidrug-resistant bacteria. *Expert Rev Anti Infect Ther*. 2012;10(7):775-790.

Laude, E.a., et al. "The Antitussive Effects of Menthol, Camphor and Cineole in Conscious Guinea-Pigs." *Pulmonary Pharmacology*, vol. 7, no. 3, 1994, pp. 179-184., doi:10.1006/pulp.1994.1021.

Lavdeep Banewal, Deepa Khanna and Sidharth Mehan. "Spices, Fruits, Nuts and Vitamins: Preventive Interventions for Myocardial Infarction." *Pharmacologia*, vol. 4, 2013, p. 553-570, doi: 10..5567/pharmacologia.2013.553.570

Lenardão, Eder J., et al. "Antinociceptive Effect of Essential Oils and Their Constituents: an Update Review." *Journal of the Brazilian Chemical Society*, 2015, doi:10.5935/0103-5053.20150332.

Leonhardt V, Leal-Cardoso JH, Lahlou S, Et Al. Antispasmodic effects of essential oil of Pterodon polygalaeflorus and its main constituent β-caryophyllene on rat isolated ileum. *Fundam Clin Pharmacol*. 2010;24(6):749-758.

Li, Hailong, et al. "Evaluation of the Chemical Composition, Antioxidant and Anti-Inflammatory Activities of Distillate and Residue Fractions of Sweet Basil Essential Oil." *Journal of Food Science and Technology*, vol. 54, no. 7, Aug. 2017, pp. 1882-1890., doi:10.1007/s13197-017-2620-x.

Magi, Gloria, et al. "Antimicrobial Activity of Essential Oils and Carvacrol, and Synergy of Carvacrol and Erythromycin, against Clinical, Erythromycin-Resistant Group A Streptococci." *Frontiers in Microbiology*, vol. 6, Mar. 2015, doi:10.3389/fmicb.2015.00165.

Marchese, Anna, et al. "Update on Monoterpenes as Antimicrobial Agents: A Particular Focus on p-Cymene." *Materials*, vol. 10, no. 8, 2017, p. 947., doi:10.3390/ma10080947.

Mckay, Diane L., and Jeffrey B. Blumberg. "A Review of the Bioactivity and Potential Health Benefits of Peppermint Tea (Mentha Piperita L.)." *Phytotherapy Research*, vol. 20, no. 8, 2006, pp. 619-633., doi:10.1002/ptr.1936.

Mckay, Diane L., and Jeffrey B. Blumberg. "A Review of the Bioactivity and Potential Health Benefits of Chamomile Tea (Matricaria Recutita L.)." *Phytotherapy Research*, vol. 20, no. 7, 2006, pp. 519-530., doi:10.1002/ptr.1900.

Mitoshi, Mai, et al. "Suppression of Allergic and Inflammatory Responses by Essential Oils Derived from Herbal Plants and Citrus Fruits." *International Journal of Molecular Medicine*, vol. 33, no. 6, 2014, pp. 1643-1651., doi:10.3892/ijmm.2014.1720.

Mulyaningsih, S., Sporer F, Zimmermann, S., et al. "Synergistic Properties of the Terpenoids Aromadendrene and 1,8-cineole from the Essential Oil of Eucalyptus Globulus Against Antibiotic-Susceptible and Antibiotic-Resistant Pathogens." *Phytomedicine*. 2010;17(13):1061-1066.

Mulyaningsih, S., Sporer, F., Reichling, J., et al. "Antibacterial Activity of Essential Oils from Eucalyptus and of Selected Components Against Multidrug-Resistant Bacterial Pathogens." *Pharm Biol*. 2011;49(9):893-899.

Mustafa, Akhlaq, et al. "Volatile Oil Constituents of the Fresh Rhizomes of Curcuma Amada Roxb." *Journal of Essential Oil Research*, vol. 17, no. 5, 2005, pp. 490-491., www.tandfonline.com/doi/abs/10.1080/10412905.2005.9698974.

Naseri, Mohsen, et al. "The Study of Anti-Inflammatory Activity of Oil-Based Dill (Anethum Graveolens L.) Extract Used Topically in Formalin-Induced Inflammation Male Rat Paw." *Iran Journal of Pharmaceutical Research*, vol. 11, no. 4, 2012, pp. 1169-1174.

Nishteswar, K. "Credential Evidences of Ayurvedic Cardio-Vascular Herbs." *AYU (An International Quarterly Journal of Research in Ayurveda)*, vol. 35, no. 2, 2014, p. 111., doi:10.4103/0974-8520.146194.

Oliveira-Tintino, Cícera Datiane De Morais, et al. "Anti-Inflammatory and Anti-Edematogenic Action of the Croton Campestris A. St.-Hil (Euphorbiaceae) Essential Oil and the Compound β-Caryophyllene in in Vivo Models." *Phytomedicine*, vol. 41, 2018, pp. 82-95., doi:10.1016/j.phymed.2018.02.004.

Ouedrhiri, W., Balouiri, M., Bouhdid, S., et al. "Antioxidant and Antibacterial Activities of Pelargonium Asperum and Ormenis Mixta Essential Oils and Their Synergistic Antibacterial Effect." *Environ Sci Pollut Res Int*. 2017 Jul 22. doi: 10.1007/s11356-017-9739-1.

Oz, Murat, et al. "Cellular and Molecular Targets of Menthol Actions." *Frontiers in Pharmacology*, vol. 8, 2017, doi:10.3389/fphar.2017.00472.

Pandey, Abhay K., and Pooja Singh. "The Genus Artemisia: a 2012-2017 Literature Review on Chemical Composition, Antimicrobial, Insecticidal and Antioxidant Activities of Essential Oils." *Medicines*, vol. 4, no. 3, Dec. 2017, p. 68., doi:10.3390/medicines4030068.

Peana AT, D'Aquila PS, Panin F, et al. "Anti-Inflammatory Activity of Linalool and Linalyl Acetate Constituents of Essential Oils." *Phytomedicine*. 2002;9(8):721-726.

Peana AT, D'Aquila PS, Panin F, et al. "Anti-Inflammatory Activity of Linalool and Linalyl Acetate Constituents of Essential Oils." *Phytomedicine*. 2002;9(8):721-726.

Piccinelli, Ana Claudia, et al. "Antihyperalgesic and Antidepressive Actions of (R)-( )-Limonene, α-Phellandrene, and Essential Oil From Schinus Terebinthifolius fruits in a Neuropathic Pain Model." *Nutritional Neuroscience*, vol. 18, no. 5, 2014, pp. 217-224., doi:10.1179/1476830514y.0000000119.

Pourghanbari, Gholamhosein, et al. "Antiviral Activity of the Oseltamivir and Melissa Officinalis L. Essential Oil against Avian Influenza A Virus (H9N2)." *Virus Disease*, vol. 27, no. 2, 2016, pp. 170-178., doi:10.1007/s13337-016-0321-0.

Raina AP, Negi KS, Dutta M. "Variability in Essential Oil Composition of Sage (Salvia officinalis L.) Grown Under North Western Himalayan Region of India." *Journal of Medicinal Plants Research*. 2013;7(11):683-688.

Rath, Cc, et al. "Antibacterial Potential Assessment of Jasmine Essential Oil against E. Coli." *Indian Journal of Pharmaceutical Sciences*, vol. 70, no. 2, 2008, p. 238., doi:10.4103/0250-474x.41465.

Ribeiro-Filho, Helder Veras, et al. "Biphasic Cardiovascular and Respiratory Effects Induced by ß-Citronellol." *European Journal of Pharmacology*, vol. 775, 2016, pp. 96-105., doi:10.1016/j.ejphar.2016.02.025.

Rivas da Silva, A.C., Lopes, P.M., Barros de Azevedo, M.M., et al. "Biological Activities of A-pinene and ß-pinene Enantiomers." *Molecules*. 2012;17(6):6305-6316.

Sadraei, H., et al. "Inhibitory Effect of Rosa Damascena Mill Flower Essential Oil, Geraniol and Citronellol on Rat Ileum Contraction." *Research in Pharmaceutical Sciences*, vol. 8, no. 1, Jan. 2013, pp. 17-23.

Santos, F. A., and V. S. N. Rao. "Anti-inflammatory and Antinociceptive Effects of 1,8-Cineole a Terpenoid Oxide Present in Many Plant Essential Oils." *Phytotherapy Research*, vol. 14, no. 4, 2000, pp. 240-244., doi:10.1002/1099-1573(200006)14:4<240::aid-ptr573>3.0.co;2-x.

Sayowan, Winai, et al. "The Effects of Jasmine Oil Inhalation on Brain Wave Activities and Emotions." *Journal of Health Research*, vol. 27, no. 2, Apr. 2013, pp. 73-77.

Sena-Lopes, Ângela, et al. "Chemical Composition, Immunostimulatory, Cytotoxic and Antiparasitic Activities of the Essential Oil from Brazilian Red Propolis." *Plos One*, vol. 13, no. 2, Jan. 2018, doi:10.1371/journal.pone.0191797.

Shaghayegh Pishkhan Dibazar, Shirin Fateh & Saeed Daneshmandi (2015) Immunomodulatory effects of clove (Syzygium aromaticum) constituents on macrophages: In vitro evaluations of aqueous and ethanolic components, Journal of Immunotoxicology, 12:2, 124-131, DOI: 10.3109/1547691X.2014.912698

Shakeel-u-Rehman., et al. "Essential Oil Composition of Rosmarinus officinalis L. from Kashmir (India)". *EC Microbiology* 14.2, 2018: 29-32.

Sharafzadeh, Shahram, and Omid Alizadeh. "German and Roman Chamomile." *Journal of Applied Pharmaceutical Science*, vol. 01, no. 10, 2011, pp. 01-05.

Soares, Pedro Marcos G., et al. "Effects of Anethole and Structural Analogues on the Contractility of Rat Isolated Aorta: Involvement of Voltage-Dependent Ca2 -Channels." *Life Sciences*, vol. 81, no. 13, 2007, pp. 1085-1093., doi:10.1016/j.lfs.2007.08.027.

Sripathi R, Jayagopal D, Ravi S. "A Study on the Seasonal Variation of the Essential Oil Composition from Plectranthus Hadiensis and its Antibacterial Activity." *National Product Research*. 2017 Aug 8:1-4. doi: 10.1080/14786419.2017.1363748.

Takaishi, Masayuki, et al. "1,8-Cineole, a TRPM8 Agonist, Is a Novel Natural Antagonist of Human TRPA1." *Molecular Pain*, vol. 8, 2012, doi:10.1186/1744-8069-8-86.

Takeda, Ai, et al. "Effects of Inhalation Aromatherapy on Symptoms of Sleep Disturbance in the Elderly with Dementia." *Evidence-Based Complementary and Alternative Medicine*, vol. 2017, 2017, pp. 1-7., doi:10.1155/2017/1902807.

Tisserand, Robert, et al. *Essential Oil Safety: a Guide for Health Care Professionals*. Churchill Livingstone/Elsevier, 2014.

Tognolini, Massimiliano, et al. "Protective Effect of Foeniculum Vulgare Essential Oil and Anethole in an Experimental Model of Thrombosis." *Pharmacological Research*, vol. 56, no. 3, 2007, pp. 254-260., doi:10.1016/j.phrs.2007.07.002.

Uyeda, Saori, et al. "Enhancement and Regulation Effect of Myrcene on Antibody Response in Immunization with Ovalbumin and Ag85B in Mice." *Asian Pacific Journal of Allergy and Immunology*, 2016, doi:10.12932/ap0734.

Valente, J., et al. "Antifungal, Antioxidant and Anti-Inflammatory Activities of Oenanthe Crocata L. Essential Oil." *Food and Chemical Toxicology*, vol. 62, 2013, pp. 349-354., doi:10.1016/j.fct.2013.08.083.

Viana, Glauce Socorro De Barros, et al. "Anticonvulsant Activity of Essential Oils and Active Principles from Chemotypes of Lippia Alba(Mill.) N.E. Brown." *Biological & Pharmaceutical Bulletin*, vol. 23, no. 11, 2000, pp. 1314-1317., doi:10.1248/bpb.23.1314.

Vidhya Unnikrishnan, and K Nishteswar. "Cardio Protective Activities of Herbal Formulation of Bhavamishra - A Review." *International Ayurvedic Medical Journal*, vol. 3, no. 2320, Mar. 2015, pp. 850-861.

Viveros-Paredes, Juan, et al. "Neuroprotective Effects of β-Caryophyllene against Dopaminergic Neuron Injury in a Murine Model of Parkinson's Disease Induced by MPTP." *Pharmaceuticals*, vol. 10, no. 4, June 2017, p. 60., doi:10.3390/ph10030060.

Yamahara, Johji, et al. "Stomachic Principles in Ginger. II. Pungent and Anti-Ulcer Effects of Low Polar Constituents Isolated from Ginger, the

Dried Rhizoma of Zingiber Officinale ROSCOE Cultivated in Taiwan. The Absolute Stereostructure of a New Diarylheptanoid." *Yakugaku Zasshi*, vol. 112, no. 9, 1992, pp. 645–655., doi:10.1248/yakushi1947.112.9_645.

Yang, Z., Wu, N., Zu, Y., Et Al. "Comparative Anti-Infectious Bronchitis Virus (IBV) Activity of (-)-pinene: Effect on Nucleocapsid (N) Protein." *Molecules*. 2011;16(2):1044-1054.

Yin, Qing-Hua, et al. "Anti-Proliferative and pro-Apoptotic Effect of Carvacrol on Human Hepatocellular Carcinoma Cell Line HepG-2." *Cytotechnology*, vol. 64, no. 1, 2011, pp. 43-51., doi:10.1007/s10616-011-9389-y.

Zalachoras, Ioannis, et al. "Assessing the Local Anesthetic Effect of Five Essential Oil Constituents." *Planta Medica*, vol. 76, no. 15, 2010, pp. 1647–1653., doi:10.1055/s-0030-1249956.

Notes

Notes

Oil Magic Protocols Are on the Droplii App!

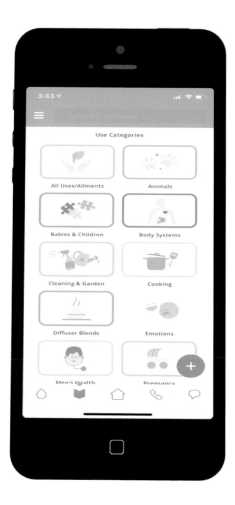

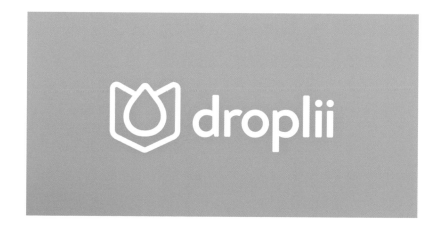

Did you notice the Droplii logo by some of your favorite recipes? Essential oil recipes are a fan favorite, and Droplii has hundreds - including recipes & protocols from Oil Magic.

Droplii is a unique essential oil resource app filled with crowd-sourced content. Whether it's an oil recipe for cooking, baby care, or just about anything else you can think of, there's a recipe for it on Droplii.

Bring your favorites right to your phone!

www.droplii.com/oilmagic

Meet the Magic of Ending Child Trafficking and Poverty.

Join Oil Magic Publishing and the LETS Empower Women foundation to help bring an end to child trafficking and poverty.

A simple bracelet made by Haitian women artisans (out of beads made from recycled trash!) is having a HUGE impact on this worldwide problem. Kristin Van Wey created the LETS fertility tracking bracelet to help women understand and track their cycles.

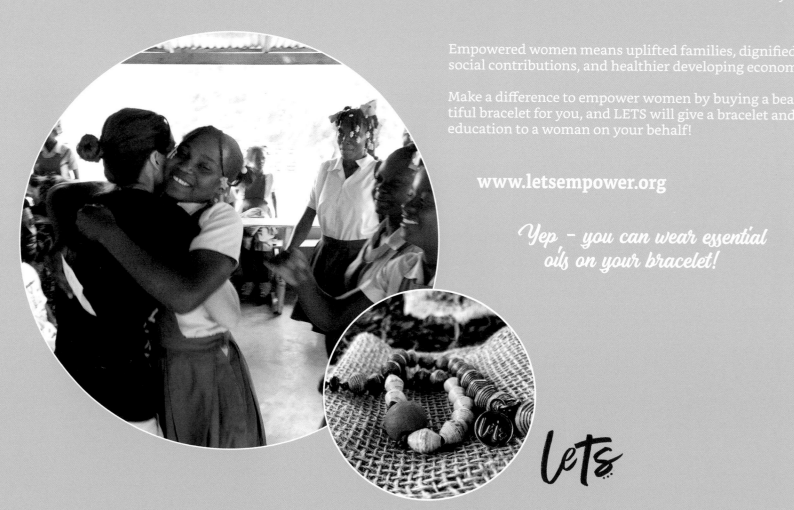

Empowered women means uplifted families, dignified social contributions, and healthier developing economies.

Make a difference to empower women by buying a beautiful bracelet for you, and LETS will give a bracelet and education to a woman on your behalf!

www.letsempower.org

Yep – you can wear essential oils on your bracelet!

LETS

"Magic is believing in yourself. If you can do that,
you can make anything happen."

-Johann Wolfgang von Goethe